43.00

D1499193

Brief Cognitive Hypnosis

Facilitating the Change of Dysfunctional Behavior

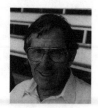
Jordan I. Zarren, MSW., DAHB is a licensed clinical social worker and a board-certified diplomate in clinical hypnosis with the American Hypnosis Board for Clinical Social Work, and in clinical social work with the National Association of Social Workers. He is a founding member of the American Hypnosis Board for Clinical Social Work and a fellow of the American Society of Clinical Hypnosis, the Society for Clinical and Experimental Hypnosis, and the Florida Society of Clinical Hypnosis. He is a Past President of the Florida Society of Clinical Hypnosis and the current President-Elect of the American Society of Clinical Hypnosis. He has over 40 years of experience as a psychotherapist.

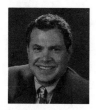
Bruce N. Eimer, PhD, ABPP is a licensed clinical psychologist and a board-certified diplomate in behavioral psychology with the American Board of Professional Psychology and in pain management with the American Academy of Pain Management. He is a member of the American Psychological Association and a fellow of the Society for Psychological Hypnosis, Division 30, of the American Psychological Association. He is also a member of the American Society of Clinical Hypnosis, the Society for Clinical and Experimental Hypnosis, and the Greater Philadelphia Society of Clinical Hypnosis. He has over 20 years of experience as a psychologist and psychotherapist.

Both authors are also certified consultants in clinical hypnosis with the American Society of Clinical Hypnosis.

NCMC
RC
497
Z37
2002

4678313

Brief Cognitive Hypnosis

Facilitating the Change of Dysfunctional Behavior

Jordan I. Zarren, MSW, DAHB

Bruce N. Eimer, PhD, ABPP

NYACK COLLEGE MANHATTAN

 Springer Publishing Company

Copyright © 2002 by Springer Publishing Company, Inc.

All rights reserved

No part of this publication may be reproduced, stored in a retrieval system, or transmitted in any form or by any means, electronic, mechanical, photocopying, recording, or otherwise, without the prior permission of Springer Publishing Company, Inc.

Springer Publishing Company, Inc.
536 Broadway
New York, NY 10012-3955

Acquisitions Editor: Sheri W. Sussman
Production Editor: Janice Stangel
Cover design by Susan Hauley

01 02 03 04 05 / 5 4 3 2 1

Library of Congress Cataloging-in-Publication-Data

Zarren, Jordan I.
   Brief cognitive hypnosis : facilitating the change of dysfunctional behavior / Jordan I. Zarren, Bruce N. Eimer.
   p. cm.
Includes bibliographical references and index.
ISBN 0-8261-1484-9
   1. Hypnotism—Therapeutic use.   2. Cognitive therapy.   3. Brief psychotherapy.
I. Eimer, Bruce N., 1953–   II. Title.

RC497.Z37 2001
616.89'162—dc21
                                                                    2001040010

Printed in the United States of America

I dedicate this book to my wife of forty-nine years, Lillian. Her patience, unwavering support and wise counsel made it all possible. Also, my daughter Marcia Schneider and her husband Marc, my son Robert and his wife Susie and their children Ella and newborn Nathaniel. Their presence has kept me young.

—Jordan I. Zarren

I dedicate this book to my loving wife Andrea and to my daughters, Marisa and Allison who make my life whole. Also, to my mother Cecile, and my father Joe, who taught me the meaning of love.

—Bruce N. Eimer

CONTENTS

PART THREE   SMOKING CESSATION AND KEYS TO CHANGE

Foreword

WILLIAM C. WESTER II

In 1961, I took my first graduate school course in psychopathology. The course was taught by George W. Kisker, author of *The Disorganized Personality* (Kisker, 1972). Dr. Kisker became my major adviser and later supervisor when I completed my clinical internship. My first exposure to hypnosis was watching Dr. Kisker use hypnosis with a hospitalized population. He became my mentor and teacher of hypnosis because there was no graduate course in hypnosis at the time. The rest is history in terms of my career in the field of hypnosis. I ended up teaching the first hypnosis course at the University of Cincinnati to graduate/medical students.

Hypnosis has been used for as long as records have been kept and originally was influenced by beliefs in the stars, magnetic fields and exorcism. The term *hypnosis* was coined in 1841 by an English physician, James Braid.

Hypnosis became more scientific and accepted and officially recognized by the American Medical Association (AMA) in 1958 as a legitimate treatment method. The last 40 years has been a tremendous growth period for hypnosis, and books too numerous to mention have been published on the subject.

Clinicians graduated from a variety of training programs, and their particular theoretical backgrounds influenced how they began to use hypnosis. Much of this early training, including my own and that of Jordan Zarren, was very psychoanalytic in nature. Clinicians took continuing education courses, and we began to see a shift to behavioral and cognitive treatment approaches. Hypnosis just seemed to fit in better within cognitive-behavioral models because of the shorter term treatment approaches that they espoused. Training programs began to change, and the advent of managed care pushed for even shorter and briefer models of treatment.

Many other health care groups have continued to recognize hypnosis, as the AMA did in 1958, as an effective therapeutic treatment modality. This has led to the need for specialized training of more licensed health care clinicians and a greater need for published material on hypnosis geared to brief treatment skills.

Books on hypnosis have continued to be published. The majority of them have been general texts, covering the whole field of hypnosis, or very specific texts, such as those addressing the use of hypnosis for pain control. Even though the cognitive treatment model has been recognized as most effective in producing change in patient behavior, there has been little written on combining cognitive techniques with hypnosis, within a brief therapeutic model—until now.

Brief Cognitive Hypnosis: Facilitating the Change of Dysfunctional Behavior is a magical addition to the field of clinical hypnosis. Two distinguished board-certified clinicians with over 60 years of combined clinical experience have provided a delightful and practical resource book for all clinicians using hypnosis as a tool in their clinical work.

The authors state that their book is for clinicians experienced in the use of hypnosis. However, after 40 years in the field myself, and having taught hundreds of graduate students and licensed professionals, it is my opinion that this book not only will add to the experienced clinician's skills but also will provide a straightforward and practical approach for the neophyte in hypnosis.

This book is a practical, well-documented, clinical volume based on solid psychological concepts and principles. As the title implies, *Brief Cognitive Hypnosis* is also consistent with the managed care model, which emphasizes brief therapy and structured treatment. Like cognitive therapy in general, the authors come from a positive frame of reference in which the patient assumes a degree of responsibility for his or her treatment. In addition to the material presented, related issues in hypnosis, such as sensory representational language, waking state reframing, and the importance of semantics, are skillfully interwoven into the framework of this book.

This book becomes even stronger with the addition of excellent case studies, brief inductions and numerous examples of specific wording to facilitate therapeutic change. Jordan Zarren even uses distraction as he mentions the appropriate use of sleight-of-hand magic in the treatment process.

The thirteen chapters are broken into three well-organized sections: Part One—Fundamental Concepts and Essential Tools, Part Two—Clinical Applications, and Part Three—Smoking Cessation and Keys to Change.

In Part One, chapters 1 through 7, the brief cognitive hypnosis model is clearly introduced and the fundamental concepts and essential tools for doing this type of therapy are logically presented. These chapters are packed full of new and alternative ideas for the experienced clinician, while providing the basics to beginners in the field who want to follow a cognitive model.

In Part Two, chapters 8 through 11, the authors get down to the specific treatment of many clinical problems, such as anxiety, dysfunctional habits, pain, and a variety of medical problems, which can all benefit from using this approach.

Part Three, chapter 12, provides a detailed single-session smoking cessation program. I learned a great deal that I can now incorporate into the single-session smoking cessation treatment approach that I have used for over 38 years.

Chapter 13, "Review: Keys to Change", pulls it all together, leaving the reader with a strong feeling of excitement for having read this excellent book. More than adequate references are given at the end of the book that support and document the brief cognitive hypnosis model.

William C. Wester, II, Ed.D., ABPP, ABPH, CEO, Behavioral Science Center, Inc., Cincinnati, Ohio. Past-President: American Society of Clinical Hyponsis.

REFERENCES

Kisker, G. W. (1972). *The disorganized personality* (6th ed.). New York: McGraw-Hill.

Preface

INTENDED READERSHIP

This book is intended for experienced health care clinicians, clinical social workers, marriage and family therapists, mental health counselors, nurse clinicians, psychologists, physicians, dentists and other licensed medical and mental health care professionals who are already using hypnosis as a tool in clinical practice. Clinicians who want to add the hypnosis tool to their practice and advanced graduate students in the medical, health, and psychological fields will also find this book valuable. We emphasize the word *tool* rather than *treatment* because we view hypnosis as an adjunctive tool that can help licensed health care professionals expedite treatment and shorten the time it takes to help their patients.

OUR GOALS

Our goals are to offer those clinicians who are already experienced in the use of hypnosis, and those who are testing it, a simpler way of thinking about patient dysfunction and a means for quickly and accurately assessing the target problem requiring immediate attention. We offer a conceptual framework for planning the treatment process, as well as ways to use therapeutic language and hypnotic procedures effectively.

This book explains which dysfunctional problems are amenable to brief cognitive hypnosis and which are not. Specific therapeutic procedures and techniques presented, along with their rationale and means of flexible application and guidelines for fitting them into an already established way of working.

Some of you may do what many of our students and those we have supervised have done. You may decide to adopt more fully our powerful and successful mode of working with hypnosis. We will address both possibilities as we proceed to communicate what we do, why we do it and how we do it. We also want to make sure that we address the interests of clinicians who are not trained in psychotherapy. Physicians, dentists, podiatrists and nurses who are generalists or specialists will find information on new skills and procedures that may be applied quickly and effectively within the domain of their professional training and previous training in hypnosis.

If you are an experienced psychotherapist, regardless of your identification with a psychodynamic, behavioral, cognitive, Freudian, Jungian, or other psychotherapeutic school of thought, you will be able to borrow, insert, and apply much, most, or all of our approach into your already familiar ways of working.

The only requirements that are needed to benefit from reading our clinically practical book are comfort with your current clinical skills, a desire to be open to new ideas, a flexible mindset and the awareness that all problem-solving requires the recognition that there is more than one way to solve a problem.

Most of the patients you see believe that they are trapped and have no choices. It is your job to open a patient's belief system to recognizing that there are other choices. It is important to modify your own belief system so that you can feel more comfortable in choosing other ways to help patients.

PURPOSE OF THIS BOOK

Our model, which we call *Brief Cognitive Hypnosis,* incorporates a unique cognitive perspective and a simple way of using change language in brief psychotherapy. It also addresses the relationship between the patient and the clinician/therapist and the continuing interaction and learning that both persons go through during the therapeutic process.

Simplifying Diagnosis and Treatment

Numerous books have been written about the assessment and treatment of specific dysfunctional behaviors that fit into single diagnostic categories. Detailed psychotherapy treatment manuals for specific psychological disorders have also recently been developed so that clinicians can implement the latest empirically validated treatments.

Traditional approaches and procedures, mostly grounded in a mainstream cognitive-behavioral perspective, do not give much attention to the significant role of *unconscious* factors in learning, as well as in the development and maintenance of symptoms. Consequently, cognitive-behavioral therapeutic rituals focus mainly on the *conscious* learning and processing of information. They place their focus on automatic negative thoughts and beliefs as the cause of patients' symptoms and emotional distress.

These are two areas where *Brief Cognitive Hypnosis* differs. While focusing on the important cognitive issue of patients' beliefs and expectations, as well as on feelings and behaviors, in *Brief Cognitive Hypnosis* we also assign great value to the role of the unconscious in the formation and maintenance of symptoms and their amelioration. We also do not ascribe sole causative value to patients' cognitions as the origin and basis of their symptoms and emotional distress.

We will discuss diagnostic categories in direct relationship to the dysfunctional symptoms and behavioral choices a patient presents when first visiting the clinician. This will help in simplifying the diagnostic process during the intake evaluation so as to identify the most urgent problem and determine the easiest way of helping the patient to deal with that problem. We will combine diagnoses involving a variety of negative coping behaviors when similar dysfunctional behavioral symptoms are manifest. This enables us to employ comparable therapeutic procedures with minor variations.

Continuing Professional Education and Enrichment

The many continuing professional education workshops we have presented over the years have brought excellent responses from hundreds of participants who have attended them. Their comments and questions have included requests for a more extensive presentation of our theories and clinical procedures in a single, concise book.

In our clinical thinking and practice of psychotherapy and hypnosis, it is often difficult to pinpoint the precise origins of many of our ideas. Over the years, as our ideas about psychotherapy and human change processes have evolved, each of us has borrowed and incorporated ideas from many sources. Our current ideas are a cumulative and interactive result of our formal clinical training, continuing professional education, personal and professional backgrounds, clinical experiences, personal interactions with colleagues and reading of the clinical, theoretical, and research literature, along with our unique personalities.

We intend this book to be a clinically practical, user-friendly guide that explains and illustrates how we work, and how we think about how we work. It is not our intention to present a scholarly review of the different bodies of literature or research that are applicable to what we do. We realize and acknowledge that our way of working clinically has been influenced directly and indirectly by many individuals whose work we have studied, heard, presented, and read. However, we think that we are presenting an original approach that we ourselves use because it makes sense and works for us.

Nevertheless, we offer our apologies to any authors who may feel that we have restated their ideas in our own words without citing them. We believe that the wheel is repeatedly reinvented. However, not all reinventions, or reconstructions, work equally well in every context.

—JIZ
—BNE

An Important Note

The clinical evaluation and treatment methods described in this book are not intended as substitutes for competent and thorough medical, psychiatric or psychological evaluation and care, nor are they intended to replace the medical or professional recommendations of physicians or other health care providers who are familiar with a given case. This book is intended to offer usable information that can enhance the effectiveness of the reader/clinician in helping his or her patients alleviate or gain control over their symptoms and change their dysfunctional behaviors.

The reader/clinician should never attempt to use psychological or behavioral or hypnotic treatment methods to mask symptoms requiring appropriate medical, surgical, dental, or psychiatric care. The clinician who intends to use the methods described in this book to treat the "emotional overlay" associated with any medical symptoms should, if possible, first consult with the patient's physicians before embarking on a course of psychological, behavioral or hypnotic treatment.

This book is intended for experienced health care clinicians and advanced practitioners and students. It is not written for laypersons. However, it is recommended that, before acting on any of the information or advice contained in this book or undertaking any form of self-treatment, the reader consult with his or her own physician, therapist or dentist.

The identities of all patients described in the clinical case examples and transcripts presented in this book have been altered to protect patient confidentiality.

Acknowledgments

I want to thank those clinicians, who as mentors, friends, and colleagues have helped me to evolve and prosper in my clinical work. Many of these individuals have also been very helpful in my attempts to have clinical social workers recognized as skilled in the use of hypnosis equally with professionals from the fields of medicine, dentistry, and psychology.

Whatever I have accomplished is mostly due to my deceased mother Jean; my dear and wise and very patient wife Lillian; my daughter Marcia, and son Robert. In fact, my wife Lillian, has been my most ardent supporter and critic. My family's patience and encouragement have been my most important nourishment over the many years.

Finally, this book could not have been written without the insistence that it needed to be done and the skill and positive compulsivity of my very bright and talented coauthor, Bruce Eimer.

—Jordan I. Zarren

First of all, I want to thank Jordan Zarren for mentoring me in the practice of brief psychotherapy and clinical hypnosis. This book primarily represents Jordan's approach to doing brief psychotherapy and clinical hypnosis, which he has termed brief cognitive hypnosis. This approach, as you are about to discover, offers a marvelous way of simplifying the diagnostic and treatment process. Given that this work is primarily Jordan's, most of the case examples reported here come from his case files.

I also want to acknowledge the many bright and creative individuals who have positively supported and influenced me over the years. These people are too numerous to name here.

On a personal level, I remain grateful for the love and guidance provided to me over the years by my dear late father Joe Eimer, and by my dear mother Cecile Eimer, who continues to mother me lovingly. I am also grateful for all of the learning, love, support, and encouragement that my wife, Andrea, has provided to me over the past 17 years. Equally, my two daughters Marisa and Allison, have taught me how to be with and be a child once again.

Last, but not least, we both wish to acknowledge Dr. Ursula Springer, our publisher, and Bill Tucker, our acquisitions editor, for their vision in seeing the value of our project and for having the confidence in us that we would deliver it as promised. We also wish to acknowledge our managing editor Sheri Sussman, and our Production Editor Janice Stangel for their help in completing this project and turning our original manuscript into a finished, well-polished product. Without these marvelous people, this book, in its current form, would not have been born.

—Bruce N. Eimer

PART I

Fundamental Concepts and Essential Tools

Introduction: Brief Cognitive Hypnosis—A Powerful Tool for Brief Psychotherapy

THE BRIEF COGNITIVE HYPNOSIS MODEL

The brief cognitive hypnosis model suggests that most behaviors that are difficult for the patient to control or change are the result of cognitive dissonance and conflict occurring between the conscious and unconscious parts of the mind. We conceptualize the conscious mind as that part of the mind that the individual has moment to moment control over. A conscious thought can initiate an immediate accompanying action, behavior or general response. A person can usually change that response by a direct thought to do so.

We conceptualize the unconscious mind as that part of the mind that controls an individual's automatic behaviors. This includes all of the actions of the autonomic nervous system, as well an individual's habitual patterns of thinking and behavior (Mutter, 1987). The unconscious mind controls the person's built-in survival mechanisms through the functions of the immune system and "fight or flight response" (Cannon, 1929) and the general adaptation syndrome (Selye, 1974, 1976). It uses inherited gene imprinting and learned environmental and social imprinting in constructing its own unique interpretation of the individual's internal and external world. Through a highly developed sensory system, the unconscious mind interprets the world by selectively filtering informational input from both internal and external sources.

The unconscious mind is also influenced by the selective interpretation of language. It is particularly responsive to extreme emotional imprinting, repetition, and suggestion through language directed to its strongest sensory representational system.

The concept of the unconscious and its evolution have played a pivotal role in the emergence of hypnosis as a tool in psychotherapy (Ellenberger, 1970; Gauld, 1992). The practice of hypnosis in psychotherapy has evolved from its common roots with the emergence of dynamic psychotherapy and psychiatry with their focus on the unconscious (Bromberg, 1959; Ellenberger, 1970; Fine, 1990). The reality of unconscious cognition is now solidly established in empirical research (Greenwald, 1992; Kihlstrom, Barnhardt, & Tataryn, 1992).

OUR VIEW OF HYPNOSIS

Hypnosis as an "Altered State"

Hypnosis is an altered state of focused attention and heightened suggestibility that may or may not include a formal trance induction. *Hypnotic trance* is an altered state that is produced by a formal hypnotic induction ritual or ceremony that serves as the focusing method. In contrast to hypnotic trances that are formally induced for therapeutic purposes, there are informal trances that occur spontaneously without any formal hypnotic induction ceremony (Bowers, 1976; Erickson & Rossi, 1979, 1981; Spiegel & Spiegel, 1987).

We view hypnosis as an alteration in internal perception, an altered state, that is initiated at the start of a unique process of communication. The communication in and of itself is not hypnosis. The altered state that we label hypnosis results from the communication process (Eimer & Freeman, 1998; Zarren, 1996a; Zarren & Eimer, 1999). We might best label natural everyday altered states as hypnoidal states, and therapeutic altered states as hypnosis states.

In the clinical setting, a *hypnosis state*, as differentiated from a *trance state,* can be induced without a formal trance induction. This occurs when a clinician communicates with a patient in a language and form that are acceptable to the patient's conscious and unconscious minds. We term this form of communication *waking state reframing.* In our view, the subsequent formal induction of hypnotic trance serves to fix the information communicated further in place in the patient's unconscious.

Hypnotic trance can be formally induced, or informal suggestions for entering into trance can be given to a patient who is already in hypnosis and ready to go "deeper" (specific examples of how to do this will be provided in later chapters). This then moves the process along so that suggestions can be given while the patient is in a trance state and *trance state reframing* can occur. This serves to fix the information communicated earlier in the waking state further in place in the patient's unconscious.

Milton Erickson (1961) and David Cheek (1994) believed that people "enter hypnosis as they mentally review sequential events" (Cheek, 1994, p. 1). Cheek (1994) wrote: "A hypnoidal state is entered when [remembering sequential events such as] recalling a tune, remembering the visual images of waves breaking on a beach, the movements of a candle flame and the words of a poem" (p. 1). Thus, a basic mechanism for inducing a *hypnotic altered state* is the review or processing of a sequence of sensory impressions or memories.

The special communication experience that initiates a hypnosis state can start as the result of an externally evoked stimulus that alerts the unconscious to pay attention. In the clinical or therapeutic treatment setting, the initiating stimulus may be the clinician's words, or the lulling sound of the clinician's voice in conjunction with the quiet, peacefulness, separateness from the outside world and feelings of safety engendered by the clinician's office environment.

Whether or not a patient enters a therapeutic altered state (i.e., *therapeutic hypnosis* or a hypnosis state) is influenced by the words the clinician chooses to use and whether or not they match the patient's primary sensory representational system. It is also influenced by the extent to which the clinician communicates the right information for that individual patient in a form that the patient can accept. The patient must be a willing participant in the treatment process.

The Role of Language

Language is inherent to how we learn. We automatically and unconsciously interpret the representational code of language to understand and apply meaning to our world. Therefore, certain language forms can affect how we feel and behave. Our sensory representational systems give guidance to these interpretations and have direct access to the learning centers of the conscious and unconscious parts of the mind. This will be discussed in more detail in chapter 3.

Clinical Hypnosis as the Therapeutic Application of Altered States

The therapeutic use of the focused altered state we call hypnosis, is seen during the delivery of waking and trance state suggestions. We view clinical hypnosis as the intentional induction and use of altered states for therapeutic purposes in the clinical setting (Eimer & Freeman, 1998; Zarren, 1996a; Zarren & Eimer, 1999).

Waking State Hypnotic Communication

This includes the state of alteration in internal perception that occurs without a formal trance induction or ceremony. It occurs during the interaction between the clinician and the patient as part of the initial contact, the intake evaluation and the discussion that follows about the problem and the treatment process. When consciously used by the clinician, it represents a large part of the therapy that provides the opportunity for most of the change to take place. The importance of the waking state to the change process will be presented in detail in chapter 3.

The Concept of Reframing

The term *reframing* refers to the purposeful verbal intervention of the clinician to assist the patient in changing the meaning of his or her beliefs that continue to propagate dysfunctional behavior. This does not change the substance of the problem, but it does change the way the patient thinks about himself or herself in relation to the problem. This will be covered in extensive detail in chapter 2.

THE HYPNOTIC TRANCE STATE

The hypnotic trance state is an intensified (more highly focused) altered state that is formally induced through some form of ritual or ceremony, which is labeled the *hypnotic trance induction.* "Suggestions involving a need to remember sensory stimuli and sequences of events are part of most hypnotic induction rituals" (Cheek, 1994, p. 8).

During the trance state, the altered ways of thinking and feeling that were accepted by the patient during the waking state, during waking state reframing, are integrated by the patient's unconscious and fixed in place in the unconscious. This is what we term trance state imprinting. Trance state imprinting is further enhanced by the delivery of additional suggestions that are more specific to the unique change needs of the individual patient. One can think of this as a "fixative process". A useful metaphor is to think of it is as if the clinician were a painter putting the final touches on his or her painting by spraying it with a fixative to make sure that it all stays in place.

20 Basic Characteristics of Hypnotic Trance

Humphreys (2000) details 20 nonmutually exclusive basic characteristics of hypnotic trance as an "altered state of consciousness" that are relevant to our discussions to follow. These include (1) narrowed focus of attention; (2) increased absorption and reduced distractibility; (3) inattention to or disinterest in environmental stimuli other than the therapist; (4) increased concentration on a particular aspect of experience (e.g., sensations, emotions, and ideation); (5) increased suggestibility; (6) reduction of critical evaluation and screening; (7) reduction of voluntary activity (mental and/or physical); (8) passive responsiveness or nonvolitional activity; (9) relative effortlessness; (10) reduction in internal dialogue or self-talk; (11) alteration of cognitive functions; (12) facilitation of atypical modes of thinking, such as "trance logic"; (13) heightened rapport with the therapist; (14) some degree of physical relaxation or comfort; (15) altered sense of one's body; (16) increased imaginal processing; (17) time distortion; (18) alteration of memory processing; (19) relative dominance of the parasympathetic branch of the autonomic nervous system accompanied by a dampening or reduction in sympathetic nervous system activity, along with attendant calming, relaxing and restorative psychophysiological phenomena (Humphreys & Eagan, 1999); and (20) relative dominance of right hemispheric cerebral functioning (see also Watzlawick, 1978).

The Concept of Imprinting

We learn from repetition and from emotionally powerful experiences. When a thought, feeling, or behavior is repeated, the unconscious part of the mind is better able to accept that which is repeated as appropriate and valid. That is how we learn and establish habits. We call this learning *imprinting*. Because the unconscious does not always discriminate between good and bad repetition, unless the behaviors and experiences are perceived as life threatening, we may learn bad habits or less functional ways of behaving, as well as good habits or more functional ways of behaving.

Most of our learning and imprinting take place in the waking state. That is, we are conscious and aware of that consciousness, and we are not asleep, or in an altered state that we label as trance. However, imprinting also occurs during highly emotionally charged experiences, such as shock, trauma, loss, and illness. These emotionally charged experiences are also altered states, and the imprints they create are often negative, uncomfortable, intrusive, and dysfunctional. The strategic utilization of therapeutic altered states (i.e., therapeutic trance) is often the best way to restructure or reframe these negative sequelae.

During the process of waking state reframing we use special change language that we refer to as *reframes* to begin the task of neutralizing negative imprinting that has become dysfunctional and that has been experienced as a problem by the patient. This will be discussed in detail later in this chapter.

Self-Hypnosis

Self-hypnosis, among other things, is a way of communicating with one's unconscious or inner mind. Most individuals do not consciously know how to appropriately communicate with their own unconscious mind. Therefore, to be effective, self-hypnosis has to be taught by someone who understands these communication factors and who is experienced in practicing self-hypnosis. This would be an experienced and well-trained health care professional who has been trained in the clinical and personal use of hypnosis. Chapter 5 addresses these issues.

Hypnosis as a Therapeutic Tool

The effective use of hypnosis as an adjunctive therapeutic tool requires that it be used within a frame of reference that contains its own well-structured system of learning and therapeutic design, such as is contained in medicine, dentistry and psychotherapy. It is a tool, in the hands of an already highly trained and skilled health care professional, for shortening the length of time required for changing and healing the patient. That health care professional should already be trained and experienced in treating a wide range of health-related problems that fall within his or her field or specialty. This means that the well-structured and researched knowledge and treatment methods in medicine, dentistry, clinical psychology and psychotherapy are the foundation on which the tool of hypnosis is added.

Hypnosis also is useful in helping the patient to accomplish change that is more permanent. It is an adjunctive tool that can improve the results of treatment and assist the patient in dealing positively with the treatment experience and the outcomes of treatment.

The many models of psychotherapy as practiced by psychologists, psychiatrists, clinical social workers, marriage and family therapists, psychiatric nurses and mental health and pastoral counselors are used as the foundation on which the tool of hypnosis is added. Because the psychotherapeutic process is essentially an interpersonal communication process, attention to sensory learning and language meaning is of paramount importance.

By reading this book, you can learn new ways of thinking about this verbal and nonverbal communication process, as the brief cognitive hypnosis model is described in extensive detail. We will offer many case studies, model scripts and specific reframes containing change language that can be blended into your current practice methods, or used as part of a new way of doing brief treatment combined with the power of a simple and interesting hypnosis paradigm.

"BRIEF" RATHER THAN "SHORT-TERM" TREATMENT

We call our model *brief cognitive hypnosis* because it takes much less time to bring about change, uses a logical cognitive frame of reference and increases the effectiveness of the tool called clinical hypnosis.

Short-term psychotherapy is the label used for therapy that takes a year or less, as compared to dynamic or psychoanalytic psychotherapy, which may go on for much longer. It is usually task rather than insight directed. Most models are precise, sometimes ritualistic designs that are taught as specific formulas to deal with specific, labeled diagnoses. They can become cumbersome in their detail and thus are often very complicated or not flexible enough. Other models of short-term psychotherapy attempt to individualize, but they are frequently nondirective, assuming the patient's unconscious already has all or most of the information it needs to solve the problem.

Brief cognitive hypnosis is usually accomplished in one to five sessions.

Verbal therapy contracts are established for five session units, when it is decided that multiple or complex problems may need to be addressed. This model is simplified and can be more generally applied to a wide range of behaviors while allowing for the needs and goals of each individual patient. It does this by logically grouping behaviors that, although expressed and experienced differently, are initiated through a common behavioral mechanism.

INITIAL COPING AND EVOLVING COMPLEXITY

Common Underlying Mechanisms of Different Dysfunctional Behaviors

We believe that there are particular cognitive, behavioral and affective mechanisms that different dysfunctional behaviors have in common as underlying factors. This will be expounded in greater detail further on. As an example, by addressing anxiety as the common underlying affective and behavioral mechanism of a number of different dysfunctional behaviors, you can often simplify the start of treatment. Instead of viewing phobias and obsessive-compulsive behaviors as separate and different problems, approach them as starting with the same basic mechanism, anxiety, and viewed them as different negative ways of coping that have become exaggerated and have evolved in an attempt to reduce anxiety.

The choice of different sets of criteria for symptoms and behaviors has been used to establish different specific diagnostic labels (American Psychiatric Association, 1994). We have conceptualized dysfunctional behavior by determining the initial emotional and physiological response mechanism that took place as the patient attempted to cope with a stimulus that was interpreted as threatening. This is in contrast to identifying the extended ritualistic behavior that evolved and became the later presenting problem as what needs to be addressed.

Our conceptual approach often allows us to start at the beginning and change the initial response that later and more debilitating negative symptoms were built upon. Thus, we can often be more focused and goal directed. It allows the patient and us to "uncomplicate" the problem into workable components. This often brings some recognizable feeling of partial relief from the intensity of the presenting symptoms very quickly. By reframing the patient's belief that he or she is trapped, we establish the possibility for new choices and change. This "untraps" the trapped feelings and fears.

By recognizing common dysfunctional behaviors that cut across a number of supposedly different diagnostic categories, you can start the change process at the very beginning by addressing the core behaviors that have evolved and have become more complex over time, by repetition.

THE THEORETICAL FOUNDATION OF BRIEF COGNITIVE HYPNOSIS

Clinical Hypnosis

The theoretical foundation of our model views clinical hypnosis as a two-faceted system:

1. A relationship-based *process of communication* that occurs from the very first contact with the patient when communication takes place with the patient's conscious and unconscious minds simultaneously. We call this process *waking state reframing*. This creates an altered state that can be viewed as an anticipatory trancelike state.
2. The *formal hypnotic trance state* that allows positive imprinting to occur in the unconscious mind and thus fixes the communications and learning in place so they can be applied automatically to create continuing appropriate changes in thinking and behavior.

Challenge Not Confrontation

We reframe the concept of confrontation and relabel it as challenge. That is, we challenge the patient's established belief systems so that the possibility of change can occur.

All patients enter into the therapeutic relationship with a number of established beliefs that tend to be expressed as absolutes. Often, the events they describe are verbalized as always happening. Patients then become trapped in particular negative behaviors because of those beliefs. The beliefs are usually not true and are invalid. That is why the patient is in trouble.

As a therapist you are responsible for helping the patient to change from believing in the absolutism of always being trapped and always feeling helpless to recognizing that this isn't true and believing that change is possible. Challenging these beliefs is the basis of the change process and the reframing process. Reframing starts to occur during the initial interview, when information is given to the patient and when the patient's questions are answered. It also occurs when you start asking the patient questions to clarify his or her beliefs.

This is all part of the process that we call waking state reframing. All of this occurs prior to any formal trance induction. The change language of hypnosis is used throughout this process.

Coping Behavior Not Defense Mechanisms

We do not talk about defense mechanisms in the brief cognitive hypnosis model. All behaviors are viewed as coping behaviors. Some are more effective and appropriate than others.

In our view, during childhood, adolescence, or early adulthood, something may have taken place that was interpreted as a threat to the continued safety or existence of the person. A minor or major fight or flight response (Cannon, 1929) may have then occurred. At that time, the first attempt to cope with the event that was interpreted as threatening or traumatic may have been a behavior that created a feeling of less anxiety and greater comfort. It may have helped at the time it was first used and thus became imprinted as the coping behavior of choice. It was then repeated when memories or feelings from that event or similar events reoccurred. Thus, it was further fixed in place by repetition. This may even happen when the chosen coping behavior is uncomfortable, painful or embarrassing, and thus dysfunctional. It is predictable and therefore is acceptable to the unconscious.

The original event is in the past. It is no longer taking place. The continuation of the initial dysfunctional coping behavior is no longer valid. It is no longer serving its original purpose. Yet it continues by repetition, as a habit. In fact, the longer it is repeated, the more it tends to feed on itself and the more it evolves. It becomes more complicated and more dysfunctional and often more generalized.

Symptoms

You need to identify invalid negative coping behaviors as such. Invalid negative coping methods are leftover dysfunctional behaviors that are labeled *symptoms*. They started as a way of coping with some stressful situation, but they continued because of repetitious imprinting and habit formation. They are no longer needed and are behavioral remnants from the past. In our view, if the patient has not responded to the more traditional approaches to treatment that have been used, this should not be interpreted as resistance, and should not be explained to the patient as a defense mechanism. It should be explained, during the waking state reframing process, as a continuing attempt to cope with an old emotional wound in a manner that is no longer needed. The cooperative and collaborative responsibilities of the patient and the therapist are to appropriately reinterpret the need for the presenting dysfunctional behavior. This can then lead to replacing it with a more appropriate functional behavior, or helping the patient accept that the behavior can be modified or eliminated without the necessity of replacing it.

DIFFERENCES REQUIRE FLEXIBILITY

We also do not acknowledge resistance as a mechanism that prevents the patient from participating in the process of change. The use of the label resistance when talking to a patient may imply that the patient is somehow responsible for the inability to do what he or she is expected to do. When we hear that the patient "can't" or is "unable to," we change what we do and suggest that because people are different from each other, different methods often work for different people. We may say, for example, "That approach (or choice, or method, or technique, or skill, or strategy) wasn't very effective for you, so let's choose another approach." We don't say, "Try harder." This allows for other choices and allows the patient to be relieved of feelings of guilt.

Patients often take responsibility for previous therapeutic procedures that may not have been helpful. They may label their inability to change as "failure," when in fact they may have been able to change had other therapeutic procedures been tried. Patients then may feel guilty, and this can further strengthen their belief that they are trapped and helpless. Being relieved of these negative feelings of failure, guilt and self-blame can help in finding an approach that can be more effective. However, this does not negate the need for the patient to take responsibility to participate in the change process.

1

Establishing the Therapeutic and Hypnotic Relationship

RELATIONSHIP BEGINS WITH THE FIRST CONTACT

All behaviors are expressions of a form of communication. Communication on a conscious or unconscious level is expressed through our verbal and nonverbal language, our behavior, our choice of coping mechanisms, even our symptoms. You need to be conscious both of your own way of communicating and of a particular patient's way of communicating. This is essential to the establishment of any relationship. A positive relationship between you, as the clinician, and the patient is necessary to bring about a positive therapeutic result. The patient must have faith in you for treatment with or without hypnosis to be effective. Therefore, from the very first contact with a patient, everything you say and do has an important effect on the relationship and the outcome of treatment.

Initial Telephone Contact with the Patient

In most cases, in our practices we make the initial appointment directly with a patient, on the telephone. During that initial telephone contact, we do a very brief intake evaluation to determine the purpose of the request for an appointment, why the patient chose to contact us, specifically what the patient's goals are, and previous treatment contacts for this problem. We explain our costs and payment options, whether the first visit is to be an evaluation only or will include some treatment components, and answer questions the patient may have before an appointment is made. This usually takes from 5 to 15 minutes. If someone else is calling to make the appointment for the patient, we inquire why the patient didn't call. We will not make the appointment unless we are satisfied that the patient is unable to personally do so for an acceptable reason.

Some problems, which will be discussed later, may be applicable to a one- or two-session treatment protocol and may be appropriate for treatment during the first or only session. As we proceed to detail the theoretical and treatment process for each type of problem, we will indicate which problems may be dealt with quickly and which may not be.

Over the telephone and face to face, it is important to be precise in the questions asked, in how the questions are worded and in the way information is given to the patient. You want to communicate to the patient that details matter. Additionally, you need to gather enough essential information during the intake evaluation so that you can formulate an appropriate treatment plan geared to the patient's specific problems and needs.

Hypnotic processes are meant to serve as agents of effective therapeutic communication and change. What you say and do in the intake evaluation will affect the patient's expectations about your skill as a clinician, the therapeutic process, and the use of hypnosis as an appropriate tool.

CONSCIOUS USE OF SELF

Throughout this book we will be talking about the clinician's conscious use of self. By this term, we mean that the clinician is the agent of change. Even experienced clinicians can fall into the pattern of reflexively and mechanically dealing with some of their patients in automatic ways. This may include categorizing a patient based on past experience and personal prejudices. This may be an unconscious reaction on the part of the clinician, who may then go into an automatic judgment and treatment mode. We all "go into automatic," learning by repetition. We and our patients develop habits that we are not always consciously aware of. When this occurs, we often stop listening to a patient and stop paying conscious attention to our own communication with a patient.

Listening to the Patient

Conscious use of self also includes paying conscious attention to the ways the patient uses his or her self. The patient's choices of language, labels, nonverbal behavior, body language, expression of strengths and weaknesses and symptoms, are but a few of the important messages he or she communicates and to which you need to consciously attend.

As an experienced clinician, you already know how to establish a relationship with a patient. Most of what you do as a professional has probably been part of the way you have practiced for many years. Recall the comment about going into automatic mode. Most of what you have been doing is probably now being done automatically and unconsciously. Most of the time it works well. However, sometimes it may work slowly, or the patient may be identified as someone you can't or don't want to work with because something just doesn't "click" between you and the patient. By learning how to use yourself consciously, you may be able to do what you already do very well, even better. This may help you to figure out what is going on when things just don't seem to be "clicking."

Listening to the Patient's Sensory Representational Language.

Listening to the sensory representational language that the patient uses to describe what he or she is experiencing and how the patient answers your questions provides essential information. You need to determine the primary types of predicates and descriptive adjectives that the patient uses:

1. Are they primarily visual, as in "When I look at myself, I see someone who is in trouble"?
2. Are they primarily kinesthetic, as in "When I feel everyone's against me, I get knotted up inside"?
3. Are they primarily auditory, as in "I keep listening to myself and hearing myself sound stupid"?
4. Are they primarily olfactory, as in "I smell something going on, and it smells fishy"?
5. Are they primarily gustatory, as in "This tastes sour to me. He's left me with a sour taste?"

Matching Predicates and Descriptive Language to Build Rapport

Once you identify a patient's primary predicates and descriptive adjectives, as well as the sensory representational systems to which they are attached, you will be aware of what primary sensory systems that patient uses most often to process information and learning. It is important to pay conscious attention to the language that you use most often, and to identify it with one or more of the five sensory representational systems. If these are different from the ones that the patient uses, you should pay conscious attention to changing your predicates and descriptive language to more often match those of the patient (Cameron-Bandler, 1978; Grinder & Bandler, 1976, 1981; Lankton, 1980; Lewis & Pucelik, 1982).

This is an important first step in establishing rapport with a patient. You may be talking the same language but be processing the information quite differently. If your sensory language is primarily kinesthetic, and a patient's is primarily visual, for example, you may have a problem understanding and relating.

For example, a patient may ask, "Can you see what I mean?, and the clinician may answer, "What you told me doesn't feel right." That's as if the patient were speaking English and you were speaking French. Neither of you really understands the other. This discrepancy can create discordance that needs to be corrected by consciously switching to the sensory representational language of the patient. Instead, you should respond with a comment such as, "Now that you have described it to me, I can certainly see it."

Unfortunately, it is not quite that simple or clear-cut. This is because most people also use sensory language in representing how they think and feel. For example, a patient may say, "When he comes near (kinesthetic) me, he looks (visual) as if he is about to do something fishy (olfactory), and that makes me feel (kinesthetic) sour (gustatory)." This is an exaggeration, of course, and is used only to emphasize the use of overlapping language relating to sensory systems. If you recognize that there is significant overlapping in the use of sensory language, pay more attention to nonverbal cues to identify the more favored processing system.

Asking Questions: Finding Exceptions to the Presenting Problem

It is important to ask questions to get more detail about the presenting problem and what has been done before. The patient usually does not express verbally what he or she is not consciously aware of. The patient does talk about his or her beliefs, and these beliefs may or may not be valid or true.

For example, the patient may be describing a problem as if it is always happening. This is an absolute. You, the clinician, know it is not always happening. So how can you help the patient recognize that there are many times when it is *not* happening? You can do this by asking more questions about possible times when it is not occurring. For example,

> Does it happen when you are asleep? Does it happen when you are busy at work? How about when you are having a good time, or when you are making love?

If you ask enough questions about other times when the problem does not happen, some of these questions will have to be answered with an "It does not happen then." When we find exceptions to the problem, we no longer have an absolute. Now the patient can be helped to recognize that he or she *is not trapped.* For example,

> So, there are times when it is not happening. Now we can help you establish a conscious and unconscious memory of those times when it is not happening, and stretch that memory, so it doesn't have to happen as often, or at all.

This is related to the following reframe:

> We only pay attention to events. We don't pay attention to nonevents. When something is happening, we pay attention to it. If something is not happening, naturally, we are not aware of it.

MATCHING OF PATIENT AND METHODOLOGY

There are a number of indicators that you can use to determine whether your treatment approaches will help patients. In our practices, most patients arrive from another health care professional's referral, a referral by a former patient or family member or friend of a former patient, or through our advertisements in the Yellow Pages. Because we are no longer associated with managed care programs and rarely accept direct payment from insurance companies, we have the flexibility to choose our patients according to our judgments of possible positive outcomes.

This reduces the number of patients we see. However, it also increases our potential success rate, and because we charge full fee for services, it balances out our income. Many clinicians are part of some type of managed care system. They will find that this approach can help reduce the number of visits a patient needs, and thus may increase their referrals and their income.

It is important to recognize that not every patient or every patient problem is going to respond to our brief therapy approach or any brief therapy approach, for that matter. Patients are screened for how appropriate they and their problem may be to how we do therapy. We cannot help everyone, so we concentrate our skills, time and energy on those we believe we can help.

Patients who call or come in expecting magic usually are not good candidates for positive treatment outcomes. These are usually individuals who are not interested in being told that they must be active participants in the change process. They generally want to be "zapped" for instant change. They want hypnosis to be an instant cure for any and all of their ailments. Often they insist, when they make an appointment, that they receive hypnosis treatment during the first session, even before we know what the real problem is. If a prospective patient is not willing to accept that formal treatment will take place only after we determine what is needed and what approach is appropriate, then an appointment is not made.

THE INITIATION OF WAKING STATE REFRAMING

A patient may express this kind of unrealistic attitude during the initial session. This is when you should interrupt the intake process and start to clarify to the patient what is real and what is not. In chapter 2 we will describe in detail the process of waking state reframing. This is when the process starts, as you explains:

> No change can occur without the active agreement and participation of the patient. The therapeutic procedures to be used are brief cognitive hypnosis and psychotherapy [or whatever your professional discipline is]. All hypnosis is not the same. Hypnosis is a tool in the hands of a clinician already skilled in his or her profession. That tool called hypnosis can help shorten the length of time it takes to help people change and can often help that change occur more easily and last much

longer. But we first need to get as much information as we can before we decide if we will be using hypnosis, and how, and I need to explain to you what it is all about.

Patients who are being pressured by someone else to seek help may be seeing you with little or no motivation to change or resolve their problem. They may be willing to pay for failure so that they can say to the pressuring person, "See? I tried and it didn't work, so get off my back." As you become aware of this possibility, this is also the time to stop the intake procedure and challenge the patient as to his or her motivation for change. Here, waking state reframing will be designed to deal with the crucial issue of clarifying why the patient wants to continue to suffer the consequences of the stated problem as opposed to wanting to be more comfortable and in charge. Often, this testing of the patient's reasoning can expose the patient's secondary gains, such as having a great deal of control over others in the family by maintaining the somewhat debilitating symptoms.

Case Study: Psychogenic Aphonia (Whispering)

Some time ago, I (JIZ) had a preadolescent boy referred to me because he was not able to talk above a whisper (psychogenic aphonia). A complete medical examination discovered no medical or physical reason for this kind of problem. The boy was seen alone, without a parent present. During the intake evaluation process, it was determined that the whispering behavior was a very powerful way for him to control his relationships with others and what he was asked to do. Others had to come close to him to hear what he was saying. Teachers, for example, had to come close to hear his answers. Because of his whispering, he was never asked to speak before the whole class. This insight was not revealed to the patient.

The patient was asked if he wanted to control the whisper and speak normally. We discussed the various pluses and minuses of the whispering problem. It was further determined that the patient did indeed want to stop whispering, but he felt that he could not do so without "losing face." The patient did not verbalize this, and it was not explained to him. He was trapped in his own controlling behavior. He said he absolutely had no control over the behavior but that he would like it to stop.

This boy enjoyed playing pinball, baseball and other individual and team sports. He was a curious and otherwise normal-appearing youngster. He was asked if he would like to play a pinball game in his head while he was hypnotized. He said he would, but that he was not sure what being hypnotized meant. It was explained that this was "like imagining some fun thing while your eyes are closed and you are very relaxed".

The patient was told that while a person is relaxed, some of the things imagined almost feel real. We reached an agreement that every time he got a ball in the hole, he would be able to verbally express pleasure without having to whisper. He said that would be great.

We did an induction (discussed in chapter 4) and proceeded to play the game. It was suggested that if he got a great score, which he alone could set, he would not have to whisper any longer. He was able to loudly express pleasure each time he got a ball in a hole, but he was not able to reach the score he had set as winning. When he was awakened, he continued to talk in a whisper. Additional attempts to win the game during hypnosis brought the same results. He rejected suggestions that he lower the score for winning. However, he did acknowledge that he no longer had to speak in a whisper all the time, because he knew now that there were times when he could in fact speak normally. He said he didn't know why he could not do it during the waking state.

It was determined that this was progress, but that we had not yet dealt with the face-saving problem. He was eventually helped to give up his whispering comfortably and save face with another strategy involving ancillary assistance (explained in chapter 6). The point to this case description is that, as the therapist, you need to determine what is possible and what is not in order to do the best therapy possible.

Motivation is important when the patient is trapped in a dysfunctional behavior. Because what the patient has done in the past has not worked, we do not repeat that approach. Instead, we try something different. This is then explained to a patient, who often expresses relief and more openness to participating in other approaches with greater intrinsic personal motivation. Therefore, it is important that you know what has been tried before that has not worked. This is part of the information that should be obtained during the intake process (see below).

To further help in patient selection, we know that, because we are dealing with cognitive function that requires reasoning and the ability to sustain concentration, severe mental impairment, either organic or psychogenic (e.g., dementia or psychosis), would suggest that the patient is not appropriate for this treatment approach.

THE INTAKE EVALUATION

During our years supervising and teaching the applications of clinical hypnosis to experienced clinicians, we became aware that the usual intake evaluations that some clinicians had been conducting were not always thorough. Clinicians needed more information to determine if the tool of hypnosis could be helpful with a particular patient. They expressed concern that their work was not as effective as they had expected or as long lasting as they had wanted. We found ourselves asking many questions about patients that clinicians could not answer. They did not have the information because they did not know to listen to a particular patient's clues that required more exploration.

You usually can get enough information in 15 minutes to address a single behavior. We may find during the evaluation, though, that the presenting problem is an excuse to make it easier for the patient to start a longer therapeutic relationship.

The patient may not be consciously aware of this as a factor in his or her decision to seek treatment. As more information is sought, the patient may say, "Oh, yes, I need to work on that, too. And that, and that, and that." This means that you are now into a much longer intake process that may require the entire session or longer.

The following is a list of the minimum information to ask for during an initial intake. Table 1.1, which follows, is a learning tool and is not to be used directly with the patient. It is not a test, just a way to help you to be aware of what needs to be asked.

INTAKE EVALUATION OUTLINE

1. Identifying information—patient's full name; address, telephone numbers (home, work, mobile), age, marital status
2. Patient's household constellation—age(s), gender(s), relationship(s) to patient, living and sleeping arrangements, significant interactional or health problems, emotional or substance abuse problems, anything else of importance to the patient regarding this area of inquiry
3. Patient's employment—status, general schedule, job satisfaction, responsibilities, relationships, worries
4. Patient's habits—smoking (brand, amount, whether it is done around children and family); coffee intake (regular or decaffeinated, amount per day (mugs or cups) and frequency/times, use of sugar or sweetener and amount); tea intake (hot or cold, caffeinated or decaffeinated, amount and frequency/times, use of sugar or sweetener); soda intake (similar details); alcohol use (types of alcoholic beverages; amount and frequency/times, comparison to past usage; patterns: nights, weekends, more when under stress; whether it is considered a problem; details about alcohol use by others in the home); prescription drugs (which ones, reasons for use, doses and number of times per day, length of use, whether they help, the physician, nonprescription drugs, include alternative medicines, e.g., herbs (amount, reasons for use, whether they help); substance abuse, both past and current, both prescription and nonprescription (when, where, how much, and for how long; reasons for use; any attempts to stop and success rate; desire to stop)
5. Patient's health and medical history—glasses; hearing aids; sleeping problems (type, frequency, longevity, treatments, success); headaches (severity, type, frequency, longevity, treatment); mouth or jaw pain, including TMJ (Temporo-Mandibula Joint Disorder) and bruxism: (severity, treatment); shoulder, neck, or lower back pain (severity, treatment); bothersome coughing; sinus problems; Allergies; breathing problems; pressure in the chest area; frequent heartburn or indigestion (severity, treatment); stomach cramps or aches; problems with bowel movements, including diarrhea and constipation; problems with urination; cramping of leg or foot muscles; major illnesses, surgeries, or hospitalizations over the past 5 years; mood swings; impulse control problems; mild or extreme

anxiety; depression; emotional problems (current or past treatment by a psychiatrist, psychologist, or other mental health professional; details)
6. Patient's family health history—obtain as much detail as necessary; this is especially important if it appears stressful for the patient or if there has been any long-term problem or intergenerational pattern of occurrence
7. Patient's referral history—professional referral (details), family member, friend, Yellow Pages, other; if a professional or person-to-person referral, ask what was specifically suggested as to the nature of the problem.
8. Patient's current expectations—details of the stated problem (description, onset, level of dysfunction); previous experiences in addressing the stated problem; previous treatment experiences for other psychological, emotional, or behavioral problems; professional fields of clinicians who have treated the patient; understanding, beliefs, and previous experience regarding psychotherapy (if applicable), hypnosis, and other treatment modalities

Patterns and Beliefs Checklist

Table 1.1 is a guide for determining that everything that needs to be asked of the patient is asked. Other topics should be addressed when dealing with specific problems, such as chronic pain, family, or substance abuse problems.

TABLE 1.1 *Patterns and Beliefs Checklist*

1. Presenting problem
2. Length of problem
3. Attempts at problem resolution
4. Ways of coping with problem
5. Present coping skills (positive and negative)
6. Identifiable or supposed precipitators of the problem
7. Degree of disability (physical and emotional) caused by the problem
8. General conscious belief systems
9. Iatrogenic belief systems
10. Beliefs about therapy and hypnosis
11. Myths
12. Primary and secondary sensory systems used for processing information
13. Representational language use
14. Patterns of thinking
15. Rituals and ritualistic behavior
16. Rationalizations
17. Explanations
18. Excuses
19. Understanding or insights
20. Social and peer influences
21. Parental and family of origin influences
22. Current family influences
23. Health professional influences
24. Role models
25. Fears and phobias
[Edit as needed]

PAYING ATTENTION TO HOW THE PATIENT COMMUNICATES

As we suggested earlier, when establishing a relationship with the patient, you need to be aware of your own way of asking for information and how you process information. We call this *conscious use of self*. Each individual has his or her own biological and psychological patterns of thinking, communicating and learning.

When you first encounter someone in whose presence you feel uncomfortable and to whom you seem to immediately respond with suspicion, distrust or even subtle or open hostility, you may think, "I don't like this person." In social situations, you can choose to avoid him or her or limit your contact. However, in your professional relationships, with both patients and colleagues, this is usually not as easy. This is why you need to develop greater awareness of your own ways of communicating and processing information, as well as those of a patient.

When your sensory processing choices clash with those of another person, you usually feel uncomfortable, and may feel dislike or distrust, or confused by the way the other person communicates to you and seems to so easily misunderstand what you are trying to communicate. This interferes with the easy establishment of rapport and can be an obstacle to communicating effectively with others, particularly with patients.

We all receive and process information through our sensory system. We see, hear, smell taste, and feel. It appears that most people process information visually. That is, they picture in their minds that which needs to be understood and learned, because this is their primary way of internalizing information. Many people experience their information intake as a kinesthetic process. They internalize their thinking to experience how that which is being communicated feels to them. Visual and kinesthetic processing seem to be the two most common and universal sensory processing systems.

A smaller number of people, often those who have perfect pitch or who have musical talent, listen very carefully to what is being said, and hear tonal cues that allow them to process information through their auditory system more effectively.

The senses of taste and smell are less often used as primary sensory processing systems. Both are important for accessing memories. The sensation of taste is triggered by a suitable stimulus applied to the gustatory nerve endings in the tongue and is imprinted early on when the newborn first exercises the sucking response and experiences the pleasure and security that sucking evokes. Smells, which are perceived by means of the olfactory apparatus, are rich in the ability to almost instantly bring back detailed memories of the past, both positive and negative in nature.

A personal experience (JIZ) demonstrates this. I was brought up in a home with my grandmother, who each year cured kosher pickles in a large wooden barrel in a pantry off the kitchen. Today, whenever I walk into an old-fashioned kosher delicatessen and smell the sharp aroma of the spices in the open pickle barrels, I have an instant flashback to my grandmother's pantry. It occurs with all the taste and pleasure of being invited to be the first to roll up my sleeve and reach into the barrel to retrieve and taste that first pickle, and give approval to that year's pickle crop.

Paying Attention to the Patient's Sensory Language

You can most easily identify patients' primary sensory systems by paying attention to the language used by patients in describing their experiences. Writing down the words a patient uses is helpful.

There are particular words that indicate sensory clues to a particular patient's way of processing and communicating information. Table 1.2 presents some predicates and adjectives for each of the sensory systems. Note that some words fit into several categories. In the table, such words are italicized. It is important to listen to a patient speak for a while in order to obtain an adequate sampling of the patient's primary sensory system.

TABLE 1.2 *Representative Predicates and Adjectives for Each of the Sensory Systems*

Visual—visualize, see, look, imagine, picture, pretty, ugly, envision, view, observe, perspective, witness, scan, scene, dim, *light, lighten,* brighten, vista.

Kinesthetic—feel, sense, touch, endure, resonate, vibrations ("vibes"), suffer, rough, hard, soft, *strong,* experience, anesthetize, numb, *nauseous, volume,* stomach, hurt, pain, *sharp,* sting, itch, ouch, gut, heavy, *light, lighten, low,* load.

Auditory—hear, listen, sound, *volume, report, rumor, voice,* loud, *lower,* tone, roar, echo.

Gustatory—taste, snack, savor, digest, flavor, sip, hungry, appetite, bitter, *sharp,* sweet, sour, tasteful, *strong,* delicious, *nauseous,* tasty, tasteless.

Olfactory—smell, nose, odor, scent, *strong,* pungent, whiff, rancid, stinks, aroma, *sharp,* stench.

The Clinician's Choice of Words

We have commented about the importance for you, the clinician, to also search his or her own sensory language. If a patient uses visual predicates and you respond with kinesthetic predicates, you may not be able to communicate with each other effectively. As suggested, one or both of you may in fact feel uncomfortable and confused about what was said, even feel unhappy about the interaction. It is easier for you to be aware and consciously change your language to match that of the patient. This will greatly improve your chance for rapidly establishing rapport (Cameron-Bandler, 1978; Grinder & Bandler, 1976, 1981; Lankton, 1980; Lewis & Pucelik, 1982).

Carefully observing the way a patient stands, walks, sits and moves can give clues. A person with a hearing problem, for example, is going to move his or her head in a certain way to aid hearing. As another example, an eye fixation induction for someone who is not visual will not be helpful in bringing about a trance state. More about these special issues later.

FORMULATING A TREATMENT PLAN

Agreeing on the Problem and the Goals

Once this information is gathered, you can begin to discuss with the patient your assessment of the problem. If it differs from the patient's presenting problem, this needs to be discussed and clarified. You may need to further refine the problem into smaller workable units that will allow for less lofty goals. The loftier the goal, the more complicated the treatment plan will be; the more complicated the treatment plan, the less observable and immediately positive the results will be.

Establishing the patient's actual goals requires some discussion that involves clarifying what the patient means by some of the things he or she says. This is all part of the process of waking state reframing. At this stage, the therapeutic objective is to agree on a reasonable (realistic and attainable) goal or set of goals. You also want to clarify what can be accomplished through the addition of hypnosis to your usual treatment approach and what may not be doable. Once goals are established, a therapeutic strategy for achieving them is needed.

Formulating a Therapeutic Strategy

Hypnosis is not the strategy or the therapy by itself. As we mentioned earlier, hypnosis is a treatment tool, in the hands of a skilled clinician that facilitates the implementation of a therapeutic strategy and shortens the length of time that therapy takes. We define brief cognitive treatment as a way to help individuals change the way they think about themselves, their world, their present, past, and future, and their behavior, relationships, and personal situation, so that change can take place. Beliefs and behavior can change, thus making it possible for a person's circumstances to change also.

Change Is Recognized Only in Retrospect

It is important for the patient to be helped to recognize that change is occurring. Usually, change is recognized only in retrospect. This means that as each small goal is realized, the patient has to be helped to be aware of it. For example, you could say:

> Have you noticed that you are no longer coming into the office all tensed up? Remember what it was like 3 weeks ago when you first came in to see me? Notice how different, how much more comfortable, you look and feel today.

A clinical diagnosis, an evaluation of the problem's severity, and an estimated time frame to solve the problem all influence your treatment plan design, as well as your verbal contract with the patient. Some patients will be seeing you with an understanding that they require only one visit, for example, for smoking cessation, or one or two visits, as for other simple habits. Others, with more complex problems, will need help in understanding that more visits will be required. While you should establish agreement with the patient about the treatment plan in advance of initiating treatment, all verbal contracts are and should be subject to reevaluation, modification and change, as necessary.

BASIC STEPS IN TREATMENT PLANNING

The following examples are meant to guide you in establishing a treatment plan. The steps outlined in each of the following two examples are not designed to be shared with the patient. Instead, you should explain to the patient what you plan to do, so that the patient understands what to expect, but what you share is not the treatment plan. Treatment planning is to help you to establish guidelines.

Treatment plans for problems that can be dealt with in only one or two sessions are very short and have only a few specific goals. They include waking state reframing but typically do not include teaching the patient self-hypnosis or self-relaxation. Treatment plans for problems that are likely to require more than one or two sessions typically require more extensive waking state reframing and usually include teaching the patient self-hypnosis or self-relaxation.

Basic Treatment Plan for a Simple Problem Requiring One or Two Visits

1. Do waking state reframing to change the patient's belief system about the problem from complex to simple. This typically involves reframing the patient's absolute beliefs about the problem behavior, to help the patient recognize that it occurs sometimes, but not always, that the problem is changeable and not permanent, that it is understandable and not mysterious and that the patient is not to blame.
2. Explain the functions of the conscious and the unconscious parts of the mind and how they are involved in controlling voluntary and involuntary behavior.

3. Discuss the nature of the hypnosis trance experience, and what the patient can expect to experience during and after the trance.
4. Determine the most appropriate induction procedure and describe it to the patient.
5. Formulate the change language and specific suggestions to be used during the patient's trance experience.
6. Decide whether to include trance in this initial session, or schedule another session for the trance work.
7. Implement the induction of trance.
8. After inducing trance, administer pertinent therapeutic suggestions, with appropriate change language and reframes, including appropriate posttrance imprinting suggestions.
9. Realert (awaken) the patient from trance, conduct a posttrance evaluation, and administer further appropriate posttrance suggestions. If asked about self-hypnosis by the patient, explain why it is NOT necessary for this particular problem.

Basic Treatment Plan for Problems Generally Requiring More Than One or Two Visits

1. Identify the negative coping behavior or symptom that is most amenable to change so that the patient can almost immediately feel some relief.
2. Determine what has been done previously to change the current evolved behavior or symptom, so as not to repeat what has not worked before.
3. Reframe the patient's absolute beliefs about the problem behavior, to help the patient recognize that it occurs sometimes, but not always, that the problem is changeable and not permanent, that it is understandable and not mysterious, and that the patient is not to blame.
4. Do a deep relaxation induction to imprint a strong memory of how it feels to be relaxed.
5. Include in this induction and trance experience instructions on how the patient can do self-relaxation to reinforce and recharge this memory of how it feels to be deeply relaxed.
6. After awakening, if the patient has been taught self-relaxation during this session, have the patient immediately relax his or her self again without the help of the clinician. This brings an even deeper level of relaxation and affirms the patient's ability to do it without help.
7. Instruct the patient to do NO self-talk during his or her own practice of self-relaxation. Suggest that this self-practice will automatically reinforce and refresh what the clinician said while teaching it to the patient. This prevents self-talk distortion that might be counterproductive.
8. Attach, through suggestion, during the trance experience, a belief that the

feeling of relaxation being experienced by the patient will be repeatable and will allow the patient to feel progressively better and exhibit fewer and milder experiences of the negative coping behavior, if at all.

9. Realert (awaken) the patient from trance, conduct a posttrance evaluation, and administer further appropriate posttrance suggestions.

10. Review the steps the patient will take in practicing self-relaxation or self-hypnosis, then discuss how this one to two times daily 10-minute practice can be inserted into the patient's daily schedule.

CASE STUDY: PATIENT TREATED FOR THE PRESENTING PROBLEM WITH A CAREFULLY TAILORED PROCEDURE

In another case, an appointment was made for smoking cessation, and it was discovered during the intake that the patient was on full medical disability from the U.S. Army. He was in outpatient treatment at the local Veterans Administration hospital with a diagnosis of paranoid schizophrenia. There were some delusional beliefs about his skills as an inventor of a very complex mechanism that he claimed to have designed for the government.

The patient was taking Stelazine three times a day and exhibited some cognitive impairment. However, he was very clear about his desire to stop smoking and talked about health as his motivation. This man knew little about hypnosis, but he believed it would not be something that would have an undue negative influence on him. He believed that hypnosis might help him stop smoking without uncomfortable withdrawal.

The patient lived in an assisted care facility in his own apartment and took good care of himself. He was neat and clean and he could get around by taxi or public transportation.

Having had experience using hypnosis with psychotic patients in the past, I (JIZ) decided that I could possibly help this patient to stop smoking without exacerbating his psychological and medical problems. I explained hypnosis as relaxation, and that he would feel relaxed and always be aware of what I was saying to him. Furthermore, I told him that he would be able to open his eyes any time he wanted to, if he wanted to. I explained that while he was relaxed and had his eyes closed, I would be talking to the part of him that controlled the smoking habit to give it information that would allow him to stop smoking.

Because of my judgment that there was some cognitive impairment, I skipped the extensive waking state reframing regarding smoking (see chapter 12). After the short explanation described above, I performed the rising and falling arms induction, (described in chapter 4). Then I verbalized the trance language material that is a regular part of our smoking cessation protocol.

After exiting from the trance, the patient stated that he felt very relaxed and heard everything. He enjoyed being hypnotized. In a subsequent telephone follow-up 6 months later, he indicated that he had not touched a cigarette since our session.

CASE STUDY: PATIENT TREATED FOR PRESENTING PROBLEM WITH ANCILLARY HELP (PSYCHOGENIC APHONIA)

Recall the case of the young boy who could not speak above a whisper, as presented earlier in this chapter. The boy loved to play baseball. A few weeks earlier, he had injured his right wrist while sliding into second base. He was told he needed surgery to correct the problem so he would be able to play baseball again. I (JIZ) asked permission from his parents to talk to his surgeon, whom I knew, about helping me help their son to speak in a normal voice.

In my meeting with the surgeon, I described what his problem was, including the need to "save face" in order to be comfortable speaking normally. I asked the surgeon if he would be willing to give certain suggestions to the youngster during the induction of general anesthesia. I explained that this state was similar to that which occurs during the hypnotic trance state. I also explained to the surgeon that suggestions from a trusted authority figure could be very powerful in establishing communication with the boy's unconscious mind to produce change. I told him that, during my next session with our mutual patient, I would set up during hypnosis the surgeon's suggestions as acceptable and effective.

I wrote out what I wanted the surgeon to say, and how to say it, and I instructed the surgeon to repeat it from time to time during the surgery. These suggestions were "When the patient is just beginning to relax during the administration of the anesthesia, say to him, 'You can rest comfortably because we are going to be able to fix everything that has been bothering you, while we repair your wrist.' Repeat these suggestions four or five times as he is going under, then every once in a while as the surgery progresses. Also, as you proceed with the repair, comment to the patient, 'This is going great and will fix everything.'"

During the next session with the boy, prior to his surgery, we talked about how he can relax himself and feel comfortable during the surgery. I taught him how to pay attention to his breathing with his eyes closed to help him feel relaxed before the surgery. I repeated this during his trance experience, and I talked about what a great doctor he had and how his doctor was "going to fix everything."

Upon awakening from the surgery, which went very well, the boy spoke in a normal voice, and he has done so ever since. Neither the medical staff nor his family, as they had been instructed, made any specific reference about this to the patient. He was congratulated on how good he had been before, during, and after his surgery and how well the healing was going.

This strategy worked because the surgeon, during general anesthesia and the actual surgery, spoke to the patient's unconscious and suggested that he, the surgeon, and the surgery would fix everything that needed fixing. This allowed the patient to psychologically "save face," if necessary, by identifying his whispering problem as "medical" and one that would be cured by medical means. The patient had been primed to accept this during the trance experience in the therapist's office.

2

The Waking State Reframing Model

The brief cognitive hypnosis model emphasizes the importance of how beliefs are established and how those beliefs create behavioral responses that can be positive or negative. We referred earlier to our view of hypnosis as an alteration in internal perception, a focused altered state that is initiated at the start of a unique process of communication. This happens in the waking state as well as in the trance state. This suggests that carefully constructed verbal communication from the clinician to the patient during the normal exchange of information can be very powerful in bringing about therapeutic change. Psychotherapy is "talk therapy." Brief cognitive talk therapy, using the language of hypnosis, when carefully and consciously crafted, can bring about positive change relatively quickly and permanently.

Waking state reframing takes place during the intake evaluation process and during the preparation for the trance experience. Most of the work in our brief therapy model actually takes place during the waking state. The clinician talks to the patient's conscious and unconscious minds at the same time. This overlapping process of communication is identified in our model as waking state reframing.

THE MEANING OF REFRAMING

The term *Reframing* refers to the intentional intervention by the clinician to assist the patient in changing the *meaning* of beliefs, rituals, patterns, labels, feelings and behaviors, to open the way for emotional and behavioral change. When initiated by the clinician, this is a conscious cognitive procedure that affects the cognitive, emotional, and behavioral systems of the patient. The reframe by itself does not produce change. What it does is change the patient's way of thinking and belief systems in such a way as to open up the possibility of change for the patient. Put in a slightly different way, to reframe something is to change the way that one thinks about something without actually changing it." The way someone thinks about something may be changed even though the facts remain the same. The original situation may in fact remain unchanged, but it can be perceived from a new point of view. How this occurs may not be obvious immediately, because even though there is a change in the point of view, the situation itself initially may remain unchanged. What is changed, as a result of the reframing, is the meaning attributed to the situation, and thus its consequences, but not its concrete facts.

Reframing operates on a different level of reality, almost like "trance logic," where change can take place even if the objective circumstances appear to suggest that they are beyond our control. When looking at half a glass of water, for example, you may perceive it as half empty at one time, half full at another. There is still only half a glass of water. Your change in perception thus changes the way you respond to the situation, not the situation itself.

CHANGING LABELS CHANGES BELIEFS

The ability of the mind to change subjective and objective realities by changing labels offers the opportunity to use therapeutic interventions that we call *reframing*. There is no single reality. All reality is our interpretation of the world and its contents based on the way we process information and what we choose to identify as our unique reality. When we feel trapped in a feeling or a behavior, we believe that we have no choices. We are caught in a dilemma. We are dammed if we do, dammed if we don't, so we may freeze and do nothing.

Successful reframing requires taking into account the views, expectations, reasons, premises, in fact, the whole conceptual framework of the patient whose beliefs and views are to be challenged. Therefore, it is essential to pay attention to everything the patient is bringing to you.

Reframing requires that you learn what a patient believes by questioning and listening and looking. It is easy to make the assumption that the patient has the same frame of reference when describing something as you do. For example, you both may be thinking about relaxing on a beach, but the patient may be thinking about a lakeside beach, whereas you may be thinking about a seashore.

An even more powerful word change involves reframing words such as *addiction* that the patient uses to identify behaviors that have so far been difficult to change. Many of these emotionally powerful negative words have been imposed on the patient by societal convention. This satisfies a societal need to label some of the most difficult dysfunctional behaviors as "disease." These problems thus are no longer considered the patient's fault, or within the patient's power to change.

These extreme labels may be accurate for some severe medical or psychological problems. Unfortunately, they often are applied to many other behaviors that are frustratingly difficult to treat, even though there may be little actual evidence to identify those behaviors in this way. For example, the label "addiction" has been applied to many dysfunctional habit behaviors that may be emotionally difficult to change. They are labeled as addictions only because they are difficult to change, not because they substantially change the biochemical structure of the brain. In other words, the label "addiction" has been used to include psychologically compulsive behaviors such as gambling, excessive sexual desire, and compulsive shopping.

This need to label some compulsive behaviors as addictive allows many treatment institutions to influence diagnoses to increase revenues, by encouraging insurance payments for longer term and more expensive treatments.

CHANGING DIAGNOSIS CHANGES TREATMENT

A good example of the effects that labels can have can be seen in the diagnosis and treatment of problems with alcohol. The problem of excessive alcohol intake is often labeled as alcoholism, even though some cases may be more accurately and appropriately labeled as problem drinking. A thorough examination of the onset, frequency and circumstances of the drinking behavior may suggest that it is not a "disease" or an "addiction," but instead a frequently repeated dysfunctional behavior. Relabeling it as such can often lead to treating the behavior or controlling it successfully. By doing so, it is being changed to a different class that is not as impossible to treat.

In our smoking cessation approach, (discussed in chapter 12), we use this concept very effectively. We change the label "addiction" to "habit," and "withdrawal symptoms" to "stress reaction." Along with other reframes, these two powerful reframes offer the patient an opportunity to reevaluate what he or she may have been hearing repeatedly from friends who could not stop smoking. These reframes also help the patient to reevaluate the messages received from advertising for commercial products to stop smoking and from the medical community, which frequently applies emotionally loaded scare labels. The emotionally loaded labels applied by these institutions to the smoking problem can in fact motivate some individuals to seek medical help if the label or classification of the problem behavior creates the belief that it is difficult to change. It may also prevent some individuals from seeking appropriate help because the label "addiction" suggests that changing the behavior may involve a very lengthy, difficult, involved and painful process.

CHOICES LEAD TO CHANGE

Reframe

We are trapped only as long as we believe we have no choices. Once we recognize that we have other choices, and we make a choice, then we are no longer trapped.

This reframe (i.e., change in thinking) can open the trap and allow for change. Similarly, we are taught from early childhood that "if at first we don't succeed, try, try again." Continuing to try again that which doesn't work will not make it work any better. However, by recognizing that there are choices and by deliberately choosing to do something different, we open up the possibility of success.

A Metaphor

Imagine yourself walking down a beautiful country path through the woods. The path leads to a beautiful lake, where you very much want to go and relax. Suddenly, you come upon a very high stone wall that cuts right across the path and into the woods on both sides of the path. You are completely blocked from proceeding farther unless you can somehow get over or through that solid stone wall. You try climbing it, but you can't. You try pushing against it, but it doesn't budge. As your frustration grows, your attempts become more frantic, and you may even bloody your hands in the process of trying. How can you get to the other side of the wall? More of the same is certainly not the answer. Yet, all too often, we do more of the same even though it is not effective, hoping that increasing the effort will work. But it doesn't.

You need to recognize, and help the patient to recognize, that there are other choices, other options, that can be applied to solving the problem. Pushing against an immovable stone wall harder and harder still will not move the wall. However, backing off and rethinking possible solutions to the problem may produce better results.

We can calmly look to the right and left of the path, near the wall, for a pathway we can follow that may take us to a door, or to the end of the wall. This makes more sense. We do so, and we notice a small clearing and path on our right near the wall. We follow it and are joyfully relieved to see an unlocked gate through the wall to the other side. There, we see a lovely flower-covered meadow leading to a serene lake on the other side. The solution to the problem is not to push so hard doing the same thing that didn't work, but to recognize that we have choices and to make a different choice.

REFRAMING IS NOT "INSIGHT"

When we talk about reframing we are not talking about "insight." Insight doesn't change behavior (Bloom, 1994). Because most of us have little conscious insight into why we behave as we do, or think about the world in the way that we do, many of us tend to *want to know why*. This desire to know the cause of our problem behavior has contributed to the development of long-term, exploratory, "insight-oriented" psychotherapies (Bromberg, 1959; Ellenberger, 1970; Fine, 1990).

In brief therapies, we are not so much interested in *why* something happened. We do not explore the past to help the patient develop insight. When we do explore the past, it is to elicit enough information to understand, not so much what happened, but what the patient did to deal with what happened.

What was the outcome of what happened? What was the choice of behavior that immediately felt good, and by repetition evolved into dysfunctional behavior? This information can help in the reframing process and in the treatment plan. By itself, this information does not change the behavior. We don't interpret meaning or decipher obscure symbolism for the purpose of developing insight.

NEED TO KNOW WHY

Sometimes we have patients who express a strong need to know why and exactly what and when something occurred that was the cause of the presenting problem. In our treatment model, we offer these patients two choices. We explain that we do not do long-term therapy that may require years of looking for meaning and cost a lot of money. So, if this is what the patient wants, choice *1* would be to help the patient find a competent therapist that does this kind of work and to make an appropriate referral.

Choice *2* is to instruct the patient to go home, and that evening, or any other time when the patient can block out an hour or two, to take a pad of paper and, in as much detail as possible, make up a reason. This can be done on a computer, if preferred. We instruct the patient to be sure to spend as much time as needed to be as complete and logical as possible in detailing all of the things he or she can imagine that led to the start of the problem, to write down what the precipitator was, how long ago it happened, where it happened, who was present and so on. When the patient is satisfied that this written narrative is complete, we instruct the patient to go over it again very slowly and make sure that nothing needs to be added or changed. This material is to be brought to the next meeting.

At that time, we review the information with the patient. The patient is then helped to believe, if only for a moment, that this information is the "true" cause of the behavior. This usually eliminates any future need to explore. The patient is helped to believe that this is the real cause in two ways. During the waking discussion, the patient is asked if the material that he or she came up with is an acceptable explanation. If the patient agrees that it is, no further discussion is required. If the patient says that it may be or is not sure, the patient is asked if it would be acceptable to do a hypnotic trance induction. During the trance experience, we encourage the patient to accept this explanation as sufficiently valid and as satisfying the patient's needs.

Our experience has been that this comes as close to the truth as the patient will get, and that it usually satisfies the patient's need to know. This is also an interesting way of using reframing.

LABELS DICTATE BEHAVIOR

Reframe

> The labels we place on the behaviors we do dictate future behavior. What we call something leads to what we do about it. If we call something a failure, then we continue to repeat the behavior as if we have failed. If we call it a mistake, we realize that mistakes can be corrected, and so we haven't failed. We have only made a mistake. So we can back off and start over again and correct the mistake.

This reframe opens up the possibility of correcting the behavior. This is a very valuable reframe that can be used when a patient has reexperienced a behavior that had been changed. Sometimes this reexperience of the behavior is called a *relapse*, such as when a smoking patient stops smoking and, in a moment of stress, lights a single cigarette, or a few cigarettes. This reframe is used during the waking state and is also one of the suggestions given during trance, to correct the mistake.

ANTICIPATION OR EXPECTATION?

When many patients talk about the future, they use the word *anticipate*. When discussing what patients mean when they choose this verb when speaking about what will happen, we find that most often it is chosen to describe a negative future outcome. A synonym of *anticipate* is *expect*. When a patient is offered the choice of using the word *expect* instead of the word *anticipate,* the general response is that this word feels better. When encouraged to explain why, the usual answer is that their previous use of the word *anticipate* always led to negative feelings that were a continuation of their current feelings of anxiety, pain, and so on. When they verbalized the word *expect*, the common expressed feeling was that, somehow, changing to a word that they had not been using to describe the future allowed them to think about the future as possibly being more positive.

Webster's dictionary lists these two words as equal choices—synonyms— with very little difference in denotative meaning. Yet many of our patients, and we ourselves, experience a different emotional response and connotation attached to each of these words. The simple choice of having a different word available to describe the future than the one the patient repeatedly used before may help the patient to interrupt the past experience of mentally creating a negative self-fulfilling prophecy.

BEHAVIOR IS AN ATTEMPT TO COPE

Most dysfunctional behaviors are the exhibited symptoms of the problem. Symptoms are a way of coping with a deeper problem. Initially, the symptoms of unconscious choice relieve some anxiety, and the patient feels better. As the symptoms become more frequent and intense, they become dysfunctional and the patient feels worse. Repetition of the symptoms imprints them, leading to further repetition and deeper imprinting.

Often the symptoms are no longer needed. They continue as a habit. So the repetitions of symptoms, which are negative coping behaviors, are then maintained as habits. A *symptom* is a coping mechanism with a negative outcome. A *habit* is a behavior, positive or negative, imprinted by repetition. Although habits are difficult to change consciously, they respond very quickly to change with reframing and an appropriate trance experience.

WAKING HYPNOSIS AND THE WAKING STATE REFRAMING PROCESS

The Waking State Reframing Process

During the waking state reframing process, the patient is helped to rethink or reframe beliefs, feelings and behaviors. This takes place during the initial intake evaluation with the patient and during the exchange of information between you and the patient. The patient's labels, belief systems, and dysfunctional coping mechanisms (i.e., symptoms) are challenged and reframed during the waking state using cognitive restructuring, suggestion, and the appropriate representational language for that patient (termed *change language* or the *language of hypnosis*).

During the waking state reframing process, the patient is being prepared consciously for a hypnosis induction and trance experience (Wester & Smith, 1984). The patient, in effect, anticipates or expects that he or she will be helped to experience hypnotic trance during the session, and waits for this to happen.

The patient's waking state reframing experience may enhance his or her acceptance of suggestions for change because it is an altered state. This altered state may be labeled an *anticipatory trance state* or an *expectation of trance state*. If you carefully observe the patient during the waking state, you may find that many of the physiological indicators that are observed during trance are already present before formal trance is induced. You can effectively use the changes in the patient that already are taking place in expectation of entering trance, to later help the patient to enter formal trance more easily and comfortably.

Be aware that we have made an exception in the use of the word *anticipatory* when applying the concept of *in expectation of entering trance*. Because this is a convenient way of thinking about it, for our purposes, we have not given a negative connotation to the term *anticipatory trance state* when used in this way.

In the brief cognitive hypnosis model, most of the change that the patient experiences occurs during the waking state reframing. The trance state is when the change is "fixed in place." A brief, carefully chosen induction is used (to be discussed in later chapters), then the fixative suggestions are given to the patient.

This way of working allows us to relatively seamlessly integrate hypnotic communication that takes place while a patient is in a waking state with hypnotic communication that takes place after a trance state is induced. We are talking about "priming" the patient's suggestibility (i.e., receptivity to appropriate therapeutic suggestions). This enhances our chances of achieving favorable therapeutic outcomes.

Case Study: Chronic Pain

A patient was referred to me (BNE) for help in coping with his chronic back pain. He had been to see numerous specialists and considered none of these contacts to have been helpful. After doing a thorough intake evaluation, I suggested to the patient that perhaps he had not really heard what one of the physicians he had visited, who I knew to be a great doctor, had been telling him. I suggested that, as an experiment, he try two of the things that this doctor had recommended. They were recommendations that could not possibly hurt. They would either help or not help.

The doctor's recommendations were (1) that the patient replace his desk chair with a more ergonomic one that better supported his posture and (2) that the patient become more aware of good versus bad posture for his back and neck. I reinforced the value of these recommendations in the waking state, then in trance. I obtained the patient's agreement to come back in 2 weeks so that he could report back to me, and so that we could decide where to go from there.

The patient canceled his next appointment because he had not been able to get a new chair until just a few days before his next scheduled appointment with me. He wanted to give it a week or two to test the strategy. The patient did call back a week later to reschedule a follow-up with me. At that next session, he reported that his back and neck didn't hurt as much after he spent several hours in his new desk chair, and that he was "minding his posture."

In this case, the patient tried something different after it was pointed out to him that perhaps he had missed something important in his earlier contact with one of the physicians he had seen. This opened up the possibility of reframing his absolute belief that none of his previous physician contacts had been helpful. It was suggested that perhaps his visit with that one doctor could turn out to be helpful if we carefully reviewed the information that the doctor had given to him. He was willing to do this. This led to his modifying several behaviors, which provided him with different feedback, and the new feedback was discordant with his old point of view that nothing was helpful. This created cognitive dissonance (Festinger, 1957), which led to his modifying or reframing his old point of view. The possibility was then opened to his reexamining several other previously fixed beliefs that, as I pointed out to him, "might not have been very helpful."

For the reader's information, the patient continued with me, and we did further work with the hypnotic trance state and self-hypnosis to help him develop greater control over his pain experience.

NONTHERAPIST CLINICIANS

This waking state reframing concept is especially applicable to those nonpsychotherapist clinicians who are treating patients with medical, physical, or dental problems. These clinicians prepare the patient for their medical or dental treatment procedures by explaining what is to be done, what to expect during the procedure, and the expected outcome. You can also talk to the patient during the procedure. Very little is taught in medical or dental school about the use of language and its effect on patients. However, much attention is paid to making sure that all negative possibilities are explained so that the risk of professional liability can be kept to a minimum.

As a physician or dentist administers a shot, a patient may hear the doctor say, "This may hurt a little." The patient tenses up in preparation of the shot because of the suggestion that it will hurt. If the doctor were to say instead, "This is nothing. You will experience only a slight pressure as I press on your arm here," then the patient would probably not tense up and the fear of the injection would be minimized.

Because you spend time talking with patients before and during procedures, why not use this time to accomplish positive expectation and change rather than imprinting negative iatrogenic suggestions? As you learn the process of waking state reframing, you can instruct your assistants and technicians on their own proper conscious use of language.

THE VALUE OF WAKING STATE REFRAMING

Waking state reframing is when intensive work is performed. The relationship is built, positive rapport and trust are established, expectations and readiness for positive change are induced, choices are pointed out and recognized, and what had previously been felt to be a trap becomes an open door to freedom and wellness.

Most patients come to you for help after they have exhausted other treatment options. During their previous attempts to find relief from their particular suffering, their repeated lack of success may have imprinted a belief that they are forever trapped. They may verbalize that you are their last resort but not really believe that you will do any better than others who have tried and failed. Previous treatment generalists and specialists may not have seemed to listen to their messages of fear, anger, depression and desperation.

These previous health care professionals may have asked few questions or given few satisfactory answers. For example, an important part of treating the "emotional overlay" associated with the persistent suffering of many chronic pain patients is to address their need for some satisfactory answers (Eimer & Freeman, 1998). It may have seemed to a particular patient that these professionals' eyes were shut, ears were covered and minds were closed.

You need to open your eyes and look at a patient, make adequate eye contact and look for cues. You need to listen carefully to a patient's language, to what a patient really is saying, and hear the hidden messages being expressed. You need to "resonate" with a patient (Watkins, 1978), so that you can feel with the patient the import of his or her emotional state and sense of helplessness. Most importantly, you need to communicate that you can be trusted, that here is an opportunity for change, that there are still choices that the patient has until now not been helped to see and that the responsibility for change will be shared between you and the patient.

INFORMING THE PATIENT ABOUT WHAT TO EXPECT

Many patients come to treatment, or are referred to treatment, because the clinician has a recognized expertise in the use of clinical hypnosis. One of your responsibilities is to explore the patient's understanding and beliefs regarding what hypnosis is and what the experience of being hypnotized will be like. Those patients who enter into this experience for the first time may have some trepidations. Those with previous hypnosis experiences that happened in the distant past or that didn't help may be concerned that you will do the same things that didn't work before. A patient may have information about hypnosis from someone who did not have a positive experience.

It is important to help the patient understand that *all hypnosis is not the same.* Hypnosis is a tool, like any other tool, in the hands of a skilled professional. The clinician does not know the credentials, background, or training of past purveyors of hypnosis that the patient has seen and therefore cannot judge others' skill or competence.

EXPLAINING HYPNOSIS

This is how you can explain hypnosis to a patient during the waking state reframing process:

> Let me explain to you how I think about hypnosis and what it is and what it is not. For our purposes, the mind is made up of two parts. One part we call the conscious mind. You have control over your conscious mind. You can look at this pen and make the conscious decision to pick it up or put it down.
>
> The other part of the mind we call the unconscious or the subconscious mind.

Both names mean the same thing. The unconscious controls all of your automatic behaviors. It controls your breathing, heartbeat, pulse rate, blood flow, all of the things that go on inside your body that keep you alive that you pay little or no attention to. They are automatically controlled by the unconscious mind.

The unconscious also controls all of the other things that you do that you feel you have little or no control of. It controls your habits, your patterns of behavior, even such things as which side of the bed you sleep on every night and which shoe you put on first when you get dressed in the morning. These are all controlled by the unconscious mind.

One of the problems is that we assume that if we know something consciously, we automatically know it unconsciously. The fact is, we may not. The reason we may not is because the unconscious part of the mind is not the memory system, although it has memory components, and it is not easily communicated with. Let me explain.

One of the ways of communicating with the unconscious is by repetition. We do something over and over and over again. The unconscious gets the idea that we want to do it. The unconscious takes charge of it and makes a habit of it. Once it is a habit, we have little or no control over it. But the unconscious hasn't asked if this is good or bad for us. So we can form a bad habit as well as a good habit. The reason the unconscious hasn't asked is because it doesn't have enough information to make that judgment. If it did, we probably wouldn't be doing it.

Another way of communicating with the unconscious is if there is a trauma, a major conflict, a death in the family, a serious illness or some other significant negative event. This can imprint into the unconscious a feeling of fear or anxiety or depression or whatever emotional response is appropriate for the particular traumatic experience.

A third way of communicating with the unconscious is the way we will be using here in the office today. That is when a person is in a deep state of relaxation, and for the moment I use the words relaxation and hypnosis interchangeably. I will talk more about that in a moment. During this relaxation, the doorway to the unconscious opens, and with your permission, I can talk to the unconscious and give it information it needs in a language and form it will accept, to change the behavior that you want to change. That is why I asked you the questions that I did, to establish the language and form specifically for you.

Once the unconscious accepts this information, it can't ignore it. It has to act on it and begin to change the behavior you want to change.

But it is not quite that simple. The reason it is not that simple is because there are two parts of the mind, the conscious and the unconscious. The conscious mind wants to change the behavior. The unconscious mind doesn't yet know it needs to change the behavior. This causes a conflict between the conscious wish to change and the unconscious control of the behavior. This conflict produces stress and discomfort. This stress is what makes it so difficult to change.

When the conscious and unconscious join together, in cooperation with each other, like my two hands folding together, without conflict or pressure or stress, the behavior changes easily and comfortably, and by repetition becomes a new and positive behavior. This cooperation between the conscious and the unconscious is very important. I can't make you do something that you don't want to do. I can help you change something that you do want to change.

The reason I talk about hypnosis and relaxation in the same breath is because I am not talking about "Zap, you are under my power." I'm talking about helping you into the kind of relaxation that you experience just before you go to sleep at night and just before you are fully awake in the morning. You are lying there, loose and comfortable and relaxed. Your mind is active. Sounds are off in the background. You know you could move if you had to, but you just don't feel like doing it. You know the feeling. We all have that experience.

That presleep, postsleep relaxed feeling is technically called the hypnogogic state. The reason it is called that is because it is very similar in brain wave function to what happens when a person is in hypnosis. You hear everything that I say. Sounds are off in the background. If your mind wanders, it doesn't make any difference, because your unconscious will hear everything that I am saying.

This is when the doorway to the unconscious opens, and with your permission, I can give information to the unconscious that it can use to help you change the behavior that you want to change. Do you have any questions?

This simple explanation about hypnosis and what to expect usually covers most of the questions a patient may consider asking. If there are other questions, you should answer them in the same comfortable, easygoing manner.

3

Change Language: General, Waking, Trance, and Posttrance State Reframing

A patient's responses are affected to a large extent by the language a clinician chooses to use. Therefore, it is important that you be consciously aware of how your choice of language and delivery affects and effects certain responses by a patient. By paying attention to the language you use with patients, you will be better able to gauge the effects you have on them. These effects are amplified by the nature of the communication interaction.

In one sense, we are talking about standardizing language. It is necessary for us as clinicians to be consciously aware of the language we use. We use specific scripts to present particular reframes and to explain certain concepts to patients, such as the concept of the conscious and unconscious parts of the mind.

In another sense, we individualize the specific language we use with each patient based on our evaluation of that patient's unique needs and perceptual processing and learning style. So, for example, with one patient, we may use visual or kinesthetic words, if those seem to be the patient's primary sensory representational systems. With another patient, we may emphasize auditory language.

Because the effects of our communications are amplified by the nature of the ongoing and unfolding interaction, we must also listen to and observe carefully the patient's responses to us. We modify our responses consciously to pace and match those of the patient (Cameron-Bandler, 1978; Grinder & Bandler, 1981; Lankton, 1980; Lankton & Lankton, 1983).

CHANGE LANGUAGE

When we talk about change language, we are talking about maintaining conscious awareness of how certain language affects, produces, and evokes certain responses in the patient and in us. We are talking about being aware of the meanings that patients attribute to both their own language and our use of language (Fourie, 1995). We are also referring to our physiological and biochemical responses to language, as well as the mind and body's ability to respond to appropriate suggestions. Language and its interpretation evoke emotion (Beier, 1966; Cheek, 1994; Ewin, 1984, 1992a; Vetter, 1969; Watzlawick, 1978). Emotion evokes biochemical and physiological responses (Rossi, 1993; Selye, 1974, 1976).

How do you know what language to use? How do you know what information to give? How do you the clinician know what labels need reframing? The answers involve assessing your own level of knowledge and recognizing how language affects all of us as individuals personally, emotionally and professionally. They also involve assessing carefully how a patient employs language, represents and constructs meaning out of experience and construes the problems that have led the patient to treatment. This requires careful questioning in order to (1) clarify the meaning of the patient's wording and expressions, (2) narrow down and establish the appropriate focus of what needs to be done to help the patient, and (3) make note of the labels the patient uses to identify his or her functional and dysfunctional world. Then you need to make conscious use of yourself as an agent of change.

Change Language Is Hypnotic Language

What we term *change language* is hypnotic language. However, this does not mean it automatically induces a formal hypnotic trance. We refer to our earlier definition of hypnosis as encompassing more than just the trance state. This means that when we use appropriate change language, we are talking to a patient's conscious mind on one level and unconscious mind on another level, without necessarily inducing a formal trance state. Consequently, a patient is likely to be more accepting of what we are saying because information is being communicated in a form that is acceptable to all parts of the patient's mind. This makes it easier to change the meaning of the patient's beliefs and experiences and ultimately bring about positive change in the patient's state.

FOUR IMPORTANT CONSIDERATIONS

There are four very important issues that relate to the effect that language has on the whole process of therapeutic change.

Sensory Representational Systems

The language forms used by a patient that express the sensory systems that patient favors for communicating and processing information represent the first aspect of communication to which you ought to attend. This can help establish good rapport. Here, we refer again to visual, auditory, kinesthetic, olfactory and gustatory sensory modalities. This choice of sensory language tells you how the patient processes information. However, sometimes there is so much crossover of sensory language that it is difficult to immediately discern a patient's primary system of sensory processing. Therefore, attention must be paid to eye movements and the subtle use of language to assist in making clinical judgments. Details are given later in this chapter.

The Patient's Labels

The labels used by a patient to describe his or her beliefs and dysfunctional behaviors further imprint the continuation of those beliefs and behaviors. We discussed this in previous chapters in some detail, and this important issue will be addressed often in chapters dealing with the treatment of various clinical disorders.

One aspect that needs to be noted pertains to the recognition of labels that imply the requirement for action versus those that do not. For example, the label *urge*, a verb defined as "exerting a force that impels to action," implies that some action to satisfy that urge needs to take place. In contrast, the label *memory*, a noun, specifically refers to the ability to revive in the mind past thoughts, images, feelings, ideas, and so on. It does not imply that some immediate action is required.

By reframing for the patient the label *urge* as the label *memory*, you can help change the patient's beliefs and expectancies about the patient's future behavior. You can do this by helping the patient redefine or relabel what he or she refers to as an urge as a memory instead. Such relabeling changes the patient's ongoing experience. An experience labeled as an urge (e.g., to smoke, to eat, to have sex) compels some sort of action to satisfy the urge. If the experience is labeled as a recalled memory, no such action is required. Memories can be interrupted, changed, or recalled at another time.

Conversely, some labels imply that no action or movement is possible. These labels typically represent dysfunctional absolutes. For example, a patient may describe certain behaviors as always happening. You can respond therapeutically by helping the patient to recognize and accept that the behavior does not always happen. This is accomplished by further questioning, and also by helping the patient to recognize the many times when this singular behavior is not exhibited—in other words, that there are exceptions to this absolute.

The Clinician's Use of Sensory and Other Language Forms

The sensory and other language forms used by a clinician that express his or her own way of communicating and processing information can help or hurt a relationship with a patient, as well as the therapeutic effectiveness of the treatment process. Therefore, it is important that you remain aware of how each of your choices of sensory and other language forms, in communicating information to a patient, is complementary or at odds with those used by the patient. This is essential to forming a good relationship with the patient, as well as a good outcome from treatment. If your and the patient's language forms are at odds, then you need to consider how to consciously alter your language to match that of the patient.

Iatrogenic Imprinting

Another factor that should be assessed is the effects that the language of other clinicians may have had in imprinting dysfunctional beliefs and behaviors. This effect can be termed *negative iatrogenic imprinting* when it inadvertently occurs as a result of what previous clinicians have said, or as a result of the negative outcomes and experiences brought about by past treatment choices and procedures that were not successful.

Unless past iatrogenically induced imprints are recognized and reframed, the current treatment can be stalled. Later, we will discuss in more detail an example of this in which a physician referred a patient to learn relaxation, but when he made the referral, he told the patient that it was impossible for her to relax. In this case, the patient was set up inadvertently for failure in learning self-relaxation until we reframed this iatrogenic imprint.

Dabney Ewin (1986, 1992a) discusses at some length an important example of the iatrogenic imprint that doctors often inadvertently create when they tell patients with persistent pain that (1) they will always have the pain, and (2) they must learn to live with the pain. The patient's unconscious, which is literal, interprets this to mean that (1) the patient will always be in pain and (2) the patient would die if he or she were to be rid of the pain. The patient's unconscious therfore is unwilling to let go of the pain.

When we talk about change language, one of the things to which we are referring is maintaining conscious awareness of the underlying meaning or deeper content of what the patient is saying and of what you the clinician are saying. Although you may both be speaking English, for example, the intent and deeper meaning of the words that are used may be interpreted differently by each of you. This divergence in interpretations can affect the therapeutic working relationship, your diagnostic judgment, and the whole treatment process. This point is especially important to consider when the patient's primary language is not English, even when the patient is fluent in English, and your primary language is English.

Words often have more than one meaning when they have to be processed and translated from one language to another. They also may have different connotative meanings if they are expressing emotional, psychological or culturally relative content. Therefore, careful questioning is required to clarify continuously the real meaning of a patient's words and expressions. In addition, the meaning of a patient's words is affected by the degree of emotionality associated with them (termed *emotional overlay*) and their centrality and commonality to that patient's habitual way of thinking.

THE PATIENT'S BELIEFS

The Patient's Expectations and Agenda

The patient comes to the treatment setting with an agenda and belief system that can be unrealistic or misinformed. This can prevent or delay a successful outcome of the treatment. As suggested earlier, it is easy to assume that you and the patient understand each other's statements, environments, and emotional, physical and visual worlds in exactly the same way, when in fact each of you may not.

The patient may have an understanding and expectations about treatment with hypnosis that are not factual or realistic. The patient also may have beliefs about the presenting symptoms that are not factual or realistic, or motivations to change based on outside influences, such as family or friends, as opposed to a personal interest in changing. The patient's previous attempts to change may have established a particular mindset that can affect the outcome of treatment. How the patient came to treatment may affect the process. What the referral source said may have negatively affected the possible outcome of treatment because of iatrogenic imprinting.

The Right Kind of Repetition Facilitates Unconscious Learning

Notice that various proscriptions and prescriptions in this book are repeated often using slightly different words. Although their meaning and purpose may be the same, namely, to help readers learn easily and effectively, the slight variations in wording are consciously designed to fit the information smoothly into a slightly different context. The right kind of repetition often increases conscious and unconscious learning, and the reality of unconscious cognition and recognition is now solidly established in empirical research (Greenwald, 1992; Kihlstrom, Barnhardt, & Tataryn, 1992).

Slight changes in the way that new and important information is repeated can allow that information to overlap previous learning comfortably without it being interpreted as too much repetition. To cite Milton Erickson, in the context of using hypnosis to treat patients with terminal illness, "Hypnotherapeutic benefits, especially in such cases as reported here, are markedly contingent upon a varied and repetitious presentation of ideas and understandings to insure an adequate acceptance and responsiveness by the patient. Also, the very nature of the situation precludes a determination of [exactly] what elements in the therapeutic procedure are effective in the individual case" (Erickson, 1980b, p. 261). The clinician's words and form of language need to be individualized to the patient's specific language and learning needs, as well as the patient's information-processing style.

In a clinician's office, this slight variation in the language used to suggest change to the patient is another important conscious use of "slightly different" language during waking state and trance state reframing. This will be discussed in more detail in chapter 4.

Most trance state change language combines reframing and direct suggestions for change, along with encouragement of the patient to give himself permission to change. Because of the hypnotic phenomenon known as trance logic, (discussed later in this chapter), direct suggestions may contain illogical content. However, the unconscious may accept them because the suggestions meet the needs of the patient and are phrased in a form that the patient can accept.

Posttrance State Imprinting

In the posttrance state, immediately after "awakening," the patient is still very receptive to suggestion. This is when change language can be used to further imprint the positive experience of relaxation by the patient and the comfortable feelings experienced during trance. At this point in the session, it is important to encourage the patient to verbalize and recognize that the good experience and pleasant way of feeling now, compared to how the patient felt when first coming into your office, are a result of trance.

It is important to be aware of the fact that we all initially recognize change in retrospect. We rarely recognize it while it is happening. Thus, helping a patient to examine how he or she feels after awakening from the trance state can promote and imprint this recognition. Once acknowledged by the patient, the experience of change can be further imprinted by suggesting continued awareness of the recently experienced change and suggesting that there will be a progressive continuation of change as the therapy process continues. This examination of the positive results and changes that continue to occur as treatment progresses is an important part of the beginning of each future therapeutic contact (this includes office sessions and all telephone calls). It establishes the future expectation of continued positive change.

CASE STUDY: UNDOING A REFERRING PHYSICIAN'S INADVERTENT IATROGENIC IMPRINTING

Earlier we discussed a patient's problem relaxing because of the referring doctor's inadvertent iatrogenic suggestion that it was "impossible" for the patient to relax. Even following a thorough intake evaluation, my (JIZ) repeated attempts were unsuccessful in helping the patient to experience this state called relaxation. The process was therefore stopped. I backed up, then asked the patient, "What were the exact words that Dr. Jones used when he 'suggested' that you come to see me?" The patient responded, "Dr. Jones said, 'It is impossible for you to relax, so I am going to send you to see Jordan Zarren to help you relax.'"

Dr. Jones was a competent physician who was highly respected by the patient. Dr. Jones's powerful iatrogenic statement, "It is impossible for you to relax," was a strong negative suggestion that was immediately and uncritically accepted by the patient's unconscious as an absolute, and thus, it was imprinted. This made it difficult, if not impossible, to accomplish relaxation, unless that negative imprint was first recognized by me and the patient was helped to change this fixed belief.

As part of the ongoing waking state reframing process, Dr. Jones's instruction to the patient was discussed, and the patient was helped to recognize that this statement, as interpreted by the patient, was not Dr. Jones's actual intent. He would not have sent her to see me, and had her spend the money for the visit, if he didn't mean for her to learn how to relax. As the patient began to process this new interpretation of what Dr. Jones had said and had really meant, she began to loosen up. She began to permit herself to accept that relaxation might be possible.

An appropriate hypnotic induction was chosen, and she was helped to experience a thoroughly relaxed state in the office. The induction included a self-hypnosis technique that she was to practice once or twice every day for about 10 minutes. Later, reports indicated that she did so with great success. Dr. Jones was then able to successfully continue to treat her for the medical problems that had been exacerbated by her constant tension and inability to experience relaxation, which created an emotional overlay.

Here we have discussed reframing a patient's imprinted unconscious belief that it was impossible for her to relax to a belief that it was possible to relax. Reframes are an important part of the concept of change language.

THE CLINICIAN'S "INVISIBLE" LANGUAGE

An interesting problem was discovered during an examination of a typed transcript of a session in which hypnosis was employed by an experienced psychotherapist who was receiving supervision in the use of clinical hypnosis. The case was that of a middle-aged woman who was experiencing mild obsessive-compulsive behavior. The patient made progress in controlling the problematic behavior, and the clinician gradually spread out the frequency of the therapy sessions from every week, to every 2 weeks, to every 3 weeks. However, by the time the patient was scheduled to see the clinician at 3-week intervals, her presenting symptoms had returned to their original intensity.

Examination of the transcript revealed that the clinician prefaced most suggestions by saying, "I want you to. . . . This was repeated over and over again using exactly the same words, or with slightly different words that meant essentially the same thing. It was suggested to the clinician that the patient's "relapse" to her earlier behavior may have been due to an unconscious situation that the therapist had inadvertently set up in which the patient was being trained to please the therapist. In other words, it was possible that the patient unconsciously had been getting better for the clinician in response to the clinician's request to "Do this for me," which is what he had been saying over and over again as read in the transcript. When the therapeutic sessions were spread out, the patient could no longer behave better for the therapist. Because the patient was not getting better for herself, the symptoms returned. This awareness allowed the clinician to change his suggestions, and the patient started to maintain her improvement without relapse.

Correcting Bad Clinical Habits

Like patients, clinicians can develop habits. We repeat things with our patients until what we say becomes almost automatic and unconscious. We can develop bad therapeutic habits as well as good ones. One of the most effective ways of becoming aware of those bad habits is by recording sessions, with the patient's permission, and having them transcribed. Just listening to the recording of the session is not enough, however. Listening to the recording while reading the transcript is much more effective. The mistakes will jump out from the page. You should review the transcripts, checking for repetitive unproductive language that is being given to the patient. By highlighting that language, you will become conscious of the language you are using, and be better able to change that language to further the patient's opportunity for change and independence.

OBSERVING BODY LANGUAGE: THE PATIENT'S BMIRS

In addition to becoming more aware of your language, it is important for the clinician to listen to the patient's nonverbal language and to observe the patient's facial and body language. These often provide additional important clues to the patient's emotional state and to how the patient accesses, processes, and learns new information. The patient's nonverbal language and facial and body language are *behavioral manifestations of internal responses* (BMIRs). The patient's nonverbal, subtle and not so subtle overt gestural responses provide clues about the patient's internal responses and experience.

These clues, or minimal cues should be noted by carefully listening to and observing the patient. However, they should never be interpreted as indicating absolutely that the patient is experiencing a certain reaction or response without verification from other sources of data (e.g., the patient's verbal report, consistencies and inconsistencies in patterns of responding, and intensity of the patient's behavioral and emotional responses). They should be used as data for forming hypotheses. There are several sources of such data.

Nonverbal Language and Voice Stress Analysis

When an individual is anxious, angry, depressed or otherwise stressed, he or she may raise or lower the volume, pitch, and tonality of his or her voice, talk faster or slower, hesitate, stutter, stammer, speak in a pressured manner or in a flat, affectless manner and consciously or unconsciously stress particular syllables or words for emphasis. The sheer quantity and volume of speech will vary as a function of that individual's emotional state. Therefore, it is important to be continuously running an informal voice stress analysis while listening to a patient.

Emotional reactions and cognitive accessing processes are often manifested by nonverbal expressions, vocalizations, and utterances. For example, patients dealing with chronic pain often exhibit signs of their pain and suffering through such pain behaviors as groaning, moaning, grunting, whimpering, sighing, grimacing, glaring, contorting, and jaw clenching (Eimer, 1988; Eimer & Freeman, 1998). As another example, someone who is perplexed or trying to remember something may repetitively say "Geez," "Hmmm," "Um, . . . um . . .," and so on, while trying to reaccess the lost material.

Breathing Patterns

When a patient is aroused, anxious, or experiencing a fight or flight response, breathing tends to be more uneven, quicker and located higher in the chest. However, the patient may begin to breathe more deeply, as if to take in more air, if he or she feels short of breath, or may begin to breathe more shallowly and hold his or her breath more frequently. The patient may begin to yawn or sigh, indicating the release of tension and stress.

Conversely, when the patient begins to enter a relaxed state, breathing tends to become more even and rhythmic, and the respiration rate tends to slow. Eventually, breathing may become more shallow, although initially, the patient may take in deeper breaths. Again, as the patient begins to settle back and relax, yawning or sighing may occur, indicating the release of tension.

Skin Color and Tone

If a patient is embarrassed or enraged, he or she may begin to redden as blood rushes to the face. However, fear may produce the opposite physiological response, making the patient appear more pale. In most states of arousal, the lips may thin and tighten. As the patient begins to enter a relaxed state, skin pallor may become more noticeable. Conversely, the lips may become more full and redden.

Muscle Tone

As a patient begins to enter a state of relaxation, muscles begin to relax. The muscles in the forehead and around the eyes, for example, may appear to flatten, and fluttering of the eyelids, if the patient's eyes are closed, may either increase or decrease. The jaw muscles may relax; consequently, the patient's lips may part and the jaw may begin to hang open. Usually, there will be less movement. The relaxed patient will appear still. Periodically, involuntary muscle twitchings, or fasciculations, may be evidenced as tension is released through the muscles. The patient also may swallow more frequently.

Conversely, if the patient is anxious or angry, facial muscles may tense. The forehead muscles may crinkle, and a frown may be evidenced. Facial tics may be observed. The patient is likely to appear restless, and the large muscles of the upper body (the neck, shoulders and chest) may tense. The arms and hands may also tense, and the patient may make fists, or tense the fingers and hands, or be unable to keep his or her hands and arms still. The patient may be unable to settle back and may appear on the edge of his or her seat.

Ideomotor Responses

The unconscious mind communicates its feelings through spontaneous and involuntary movements of the voluntary muscle system, that is, skeletal muscles. This expression or conversion of ideas and emotional reactions and feelings into automatic, largely unconscious motor responses is termed *ideomotor responding.* For example, we may automatically nod our head or smile without being aware of it when something feels good and we may automatically shake our head no, or frown when something does not feel right. These observable ideomotor responses are minimal cues to the patient's internal emotional reactions and states. It is important to watch for the occurrence of these cues in patients.

Physiological and Visceral Responses

The unconscious mind also communicates its feelings through automatic changes in the autonomic nervous system (ANS). The ANS controls all of the physiological functions that keep us alive. These functions include heart rate, blood pressure, breathing, digestion, bowel and bladder functions and hormonal responses.

When a person experiences some form of the fight or flight response and becomes anxious, scared, angry, enraged or otherwise aroused, heart rate, respiration rate and blood pressure usually increase. Breathing may become centered mostly in the upper chest; and the bladder and/or bowels may become stimulated, with a consequent increased need to visit the bathroom. The individual also may experience stomach pain or nausea if the stomach is relatively full of food and the digestive process is not stimulated. As the hypothalamic-pituitary-adrenal (HPA) axis, the body's physiological stress response system, is also activated, certain hormones and neurotransmitters are produced in larger quantities as compared to when the mind–body system is unaroused. These hormones and neurotransmitters, such as norepinephrine, adrenaline and cortisol, set the body's instinctive fight or flight reaction in motion.

Conversely, when an individual enters a relaxed state, certain opposing autonomic and visceral responses to those mentioned above may occur. The individual's heart rate, respiration rate and blood pressure usually decrease. Breathing may become more centered in the middle chest area and the abdomen. The bladder and bowels tend to relax. There may be an increase in flatulence. Stomach contractions or spasms may increase if the hunger response or digestive process is stimulated and stomach acids are secreted. When the brain sends a message that all is safe to the HPA system, the body's physiological stress response system is deactivated and the production of stress hormones and neurotransmitters is turned off.

Observing Eye Movements

It has often been said that the eyes are the windows to the soul. A patient's physiological ophthalmic responses (e.g., dilation of the pupils, tearing and blinking), eye movements and eye scanning patterns may also serve as BMIRs. The eyes can often convey clues to a person's emotional state and thinking processes.

When people are thinking and talking, they tend to move their eyes in regular, repeated patterns as they scan their memory. These eye movements are the accompanying physical expression of their attempt to gain access to internally stored information. A patient has to go inside to access information and develop thoughts that he or she wants to express. You can observe these BMIRs, especially if a patient is not very verbal, to further ascertain that patient's way of processing. These eye movement patterns often provide clues to a patient's primary or dominant sensory representational systems for accessing and processing information (Bandler & Grinder, 1979; Cameron-Bandler, 1978; Lankton, 1980; Lewis & Pucelik, 1982). Therefore, it is useful to carefully observe the patient's eye movements when he or she is answering your questions that require memory recall.

Again, it is important that you not rely on just one source of sensory data for drawing conclusions about a patient's dominant processing systems. The reliability of your hypotheses will be bolstered when information is obtained from several sources (e.g., the patient's language forms, eye scanning patterns and physiological responses).

Eye Scanning Patterns

Eye scanning patterns are perhaps the most easily recognized BMIRs and are clues to a patient's cognitive and emotional accessing and processing behaviors (Bandler & Grinder, 1979; Cameron-Bandler, 1978; Lankton, 1980; Lewis & Pucelik, 1982). However, like all of the other BMIRs described above, the data they provide should not be taken as conclusive without additional sources of confirmatory data that can be obtained by talking with the patient, listening carefully to the patient's language and noting and observing all of the patient's behaviors, both overt and covert, gross and subtle.

Most people are right-handed, so we will describe patterns that are usually (but not always) shown by right-handed people, most of whom are left hemisphere dominant. The patterns are reversed for some, but not all, left-handed individuals, some of whom may be right hemisphere dominant or of mixed cerebral dominance.

Some individuals may be ambidextrous, or do some things with one hand and other things with the other hand. Often, a left-handed individual whose inherited hand dominance was changed from writing with the left hand to writing with the right hand in his or her early school years will have developed superior fine motor skills with the learned dominant right hand and superior gross motor physical skills with the once dominant left hand. Such a person may bowl as a "lefty" and draw or do fine needle work as a "righty." These persons may have well-developed multiple accessing systems and may not fit the Generalizations to follow. Therefore, this information is important to obtain during the intake evaluation.

The word *looking* in the following descriptions refers to the eye movements of the person in the direction indicated. *Left* means toward the person's left; *right* means toward the person's right.

Looking Up and to the Right: Constructed Visual Images

This eye movement pattern is understood to reveal that visual images or pictures are being created by the individual. These images may be made up of previously experienced and remembered visual input newly created visual representations. They also can be created images that are responses to other sensory stimuli or the clinician's questions. Because these are transitory images, they usually are without depth or vivid color. From a neuropsychological perspective, this accessing pattern is thought to involve left hemisphere occipital, parietal, and temporal cerebral activity.

Looking Up and to the Left: Eidetic Images

This eye movement pattern is understood to reveal the accessing of stored or remembered visual images of past events and other previously experienced visual stimuli. They may include dreams, fantasies and other constructed memories that have been imprinted by emotion or repetition. They may have depth, color, even motion. From a neuropsychological perspective, this accessing pattern is thought to involve right hemisphere temporal-parietal and occipital cerebral activity.

Staring Straight Ahead: Visualizing Both Constructed and Remembered Images

This eye position is understood to reveal the simultaneous accessing of both remembered and constructed images or the combination of remembered images in a new way. For example, it may reveal that the perceiver is imagining what a person he or she knows (visually remembered) would look like (and perhaps even "feel" like) dressed in a manner uncharacteristic for that person. Neuropsychologically speaking, this accessing pattern is thought to involve bilateral occipital and more whole-brain cerebral processing.

Looking Level and to the Right: Constructed Speech

This pattern relates to the process of creating spoken language. The person is putting into words what he or she wants to say next. This eye movement pattern is often used extensively by individuals who have a different first language than English. They often have to switch from their native language into English as a second language. This accessing pattern is thought to involve left hemisphere temporal cerebral activity.

Looking Level and to the Left: Remembered Sound

This eye movement pattern includes jingles, melodies, the words of songs, the childhood "alphabet song," slang and swearing. It also includes accessing of sounds and auditory messages that are short, repeated, rote reminders of tasks to be done, such as "Stop at the store on the way home," that have been repeated and then dropped from conscious awareness. It is thought to involve right hemisphere temporal-parietal-occipital cerebral activity.

Looking Down and to the Right: Feelings

This eye movement pattern allows a person to access emotions and stored kinesthetic memories. Depressed persons, who are very "into" their feelings of sorrow and despair, even downright depressed, often are viewed with head down, shoulders rounded, and their body drawn in. This emotional state accessing pattern is thought to involve left hemisphere frontal-temporal and parietal cerebral activity.

Looking Down and to the Left: Internal Dialogue

When a person is in deep thought, he or she may access words and sounds that are invoked internally during this state, and gaze down and to the left. Often, when a person is mumbling something, not even aware that words are being expressed out loud, that individual is accessing internal dialogue. This is referred to by traditional cognitive therapists as "self-talk" and "automatic thoughts" (Beck, 1995; Eimer & Freeman, 1998; Ellis, 1996; Meichenbaum, 1977). Usually, internal dialogue is a running commentary on current experience. This eye movement pattern is thought to involve right frontal and temporal cerebral processing.

Other ways that the patient accesses and processes information may be expressed through shallow breathing, when the patient is constructing or remembering visual images and head cocking at an angle to hear what is being said better. This head positioning may also suggest a hearing problem that may need to be looked into further and assessed. This could require changing the seating positions of the patient and clinician.

These nonverbal accessing cues are offered as additional ways of learning the patient's cognitive-perceptual processing patterns. They may be very apparent or not apparent at all. We consider these ancillary and complementary to the verbal cues discussed earlier.

GENERAL REFRAMES

Labels Reframe

The labels we place on the behaviors we do dictate future behavior. For example, if we call a reoccurrence or temporary relapse of a previously changed negative behavior a failure, then we may tend to repeat that behavior again because we have invoked implicitly the belief that we are "trapped" in it.

Alternatively, if we call it a Mistake, then that verbal label suggests that the behavior can be corrected and we can then proceed to correct it. Thus, the reframing of a belief that expresses failure to the recognition and belief that it was only a mistake can allow an individual to further believe that the behavior does not have to continue, because mistakes are errors and errors can be corrected. Clinically, the correction can take place during waking state reframing or during a subsequent trance experience through trance state reframing.

As an interesting aside, a new computer software program has been released called GoBack (Gateway & Cogates, 1998). This program allows the user, directly after a computer system crash, infection by a computer virus, or simple mistake that causes data to disappear or be deleted, to go back to before the problem happened and reinstall or undelete the correct information, to allow the computer to behave correctly. In other words, the program allows the user to correct the mistake. Memory of the functional system contents is retained long enough to be accessed, if done immediately, to allow the computer to return to full normal function.

If a patient has called because a problem has reoccured, and is not scheduled soon for another appointment, you can suggest that the next time he or she practices self-hypnosis, the experience of going into relaxation (trance) will automatically correct the mistake. You can tell the patient that self-suggestion (self-talk) during relaxation will not be necessary, because the relaxation experience by itself will correct the mistake by bringing back the memory of not having the behavior.

Events/Nonevents Reframe

This is an ideal lead-in to the following reframe:

> We only pay attention to events. We don't pay attention to nonevents. That is, we pay attention to things that are happening or have happened. When something is happening or has happened, it is an event. On the other hand, we don't pay attention when something is not happening. After all, how can we be aware of something if it is not happening? So, when something is not happening, there is no event.

The "Absolute" Reframe

The patient who comes in talking about always feeling afraid or anxious needs to be helped to recognize that always is an absolute. Using another general reframe can help to refute this belief. That reframe is the fact that the only absolute is that there are no absolutes.

Further questioning the patient about times when the patient is not afraid, such as when sleeping, with family or friends, or during other pleasant, secure times, can do this. The only agreement needed from the patient is that there has been at least one time when the patient was not afraid. The acknowledgment of this exception can allow the patient to change the label from always to sometimes. This change in belief can open up the possibility that less frequent repetition and eventual elimination of the fear, the fearful thoughts and the fear-based behavior are possible.

Posthypnotic Suggestions versus Posttrance Imprinting

Posthypnotic suggestions usually have a short lifespan or psychological half-life. Therefore, they usually have to be reinforced by you or the patient to maintain effectiveness.

By way of explanation, recall our earlier discussion about the major ways of communicating with the unconscious part of the mind. One of the major ways is repetition. When we repeat something over and over again, that behavior or thought tends to become automatic and unconscious. *Posthypnotic suggestions* are suggestions delivered in the trance state for certain behaviors, thoughts, or feelings to occur after the trance state is terminated in the presence of specific cues or stimuli, but which are outside the patient's conscious control and aware-ness—hence, unconscious. In order for these types of unconscious associations to last, they have to be repeated over and over again without the patient's feeling that the posthypnotically suggested behavior or feelings are being delib-erately or consciously invoked.

Posttrance imprinting means instructions given to the patient during trance, and rehearsed in the trance state, that require consciously evoked actions by the patient. Self-relaxation and self-hypnosis practice, for example, are posttrance imprinting behaviors. The actual behavior is evoked by a conscious decision. The experience of the consciously evoked behavior further communicates to the unconscious change and unconscious automatic control. Consciously choosing to do an instant relaxation procedure to interrupt stressful feelings is another example of this that will be discussed in detail later. By repeatedly consciously accessing instant relaxation, it becomes automatic by repetition.

4

Trance Induction: Design, Choice, and Administration

DEFINING *HYPNOSIS* AND *TRANCE*

The APA Division 30 Definition of Hypnosis

The Division of Psychological Hypnosis (Division 30) of the American Psychological Association (APA; Kirsch, 1994, pp. 142–143) defines and describes hypnosis as

> a procedure during which a health professional or researcher suggests that a client, patient, or subject experience changes in sensations, perceptions, thoughts, or behavior. The hypnotic context is generally established by an induction procedure. Although there are many different hypnotic inductions, most include suggestions for relaxation, calmness and well-being. Instructions to imagine or think about pleasant experiences are also commonly included in hypnotic inductions.

Regarding the issue of responsivity to hypnosis, the Division 30 description goes on to state that

> [people] respond to hypnosis in different ways. Some describe hypnosis as a normal state of focused attention, in which they feel very calm and relaxed. Regardless of how and to what degree they respond, most people describe the experience as very pleasant. Some people are very responsive to hypnotic suggestions and others are less responsive. A person's ability to experience hypnotic suggestions can be inhibited by fears and concerns arising from some common misconceptions. Contrary to some depictions of hypnosis in books, movies or television, people who have been hypnotized do not lose control over their behavior. They typically remain aware of who they are and where they are, and unless amnesia has been specifically suggested, they usually remember what transpired

during hypnosis. Hypnosis makes it easier for people to experience suggestions, but it does not force them to have these experiences.

Finally, the Division stresses that

[hypnosis] is not a type of therapy, like psychoanalysis or behavior therapy. Instead, it is a procedure that can be used to facilitate therapy. Because it is not a treatment in and of itself, training in hypnosis is not sufficient for the conduct of therapy. Rather, clinical hypnosis should be used only by properly trained and credentialed health care professionals (e.g., licensed clinical psychologists), who have also been trained in the clinical use of hypnosis and are working within the areas of their professional expertise.

Note that although this definition is one offered by a psychological organization, it is general enough in nature to be acceptable to all health care professionals who use hypnosis as an adjunctive treatment tool.

Our Definition of Hypnosis

We agree with the APA's theoretically neutral definition and description of hypnosis. From our perspective, however, as we explained in the introduction to this book, we view hypnosis as an alteration in internal perception, an altered state, that is initiated at the start of a unique process of communication evoked by an external stimulus that alerts the unconscious mind to pay attention.

The Trance State

As we discussed earlier, the trance state is a further intensification and focusing of this alteration in internal perception. It can occur spontaneously, or be purposely induced by the clinician or by the patient (self-hypnosis). Earlier, we listed nonmutually exclusive basic characteristics of hypnotic trance as an "altered state of consciousness," which has been delineated by Humphreys (2000).

Deep Relaxation, Involuntariness, and Automaticity

In our view, therapeutic trance also involves a component of deep relaxation fostered by parasympathetic activation or dominance in the continuing homeostatic balance between the parasympathetic and sympathetic branches of the autonomic nervous system (Benson, Arns, & Hoffman, 1981; Edmonston, 1981; Eimer & Freeman, 1998; Humphreys, 2000). There is also an element of what is termed *involuntariness* or unconsciously mediated automaticity involved. Thus, the experience of hypnotic phenomena is felt to be effortless as opposed to effortful and consciously willed (Eastwood, Gaskowski, & Bowers, 1998; Holroyd, 1996; Spiegel & Spiegel, 1987).

Facilitating Communication and Therapeutic Learning

The above characteristics of the trance state may allow certain important therapeutic learning to take place much more quickly on cognitive, emotional and physiological levels during psychotherapy, or during any other form of medical or dental treatment in which the clinician uses hypnosis as an adjunctive tool. Drawing on Milton Erickson's work, as reported by Erickson and Rossi (1979, 1981), and further developed by Rossi (1993) and Rossi and Cheek (1988), in trance, the patient can be helped to access inner resources and potentials for healing. More recently, McNeal and Frederick (1993) developed the concept of inner strength (Frederick & McNeal, 1999) from the standpoint of ego state psychology (Watkins & Watkins, 1997). They defined *Inner Strength* as a helpful ego state (i.e., aspect of the patient's personality) accessed in trance that can help the patient get in touch with inner resources and strengthen the patient's ego (i.e., the patient's self-confidence and self-efficacy).

Hypnosis facilitates communication and development of a relationship with one's own unconscious. In a state of deep relaxation, a "doorway" into the patient's unconscious is somehow opened and with the patient's cooperation and permission, therapeutic information can be provided in a language and form that are acceptable to the patient (Eimer, 2000a, 2000b; Zarren, 1996a; Zarren & Eimer, 1999).

In psychotherapy, and both before and during treatment in health care settings other than the psychological (e.g., medical and dental), the clinician skilled in the use of hypnosis facilitates the redirection and narrowing of the patient's attention toward a therapeutic goal. This hypnotic communication process takes place during the waking state (i.e., waking state reframing) and during formal hypnotic trance work. It is grounded in a positive therapeutic relationship based on trust, faith, necessity and positive expectancy. It promotes the patient's comfort, cooperation, suggestibility and ease of compliance with the treatment procedures.

From Waking State Reframing to the Hypnotic Trance State

In brief cognitive hypnosis, we go through the process of waking state reframing, during which we communicate with the patient's conscious and unconscious minds simultaneously to start the change process. However, we have not yet fixed the change in place. We then purposely induce the therapeutic trance state and the "doorway" to the unconscious mind opens. Next, we give the unconscious further information, in a form and language it will accept, to fix in place the desired change.

When using a trance induction procedure as part of the ongoing therapeutic process, we are dealing with the further changing of the patient's belief system. Because one of the unique phenomena of the hypnotic trance is a suspension of some critical judgment, termed *trance logic*, the patient can more readily accept suggestions of change without having to examine these suggestions critically as to their logic or difficulty.

HYPNOTIC INDUCTIONS

Inductions are the beginning of, or entrance to, the trance experience. The body of the trance experience follows the induction procedure. This is a continuous flow experience. We may only spend a few minutes on the induction and many more minutes verbalizing the suggestions for change during the extended trance state.

Readers may think that this simple statement doesn't require much attention. However, it does. That is because most hypnosis training emphasizes the teaching of induction procedures. There is usually little discussion about what we do with the trance state once we have induced it. The bulk of this information will be contained in Part Two of this book, which deals with specific procedures for specific problems.

During the induction and the trance state, the language used by you as the clinician is critical in helping a patient's unconscious mind to accept specific or even general suggestions. You are further imprinting or fixing change in place during the trance experience. The trance functions as a catalyst and a fixative, but it does not initiate the change. The change is initiated in the waking state.

The trance experience by itself, however, can create a memory and atmosphere for general change by creating an experience and memory of deep relaxation. This deep relaxation experience may feel new and different to the patient. This is because it reduces or temporarily eliminates most of the physical tension generated as the result of the emotional overlay created by the dysfunctional behavior or symptoms the patient has been experiencing. As we further explain our views of the meaning and value of the trance state, we will offer details and scripts for using trance-produced relaxation as a powerful starting point for more permanent change.

Choice of Induction

Several considerations will affect your choice of an induction procedure. One consideration that we have already discussed in chapter 1 is the patient's way of processing information. You need to consider the individual needs, personality style and learning systems of the patient, as well as the clinical problems we are addressing here. For example, long inductions may not be suitable for most pain patients. These patients need to begin to experience a reduction in tension very quickly during induction to distract them away from the area of concentrated discomfort (Eimer & Freeman, 1998).

Frequently, a long progressive relaxation induction may get "hung up," because the progressive relaxation gets stuck at those body locations where the pain is experienced the most. Unless there is some form of immediate feedback from the patient when this happens, you will be unlikely to know whether or not the patient is keeping up. If the patient is not keeping up, then continuing the progressive relaxation induction may lead the patient to believe that he or she cannot be helped. This is especially likely to result if the patient's attention to the pain becomes intensified instead of reduced. If this occurs, it will probably interfere with the induction of a suitable trance state that is deep enough to facilitate therapeutic change. It may even make both you and the patient believe that hypnosis is not appropriate.

Internal versus External Focus of Attention

Some patient complaints require induction methods that are externally focused because of extreme somatic (i.e., internal) symptoms. In such cases, the patient's focus of attention may need to be redirected away from the experienced internal locus of his or her symptoms and discomfort. Inductions that use eye fixation or holding on to an object such as a marble would be appropriate. Others require an internal focus because of strong emotional feelings the patient is experiencing that may be exacerbating the patient's physical discomfort. In this case, attention to breathing or awareness of arm rigidity may be used.

Brief and Direct Rather Than Long and Drawn Out Induction Procedures

In the practice of brief cognitive hypnosis, we favor relatively short and direct induction procedures. Long and Drawn out relaxation, metaphoric or confusion inductions tend to get in the way of the brief cognitive hypnosis paradigm and therapeutic agenda. Thus, whatever induction procedures the clinician likes best are generally acceptable as long as they are quick and direct and are chosen based on the patient's individual needs and the nature of the problem being treated. In the remainder of this chapter, we will script some original inductions and some traditional inductions that have been modified to meet the goals of the brief cognitive hypnosis model.

The Assessment of Hypnotizability

In brief cognitive hypnosis, we do not routinely test for hypnotizability. The single exception to this rule may occur when working with patients dealing with chronic or persistent pain. In such cases, the assessment of hypnotizability can inform the clinician in choosing effective methods for inducing hypnotic analgesia and developing individualized pain coping strategies (Eimer, 2000a, 2000b; Eimer & Freeman, 1998; Eimer & Hornyak, 2001). It can also guide the clinician's choice of direct suggestions, cognitive reframes, hypnotic metaphors and pain relief imagery. These issues will be discussed in chapter 11.

Although some clinicians always test for hypnotizability as a regular part of the intake process (Council, 1999; Spiegel & Spiegel, 1987), we do not do so for two reasons:

1. If a patient tests with low hypnotizability, this often leads the clinician to work with that patient with the preconception that hypnosis and trance work will not be effective. This can become a self-fulfilling prophecy, as clinicians' expectations influence patient's expectations, and patient's expectations influence treatment outcomes (Coe, 1993; Kirsch, 2000; Shutty, DeGood, & Tuttle, 1990). In such cases, patients are often deprived of the benefits of hypnosis as a tool for making treatment more pleasant, quick, and efficient, and thus therapeutic results may be compromised.

2. Experimental and laboratory research on hypnotizability do not necessarily or specifically translate into clinical practice (Barber, 1996; Eimer & Hornyak, 2001; Woody, Bowers, & Oakman, 1992). This is because valid experimental research requires standardized, fixed, inflexible and replicable procedures. Clinical work, in contrast, requires flexible, adjustable, and adaptable procedures based on individual differences among patients in personality, dissociation potential, cognitive style and the flexible control of cognitive processes (Bates, 1993; Evans, 1991; Spiegel & Spiegel, 1987).

Early in our work, we did test for hypnotizability. We found that even those patients testing as "low hypnotizables" could benefit from brief cognitive hypnosis when it was carefully tailored to meet their individual needs and when appropriate reframes were put in place during the waking state reframing process.

The Issue of Trance "Depth"

We do not worry about how "deep" the trance experience is. Although we use the term *deep*, we are not referring to "distance traveled," but rather to the quality of the trance experience. This is often explained to the patient. Although we use "deepening procedures," and teach them to our patients, our only test of "depth" is the subjective report by the patient of how comfortable he or she feels. Patients experience different levels of subjective relaxation throughout the trance experience (Wester, 1981; Wester & Smith, 1984). That is, patients typically feel either very relaxed or less relaxed at different times during their trance experience.

The trance induction scripts that follow in this chapter are generalized. They do not present the language that may be added during the trance state to meet the needs of individual patients. They also do not include reframes or suggestions specific to the particular dysfunctional complaints of patients. However, our sample trance induction scripts may use some specific suggestions and reframes as examples. In Part Two we address specific clinical problems and our flexible but directed approach to trance language. We also discuss trance states with the patient's eyes open and with the patient actively involved in dialogue with the clinician.

INDUCTION CATEGORIES

We divide induction procedures into three categories: (1) instant spontaneous inductions that flow from the patient's readiness to enter into trance, (2) inductions that include the teaching of self-hypnosis, and (3) inductions that do not include the teaching of self-hypnosis.

Instant Spontaneous Inductions

There are some patients who exhibit trancelike behavior during the waking state reframing process. They may blink very fast and frequently or have difficulty keeping their eyes open. Their body posture and breathing may suggest that they are already very relaxed. Their facial complexion may deepen, and their eyes may be fixed on some object in front of them or look "glazed over."

Instant Spontaneous Induction Trance Script

When these behavioral manifestations of internal responses become obvious, you can say:

> You are already feeling very relaxed, so why don't you just close your eyes and allow yourself to relax even more?

Usually, the patient does just that. That is, the patient closes his or her eyes and formally enters trance. You may then say:

> This is what it feels like to be in hypnosis. You can enjoy it even more by paying attention to your breathing without trying to change it. If your mind wanders, the moment you realize that you are thinking of something else, bring yourself back to concentrating on your breathing and feel yourself going even deeper into relaxation and hypnosis—deeper with each normal breath that you take, and deeper with each word that I say, regardless of the meaning of my words. As you go deeper and deeper into relaxation and hypnosis with each breath and each word, the doorway to your unconscious opens. With your permission, I have the opportunity to talk to your unconscious and give it information it needs to help you change the behavior that you want to change.

A Therapeutic Double Bind

If the patient does not close his or her eyes when initially suggested, you can say:

> That's fine. You can close your eyes whenever you are ready to feel more relaxed. When you do, you will know what it feels like to be in hypnosis. Meanwhile, just pay attention to your breathing and enjoy how it feels to be relaxing more and more.

This is a suggestion that can be interpreted as a therapeutic double bind, because whatever choice the patient makes is acceptable to the clinician. The patient usually will close his or her eyes shortly if you remain silent. When that happens, you can pick up on giving suggestions by saying:

> Now that your eyes are closed, continue paying attention to your breathing without trying to change it."

Adding Therapeutic Suggestions After Instant Trance is Induced

At this point, you can proceed to add appropriate suggestions and slightly altered reframes to further imprint and fix in place the desired beliefs and therapeutic changes. If you planned on teaching the patient self-hypnosis, you should not do it during a session when an instant trance occurred. Instead, suggest to the patient, while in trance, the value of this deep relaxation experience that can build a "memory" of what it feels like to be deeply relaxed and that can be used next time to teach self-hypnosis.

We will discuss posthypnotic suggestion and posttrance imprinting shortly. Teaching self-hypnosis combines elements of both. Self-hypnosis is taught during trance, so it includes unconscious posthypnotic responses to suggestions to fix the experience in place for future use. It also is further imprinted outside the initial trance experience. It becomes something the patient consciously does to feel better. By regular repetition, it becomes a part of daily ritual, and is done almost automatically.

Inductions That Include Teaching Self-Hypnosis

Eye Fixation With Attention to Breathing Induction Trance Script

The following induction fits the brief cognitive hypnosis paradigm in that it is brief, direct, and conducive to teaching the patient self-hypnosis:

> Sit comfortably in the chair, with your feet flat on the floor and your arms comfortably on the arms of the chair or in your lap and look at some small object in front of you. Here in the office you can look at the hands of the Buddha in the

picture on the wall or at the crystal ball in the stand on the windowsill in front of you. As you continue to look at the object, pay attention to your breathing without trying to change it. Just let yourself breathe normally while you pay attention to your breathing. Let your breathing become the center of your thoughts and attention while your eyes stay focused on the object you chose in front of you. If your mind wanders, and it may, the moment you realize that you are thinking of something else, bring your mind back to concentrating on your breathing.

As you do this, you will notice that you begin to blink more frequently than usual, and that your eyelids may feel heavier. This more frequent blinking and the way your eyelids feel are a part of the hypnosis experience. Shortly you will find your eyes closing. When they do, just leave them closed until I ask you to open them. Do not squeeze them tight. Just leave them closed lightly and comfortably. You may notice a fluttering of your eyelids. That is also part of the hypnosis experience. After a while, you will pay no attention to them. Meanwhile, your breathing has begun to change as you become more relaxed. Notice how comfortable your breathing feels, and how much more relaxed you have become. Allow your more comfortable breathing to take you deeper and deeper into relaxation and hypnosis. As you continue to go deeper with each breath that you take, and with each word that I say, regardless of the meaning of those words, the doorway to your unconscious opens and with your permission, I have the opportunity to talk directly to your unconscious and give it the information it needs to help you change the behavior that you want to change.

Here you might add appropriate suggestions and rephrased reframes to complete the imprinting process and fix the desired changes in place, if you have decided that teaching self-hypnosis is not essential to accomplishing the therapy goals that you have established. However, if you have decided that teaching self-hypnosis is essential, then you can say the following:

Today, you are learning what it feels like to be comfortably relaxed. You are building a memory of deep relaxation that you can borrow to relax yourself. When you are relaxed, you can't be angry or upset, anxious or afraid, frustrated or stressed, because relaxation is the physical and emotional opposite of those feelings.

When you want to practice your own self-relaxation, your own self-hypnosis, you will do what we did here in the office today, by yourself. Ideally, that would be first thing in the morning before breakfast, and again late in the afternoon or sometime before dinner. Find a comfortable chair to sit in, off by yourself, look at some object not too far away to fix your gaze and pay attention to your breathing. Don't try to change your breathing. Shortly, your eyelids will begin to feel heavier, you will notice that you are blinking more frequently than usual and you will gently and comfortably close your eyes without squeezing them tight. Continue to pay attention to your breathing without trying to change it. Your breathing will change by itself. If you find your mind wandering, the moment you realize it is wandering, bring your attention back to your breathing, and allow yourself to relax even more.

After a while, when you choose to awaken yourself, as we will be doing shortly here in the office today, you will feel very good, very relaxed, and very comfortable, yet wide awake at the same time. You will feel better for some time after you awaken yourself from your own self-relaxation. You will do that by counting slowly from 1 to 5. With the number 5, open your eyes and be wide awake, yet still feel a great deal of relaxation. But don't do that yet. I will help you do that today shortly.

If you have decided that it is appropriate to teach the patient a coping skill for instantly managing stress, then you can say the following:

I am going to teach you a whole new way to relax yourself instantly to deal with stressful situations whenever you need to, wherever you are, in seconds, without closing your eyes and without anyone knowing you are doing it.

Stress is usually experienced as a pressure or feeling in the chest or shoulders, or in the back of the neck. When this begins to happen to you, and you may be more aware of it more quickly, just look at something, not too far away, to focus your attention. Then take two or three very slow, deep breaths. Breathe in through your nose and let out the tension slowly through your mouth, all the way down to your stomach. Immediately, you will bring back a part of this feeling of relaxation, enough to melt away, dissolve away, any feelings of pressure, or tension, or stress.

You are sitting here in the chair already very relaxed. Take a few very slow, deep breaths. Breathe slowly in through your nose and breathe out the tension slowly through your mouth, all the way down to your stomach. Very good. Now, take another slow, deep breath, but slow it down even more. Excellent. Let yourself breathe normally. That's great. That helped you to feel even more relaxed, didn't it? If it did, just nod your head for me. Thank you.

Now, when you are ready to awaken yourself, count slowly and silently to yourself from 1 up to 5. With each number you count, you will feel more and more alert while still feeling relaxed. With the number 5, open your eyes and be wide awake. How do you feel? How was that? You did feel more relaxed from the deep breaths, didn't you? That's great.

While discussing this in a workshop, someone once asked us, "Why don't you just automatically teach self-hypnosis to every patient?" There are some behaviors that we refer to as simple habits, which we treat as single-session procedures. Once the behavior has been extinguished, we do not want the patient to do anything that would become a ritual that is necessary to continue to prevent the behavior from returning.

That would be like trying *not* to think of a pink elephant. The harder you try not to do something, the more difficult it becomes, and the more obsessed you become with what you are trying not to do. This is what often happens when people try to stop smoking "cold turkey." It creates a stress reaction that can increase thoughts of smoking and that can make the desire to smoke even stronger. Therefore, we usually do not teach self-hypnosis for single-session procedures. Sometimes, however, we teach instant relaxation, such as deep breathing, for general stress control. We also may use playing with a marble as a distractor, for immediate stress control (see the next section).

Zarren's Marble Induction Trance Script

This is an ideal way to externalize physical discomfort and somatic ideation. It combines visual and tactile-kinesthetic systems. It is excellent with children, because they can be taught to make the marble disappear as part of an ego-building process. Adults also enjoy learning a little magic to give themselves an ego boost.

I am going to give you something that you can use to help yourself into hypnosis and relaxation. You will learn to do this here in the office today, and you will be able to do it without my help at home or almost anywhere. There is a large jar sitting on the table containing many beautiful marbles of different sizes and colors and textures. Reach into the jar and choose a marble that you would like to be your marble. Choose one that looks and feels most comfortable for you. Try them out. Pick up as many as you want until you find the one that you like the most.

Now, sit back in the chair with the marble in your hand and notice that just holding the marble brings a smile to your lips and a nice feeling inside you. This is because marbles somehow instantly bring us back to a time in childhood when we were enjoying ourselves. Hold the marble between your thumb and fingers and feel it by rolling it around. Look at the way the light changes the colors embedded in the marble. Feel the slight imperfections in the round glass globe that you are holding. Realize that something this beautiful doesn't have to be perfect and yet can still be very special.

As you do this, you are aware that you are feeling much more relaxed and you are blinking more frequently than usual. When your eyelids get very heavy, or when the marble begins to go out of focus, gently close your eyes and close your hand around the marble so that it doesn't fall out of your hand. As you do this, you immediately go very deeply into relaxation. Pay attention to the feel of the marble in your hand. Notice how much warmer it feels. If you want to, you can even see the changing colors and swirls of color in the marble with your eyes closed. As you continue to concentrate on the marble, you will go much deeper into relaxation and hypnosis. If your mind wanders, the moment you realize you are thinking of something different, just bring your mind back to concentrating on the marble in your hand.

You control the marble. You are in charge of it, and the marble helps you to experience very deep relaxation, without pressure or tension or stress. It helps you to feel very comfortable. Even just holding the marble can help you to feel very comfortable.

Now your concentration on the marble is even stronger and your feeling of relaxation is even deeper. When you are relaxed, you can't be angry, you can't be anxious and you can't be uncomfortable. These are physical and emotional opposites of each other. Relaxation is your first goal, leading to changes in how you feel, how you think and how you behave. You are building a memory of deep relaxation that you can use to help yourself relax on your own.

To teach self-hypnosis:

Plan to use this marble, your marble, a few times a day to relax yourself, the way we did here in the office today. Hold the marble in your hand, look at it, roll it between your thumb and fingers, feel it, see the colors change, the reflecting light and relax. Close your eyes gently, close your hand around the marble and relax much deeper. Stay in relaxation for a while and enjoy your freedom from physical and emotional discomfort. Then awaken yourself by counting from 1 to 5, turning your hand face up, slowly opening your hand, then your eyes, as we will be doing shortly. The opening of your eyes will allow you to continue to feel very relaxed yet energized.

In addition to using the marble to help yourself go deeply into relaxation, from now on, you will be able to use this marble to relax yourself, in seconds, whenever you need to most, wherever you are, without closing your eyes, without anyone knowing you are doing it. Just holding the marble in your hand brings back a feeling of relaxation. This almost instant relaxation technique is a very valuable tool that you can have available to deal with stressful situations no matter when or where they may occur.

1—2—3—4—5. Now, open your eyes and look at the marble, and really feel great—wide awake, yet relaxed at the same time.

When working with children, or even adults, we teach them to use their chosen marble for self-hypnosis. Often, we also teach them a magic trick, such as the "French Drop," the "Top-of-Fist Vanish," or the "Bottom-of-Fist Vanish," to make the marble disappear. These fascinating and amusing tricks are easily learned from a book on magic, such as one by Tarr (1976). Tarr's book is an excellent illustrated guide containing clear step-by-step illustrated explanations of the above tricks and many others that are not difficult to learn with a little practice.

The marble induction is also very good for patients who are dealing with serious illness or chronic pain. It encourages patients to externalize their attention while holding on to something that is outside (held in the hand) and under their control. We often use this induction when working with patients with alcohol and substance abuse problems, as well as problems related to side effects from prescribed medications. During the body of the trance, medication side effects can be externalized to the marble and rubbed away. The marble also functions as a powerful talisman that can bring about instant relaxation.

The marble induction combines the two primary sensory systems that most people use to process information, visual and tactile-kinesthetic. Tactile-kinesthetic inductions are very powerful when dealing with medical and physical problems, as well as feelings of helplessness. Patients trained to use the marble, for example, can interrupt a rage reaction by reaching into a pocket or purse and holding the marble.

The marble carries the value of worry beads, the holding or rubbing of a religious symbol, or the same kind of security that is associated with a New Age crystal. The marble is like an adult "security blanket" that can be kept easily and, when combined with learning to do magic, contains an implied suggestion that the marble itself is "magical." More details follow in Part Two.

Inductions That Do Not Include Teaching Self-Hypnosis

All of the inductions can be used without teaching self-hypnosis when the clinician is doing a single-session change procedure. However, the one we use most often is detailed below.

Rising and Falling Arms Induction Trance Script

This induction is a combined adaptation of arm levitation and reverse arm levitation and contains a self-ratification of the trance experience. We use this induction most of the time during our single-session smoking cessation program. It is fast, it redirects the patient's attention to his or her arms, and it creates an immediate feeling that something uniquely different is happening as the rigidity and changes in arm position occur.

> In a moment, I am going to ask you to close your eyes, but not yet. When I do, leave them closed until I ask you to open them, and don't squeeze them tight. Just let them close comfortably and easily. Meanwhile, lift your two arms up like this. (Demonstrate by raising and extending your two arms straight out and rigid, palms down, parallel to the floor and about chest high.)
>
> Turn one hand over, palm up. That's good. Now, when you close your eyes, but not yet, I am going to attach a string to this wrist. (lightly touch the wrist with the palm facing down) attached to a large make-believe helium-filled balloon. (Slowly move the finger, touching the wrist face up and then in a circle, simulating the outline of a large round balloon.) If I really did attach a helium-filled balloon to this wrist, this arm would move slowly up, wouldn't it? I am also going to place a make-believe small book in the palm of this hand. (Lightly touch the palm of the hand face up.) If I really did that, this arm would get heavier and move down, wouldn't it? But don't move your arms on purpose. Let them move by themselves.
>
> Now, gently and comfortably close your eyes. I am tying the string attached to the balloon to this wrist (lightly touch the wrist), and this arm will get lighter and lighter and slowly rise. I am placing the small book in the palm of this hand (lightly touch the palm of the hand facing up), and this arm will get heavier and slowly move down. One arm is slowly rising, and the other arm is slowly moving down. But something else is also happening. Both arms have become stiff and rigid. I am going to lightly press a finger on each wrist. (Lightly press down on each wrist with your fingertips simultaneously.) As I press lightly down on your wrists, notice that both arms tend to bounce. That is not usual. It only happens when someone is going into hypnosis. So it tells us that you are in going into hypnosis.
>
> Keep this arm floating in the air. (Lightly tap the wrist of the hand facing down.) (Lightly turn over the hand facing up as you say the following:) Now, with your permission, I am going to turn this hand over and slowly lower it down to the arm of the chair (or, if the chair is without armrests, say *to your lap*), without your help, while you go even deeper into relaxation and hypnosis. Very good. I am going to put a small hole in the helium-filled balloon tied to this wrist, and slowly guide this arm down to the other arm of the chair [or lap] as you go even deeper

into relaxation and hypnosis. Very good. The eyelid fluttering that you are experiencing is a part of the hypnosis experience. After a while you will pay no attention to it.

As you are sitting in the chair, already relaxed and breathing normally and listening to the sound of my voice, you will find yourself going even deeper into relaxation and hypnosis—deeper with each breath that you take and deeper with each word that I say, regardless of the meaning of those words. As you go deeper with each breath and deeper with each word, the doorway to your unconscious opens. With your permission, I have the opportunity to talk directly to your unconscious and give it information it needs to help you change the behavior that you want to change. (Name the behavior, such as *"to be a nonsmoker."*)

This brief induction actually takes longer to describe than it does to carry out. Specific trance language for specific problems will be discussed in later chapters. Toward the end of this trance experience, we often attach the instant, eyes-open relaxation using three deep breaths, which can be used by the patient as a "stress interrupter" without anyone knowing that it is being done. Refer to the eye fixation with attention to breathing induction described earlier.

TRANCE-DEEPENING METHODS

There are a number of very comfortable trance-deepening procedures, some included in the trance inductions described above, and others that can be added to any trance process to create a feeling that the relaxation (trance) experience is deeper and more satisfying. We find this is usually not necessary when doing a single-session behavior change procedure. However, with ongoing treatment, and when helping a patient to learn self-hypnosis, we usually teach the patient to experience a more comfortable feeling of being relaxed. These are some specific situations when it may be appropriate.

If, during the first trance experience, the patient comments that he or she did not feel very relaxed, or not much different than usual, a deepening procedure is appropriate. Here, we usually use a simple, slow countdown from 20 to 1, after the hypnotic induction procedure is completed and we are into the body of the trance experience. We might say:

Now that the doorway to your unconscious is open, I am going to help you to go even deeper into relaxation and hypnosis by my counting slowly down from 20 to 1. With each number that I count, you will find yourself going deeper and deeper into relaxation and hypnosis. So just listen to the numbers and let yourself go, and enjoy the experience of going deeper into relaxation and hypnosis. As you go deeper, you will feel better with each number that I count. 20—19—18—17—16—15—14—13—12—11—10—9—8—7—6—5—4—3—2—1."

Because of its simple application, this deepening procedure can be used before the application of direct suggestions for change and learning. After you have taught the patient to do self-hypnosis and the patient has been practicing between therapy sessions, have the patient place himself or herself into trance as he or she has been doing at home. Then ask the patient to signal with a head nod or hand or finger lift when he or she is ready to be taken deeper. Do the countdown with the dialogue above, then suggest that the patient also count down silently when he or she does his or her own self-hypnosis, to further deepen the experience of relaxation and hypnosis.

Although we will be dealing with this next comment in extensive detail later in the book, it is important to note here that we do not have the patient verbalize self-suggestions during the early learning of self-hypnosis. The patient is instructed as follows:

> When you regularly practice your own self-relaxation or self-hypnosis, do not talk to yourself. Just enjoy the deepening feeling of relaxation. As you do this, the things that I say to you when we are working together here in the office will automatically be reinforced during your own self-hypnosis.

Fractionation

After an induction and deepening procedure, the patient can be "awakened," then helped to go back into trance a second time. If the patient has been taught self-relaxation or self-hypnosis, the patient can be asked to put his or her self back into hypnosis without the clinician's help. This immediate reinduction of the trance state is called fractionation. It is a very powerful deepening procedure and helps the patient to recognize that, in fact, the patient can accomplish self-hypnosis on his or her own.

CHOOSING THE RIGHT INDUCTION TO MEET THE NEEDS OF THE PATIENT

We all have favorite inductions. We have offered some of ours in this chapter. Choosing the induction best suited to a patient's needs is important because it often prevents what is frequently described by others as "resistance." The following general guidelines of dos and don'ts apply to induction choices involved in brief cognitive hypnosis.

1. Choose short inductions.
2. Don't teach self-hypnosis for single-session procedures. If a behavior can be successfully changed in one or two visits, why do anything that may suggest otherwise? (Exceptions will be discussed later.) Stress control skills, such as taking a few deep breaths or holding the marble, can be taught for instant relaxation.
3. Avoid using an induction procedure that stresses visualization with someone whose primary sensory processing system is not visual.

4. If you decide to use visual images for a visually oriented patient, make sure that what you are suggesting the patient visualize is in fact what the patient is seeing. The fact that people construct their own interpretations and images in response to the suggestion to visualize something was nicely illustrated in "The Family Circus" by cartoonist Bil Keane. The cartoon pictured the father of four children of different ages reading a story to his children. The father says: "You're standing by the water's edge and . . .". The older boy visualizes a beach on the seashore. The daughter visualizes walking along the shore of a mountain lake. The younger son visualizes standing by a river, and the toddler sees himself looking at a small creek behind his house.

5. The concept of visualization, which emphasizes seeing in the context of trance, includes all of the sensory systems. When suggesting such things as "feeling the texture," or "smelling the rose," or "hearing the rushing water," or "tasting the apple," we are tapping into the other primary sensory systems. We consider these activities to be forms of visualization.

6. Choose an induction and trance experience that helps the patient to externalize thinking when dealing with pain or other physical, somatic, and medical problems. (Exceptions will be discussed later.) The marble induction is an example.

7. When dealing with anxiety-related problems, or with patients who have difficulty appropriately identifying or interpreting body messages, choose an induction that encourages the patient to focus inward. The patient's difficulty in appropriately recognizing and interpreting the meanings of normal body messages may require extensive reframing in and out of the trance state. (Body message identification and interpretation problems will be discussed in more detail when we address anxiety disorders, eating disorders, sleep problems, and other physical dysfunctions.) Appropriate inductions include concentrating on breathing, arm extension and the fluttering of the eyelids. An eye roll with the eyes closed may also be an excellent initial trance induction or trance-deepening technique (Ewin, 1984, 1998).

8. If one induction does not seem to be working, choose another, then tell the patient:

> Everyone is different. All hypnosis is not the same. Some approaches work better with some people and other approaches work better with others.

I (JIZ), once observed a clinician doing an induction that involved an arm levitation. The patient's arm did not rise very high, and the clinician kept trying to get the arm to rise higher. Almost a whole session was used without success. When the patient was asked afterward what had happened, she said, "I wanted to tell you that my arm was high enough, but I didn't know if I should talk, so I didn't say anything." When I discussed this with the clinician, after the patient left, he admitted, realizing too late, that he had been afraid of failing to induce hypnosis with the patient and felt trapped in what he was doing.

The patient should feel comfortable with the induction being used. If there seems to be a problem, give the patient permission to tell you what is going on. If the patient has physical limitations, such as a sore neck or shoulder, an arm extension induction would not be appropriate because of possible strain on the affected area.

9. Avoid asking the patient to do it for you, the clinician (e.g., "I want you to . . .").

GUIDELINES FOR EFFECTIVE TRANCE STATE SUGGESTIONS

As stated earlier, during the trance induction and the trance state, the language used by the clinician is critical in helping the patient's unconscious mind to accept specific or even general suggestions. The clinician further imprints or fixes desired changes in place during the trance experience. In the practice of brief cognitive hypnosis, we follow a number of basic principles, or guidelines, in our verbal delivery of suggestions to the patient in trance.

1. Linking Ideas

Trance state suggestions are meant to reinforce positive behaviors and promote positive expectations for continued positive change. You do this by linking positive changes already accomplished to the expectation of continuing positive change. One thing that has already been accomplished can be suggested as the basis for accomplishing something else that is related but not yet accomplished. For example, you might suggest:

> You did very very well. You succeeded in staying calm when you were riled, which is proof of your progress in taking charge of how you feel and how you behave. Now that you know that you can do this, you can continue to gain greater control from now on. As we continue to work together, [or, *As you continue to experience progress,*] you will continue to experience more and more control over your feelings and behaviors.

2. Verbalizing Confidence and Positive Motivation

When you give suggestions for behavior change, they should be linked to the patient's key motivations for changing, to facilitate their acceptance by the patient's unconscious. Also, verbalize confidence that the desired changes will take place. For example:

> "When you stop smoking today, as you will, your body immediately begins to heal itself and repair itself. You find that you feel better and enjoy your life more with your improved state of health.

Another example:

When you're in deep relaxation, self-hypnosis, using the marble as the focus of your attention, you're enhancing your body's ability to do what needs to be done, to send the necessary signals and messages and biochemistry to the areas that need to be helped to heal within your body, your mind and system.

3. Appropriate Amount of Repetition

Repeat suggestions several times, at different points during the trance state, with and without slight modification, to facilitate their imprinting into the patient's unconscious.

4. Positive Phrasing

Phrase suggestions in positive, as opposed to negative, terms. Tell patients what will happen, or what is happening, as opposed to what they do not or will not experience. For example, it is therapeutically effective to suggest:

Every day, as your body continues to heal, you will notice that you are feeling better and better and more and more comfortable.

It would probably be less effective to suggest:

You will not feel as much pain.

The latter suggestion might be interpreted by the patient's unconscious as "*I will feel pain*," minus the *not*.

5. Time Frames

It is useful to place suggestions in a time frame, especially when you want to suggest the lessening or end of a behavior or experience. For example, it may be therapeutically effective to suggest:

You no longer need to clench your teeth to release tension. You now have other, more effective ways of releasing tension."

On the other hand, to suggest "You don't need to clench your teeth to release tension" could be interpreted by the patient's unconscious as "I do need to clench my teeth to release tension" (minus the *not*) because the dysfunctional coping mechanism of clenching had been imprinted in the unconscious.

6. Expectant Time Markers

It is also useful to use time markers to prime, or prepare, the patient's unconscious for the next suggestion, to build expectation, as in saying,

In a moment, but not just yet, I will ask you to allow your eyes to close.

7. Present and Future Tenses

Related to the issue of time frames, it is useful to make suggestions in the present tense and to link these with suggestions of what will happen, as long as these suggested changes are believable and desirable, hence, acceptable. For example:

> You are feeling more enthusiastic about exercising your new skills, and you have more energy as you do your job. You will enjoy your job more and more as you exercise these new skills.

8. Precision

Be as precise as possible in delivering suggestions. This makes them easier to follow. The less wordy suggestions are, the better. In trance, the patient does not think critically or analytically. The patient's unconscious processes not just the words themselves but also the entire flow and the feelings created by the suggestions. Therefore, be selective about your choice of words. This is what we meant when we talked earlier about the "conscious use of self."

9. Keep It Simple and Concise

Related to this last point, in the trance state, give direct suggestions that repeat your waking state suggestions in a simpler and more concise form. Suggestions should be limited in their scope. Do not try to tackle too many problems at once. Do not introduce entirely new areas for suggested changes during the trance state. The patient's attention is narrowed. Trance is a focusing mechanism. Too much at once tends to unfocus, and bring the patient "up" out of trance.

10. "Don't Try. Do It!"

That brings us to the issue of the use of the word *try*. *Try* is not a good word to use in either waking state or trance state suggestion. To try implies effort and strain. One of the advantages of hypnosis and trance work is that they can bypass conscious processing. To draw the patient's attention to "trying" therefore defeats this built-in advantage of using the hypnosis tool. Trying also implies "to attempt" and "to test." Thus, it implies the possibility of failure. You certainly do not want to direct the patient's attention to the possibility of failure on either a conscious or an unconscious level. Do not suggest "trying." Suggest "doing it."

11. Remove Unwanted Suggestions

One final point: Don't forget to remove unwanted suggestions. Be sure to suggest that when the trance state is ended, and the patient is awakened or "realerted," that the patient's desirable, normally alert state of consciousness or "prehypnosis" state will be restored. Suggested sensory or motor changes that had been used for trance ratification or deepening need to be removed. You don't want your patient leaving your office with an arm that feels "stiff as a board," or "light as a feather," or "buoyant like a balloon," or with a totally numb and unfeeling hand. Don't forget to restore your patient's pretrance sensory motor status. However, this does not include removing desirable, ecologically valid positive changes in the patient's experience and behavior that are intended to continue after the trance state is terminated. Here we are referring to both posthypnotic suggestions and posttrance imprints. You can suggest that the patient will continue to experience some comfortable relaxation for some period of time, while still active and alert.

5

Self-Hypnosis for Continued Problem Resolution

WHAT IS SELF-HYPNOSIS?

Following the extensive discussion on hypnosis, trance, and hypnotic and trance language in the preceding chapter, which included reference to self-hypnosis procedures, we need to further clarify the many facets of hypnosis initiated by the patient. We define *self-hypnosis* as the process by which a person intentionally initiates a hypnotic trance state by himself or herself. Thus, it refers to the means, or the procedure that is self-initiated by an individual to induce a hypnotic trance state, as well as the self-initiated hypnotic trance state itself. We may label the experience the patient initiates as self-relaxation or self-hypnosis, or both. We consider the simple practice of self-relaxation to be self-hypnosis.

"It is virtually impossible for people who have never experienced hypnosis to teach themselves hypnosis" (Cheek, 1994, p. 58). Therefore, self-hypnosis is usually taught to a patient during a formal trance state experience. As David Cheek pointed out, "We have all been heavily indoctrinated since birth with the idea that no new learning can occur unless someone teaches us. Any effort to try [e.g., learning self-hypnosis] without training seems to evoke Coué's Law of Reversed Effect" (p. 58). This law states that the harder we try to do something that needs to be natural and spontaneous, such as falling asleep, the harder it becomes to accomplish. Likewise, the harder we try not to do something, such as, trying not to think of a pink elephant, the more likely we are to get the opposite result, in this case, to keep thinking of a pink elephant.

James Braid (1795–1860), a Scottish surgeon, coined the term *hypnosis* as a replacement for *Mesmerism*. He wrote that "patients can throw themselves into the nervous sleep (hypnosis) and manifest all the usual phenomena of Mesmerism through their own unaided efforts" (Braid, 1843). In fact, it has even been reported that Franz Anton Mesmer (1734–1815) a German physician who is considered to have been the father of hypnosis, and who was the inventor of the concept of animal magnetism, even "mesmerized" himself to treat his own ailments (Gravitz, 1994).

The father of modern self-hypnosis is considered to be Emile Coué (1857–1926), a French pharmacist who taught patients "Self-mastery through conscious autosuggestion" (Coué, 1922). Coué established some basic laws of autosuggestion, including the Law of Reversed Effect, defined above. Coué's student C. Harry Brooks (1922) further wrote: "Every idea which enters the Conscious mind, if accepted by the unconscious, is transformed by it into a reality and forms henceforth a permanent element in our life." (pp. 54–55). He conceptualized the process of "autosuggestion" as consisting of two steps: (1) the acceptance of an idea and (2) its transformation into a reality. He believed that this could happen through the process of repetition.

Note Coué's title. He specifically called his approach to self-suggestion "conscious autosuggestion." That means that the conscious mind, during the waking state, is giving suggestions repetitively so that the unconscious mind will accept them and make them a part of the unconscious. He further believed that "*all* suggestion is autosuggestion." Thus, the clinician can give the patient suggestions for change, but in order for that change to occur, the patient must take possession of the suggestions and make the suggestions his or her own. All suggestions that are accepted therefore become autosuggestions. This may not require the patient to frequently repeat these suggestions through self-talk, but only to accept the suggestions as the patient's own.

Coué was the originator of the much quoted phrase "Every day in every respect, I am getting better and better." (Coué, 1922, p. 23). It is often rephrased as "Every day, in every way, I am feeling better and better."

The acceptance of an idea and that idea's transformation into reality, according to Coué, were accomplished by the unconscious. He wrote that whether or not an idea originated in the mind of the patient or was presented by an external event or another person (waking state reframing or trance state) made no difference. In both cases, the idea is submitted to the unconscious and either accepted or rejected. Thus, the distinction between "autosuggestion" and "heterosuggestion," or therapist-given suggestion, was seen to be arbitrary and superficial. More than just a few modern hypnosis clinicians, researchers, and scholars have maintained that all hypnosis is essentially self-hypnosis—that is, self-induced (Cheek, 1994; Erickson, 1948; Kroger, 1977; Sanders, 1991; Teitelbaum, 1965).

Whether or not the hypnosis state, induced in the communication process between the clinician and the patient, is essentially self-hypnosis depends on whether or not the ideas submitted to the patient are accepted by the patient's unconscious. For this to be so, the clinician must use language in a form that can be accepted by the patient's unconscious. When the clinician uses the right language, it makes the hypnotic communication process much more effective.

The most comprehensive review of research studies on self-hypnosis was done by Fromm and Kahn (1990). The reader is referred to this volume for a detailed exposition of scientific studies on this subject.

When Is Self-Hypnosis Taught?

Self-hypnosis is not taught to the patient who is being seen for a single visit. It is usually taught to the patient who is to be seen for a minimum of three or more visits. The major purposes of teaching self-hypnosis are (1) to give the patient self-control that can be continued through self-administration, and thus reduce the patient's dependence on the clinician, (2) to help the patient experience a greater sense of personal power over something that the patient has felt power-less about, and (3) to reduce the cost of treatment by assisting the patient to continue self-treatment.

SOME IMPORTANT CONSIDERATIONS

There are four progressive processes and considerations that relate to the patient's initial learning and immediate and ongoing utilization of self-hypnosis. They are (1) the choice of trance induction, (2) helping the patient experience and build a memory of simple relaxation, (3) the types of suggestions the clinician should administer during the initial teaching and patient learning of self-hypnosis, and (4) how the patient can later use self-suggestions once he or she is comfortable with self-initiating and deepening the self-hypnotic trance state.

Choosing the "Right" Trance Induction

We prefer choosing simple procedures for the induction and teaching of self-hypnosis. They should be short and easy to learn without complicated instructions. They should induce a trance experience that the patient will be able to repeat during his or her own self-hypnosis.

The procedure should be practiced in a sitting position, with the patient's head supported if needed. We do not encourage patients to practice self-hypnosis lying down. We generally avoid doing hypnosis work in the office with the patient in a prone position. We use a comfortable armchair that can have a pillow placed to allow the patient to put his or her head back if that is most comfortable. The patient sits back without slouching, with the feet flat on the floor. Lying down, on the other hand, usually leads to sleep. So we discourage using a bed, sofa, or recliner for self-hypnosis sessions. If a recliner is used, we suggest that it should be in an upright position.

As usual, there are exceptions to the above. Some patients are more comfortable in other positions. For example, a patient with a bad back requested that she be allowed to lie on the floor and look up at the ceiling while experiencing hypnosis. The hard carpeted floor was more comfortable for her. We used an eye fixation induction with added specific suggestions that

> your unconscious mind will know if you are about to fall asleep. If that happens, your unconscious will move your body slightly to alert you enough to maintain the trance state and not fall asleep.

This is usually enough to prevent a sleep state from occurring. This same suggestion can be used if the patient is sitting up during trance, and the clinician or the patient is concerned that the patient will fall asleep.

Another patient who had fibromyalgia had a difficult time finding a comfortable position for the trance experience. She asked if she could hug a pillow and curl up on the small couch in my (JIZ) office, with her head against the back of the couch. This felt more protective to her, and she could move as much as she wanted. She also tended to be very restless, and she would often feel the need to get up and walk around during waking state therapy. She was pleasantly surprised that she could stay still so long while she was in trance.

We find that patients who tend to be restless, who may often need to get up and move around during talk therapy, are quite pleased with themselves and the hypnotic trance process, when they find that they are able to stay seated for so long during trance.

Case Study: Stress Control

A 63-year-old female called me (JIZ) about smoking cessation. Her dentist had referred her. During the intake evaluation, she stated that she had been widowed for a few years. She had a constant cough, shoulder pain and chronic lower back problem that she reported did not respond to any pain medication. She was leaving in a week to go back up north for the summer and felt she needed to control her smoking behavior.

Because of the pain issues, I decided to use the marble induction (see chapter 4) to help her externalize her physical discomfort. She also would be able to use the marble as an instant relaxation tool. This approach seemed to work well for her. She called me a few days before she was to leave and told me that she was not smoking, but that the marble was not helping her with the stress because both of her hands were in constant motion. She had responded well to the smoking cessation protocol but continued to feel stressed and in much pain.

Individualizing Self-Hypnosis to Meet the Patient's Unique Needs

We set up an appointment for the next day to find a way to help her deal with stress. During that session, after discussing the problem of her hands being constantly in motion, I decided to focus her attention on her hands as a self-hypnosis procedure. I gave her the following directives:

> Your hands are an expression of the stress and discomfort that you are feeling. Your hands can also help you to control the stress and feel more comfortable by helping you to feel relaxed. Sit up comfortably in the chair and place your elbows on the arms of the chair. Hold your hands about 8 inches apart with your palms facing toward each other, like this. [I demonstrated the position.] Look at your hands, and feel them slowly moving toward each other like magnets being attracted to each other. Don't do this on purpose. Recognize that this is happening without your help. As your hands move closer and closer, you feel more and more relaxed. When your fingers touch each other, you will gently close your eyes while you fold your hands together. When they are folded together, you will feel very relaxed and lower your folded hands down to your lap. That's very good. You really are so much more relaxed and more comfortable. Most of the feelings of stress and discomfort are gone and you feel very good. Your hands now know how to help you to control your stressful feelings. Your hands now know how to help you to experience greater comfort. Once or twice a day, you can sit down in your most comfortable chair, and let your hands relax you and relieve you of stress and discomfort, the way they did here in the office today. It won't take long. Concentrate on the good feeling of relaxation. When you are comfortable enough, you can open your eyes, unfold your hands and continue to feel good.

This patient left the office feeling comfortable both physically and emotionally, and said she looked forward to using her hands to help her feel good. She called me 2 months later from her summer home and reported that she was "doing great." Her hands were helping her to deal with the stress, and that there was much less stress. She also reported that her pain had diminished and that she was looking forward to coming back to Florida in a few months. She stated that she would call me then to check in.

The above example illustrates that, although there are preferred approaches to trance induction and self-hypnosis, continued flexibility remains an important ingredient in the practice of brief cognitive hypnosis. Even though our favored inductions for those patients who are taught self-hypnosis are the eye fixation with attention to breathing induction and the marble induction, we are always ready to adjust our approach based on the patient's ongoing feedback. The above anecdote provides a good example of how to be flexible in the design and choice of trance induction procedures in the office and in the teaching of self-hypnosis.

Simple Relaxation

We can't emphasize enough how important simple relaxation is for the immediate effect it has on the patient as an important experiential reframe allowing the patient to feel different and better. This initial experience of physical and emotional relief is often the first good feeling the patient can identify with in a long time. Patients often verbalize that they have not felt so relaxed for many years or even ever. Because of this, the simple experience of relaxation may appear exaggerated. However, this allows for the fixing in place in the patient's unconscious of a powerful memory imprint that opens up further possibilities for change and symptom relief.

Simple relaxation is the first and primary goal, sometimes the only goal, in teaching self-hypnosis to the patient. When self-hypnosis is initially taught, it is usually labeled "self-relaxation." It is described to the patient as the beginning way to (1) reduce the emotional overlay that has made the patient's problem worse, (2) imprint a memory of relaxation that can be repeated for continuing progressive relief, (3) establish workable skills for evoking instant relaxation whenever the patient feels the need, (4) interrupt the belief that the patient is "trapped" in dysfunctional feelings and behavior, and (5) choose one or two 10- to 15–minute periods during the day when the patient can enjoy treating himself or herself to a comfortable quiet time.

The values of self-relaxation should be discussed with the patient during the waking state as part of the waking state reframing process. It should be explained that the patient is to do no self-talk, and not give self-suggestions, during this learning and practice of self-relaxation. The only immediate goal is to learn how to relax. Being able to imprint and increase the feeling of relaxation establishes a foundation for future change. When the patient is very relaxed, he or she cannot be tense, upset, uncomfortable, anxious, afraid, stressed or angry. All of these feelings are physical and emotional opposites of the feeling of relaxation.

Clinician-Administered Suggestions

When we teach self-hypnosis, after the initial simple relaxation period of learning, we may further instruct the patient not to attempt to give suggestions to himself or herself when continuing to practice what we now label self-hypnosis. Our rationale for this is that we want to avoid a situation where the patient unknowingly distorts our suggestions when he or she self-administers them during self-hypnosis. The effort involved in remembering what to say to oneself while in self-hypnosis can often be counterproductive.

We explain that now that the patient has successfully learned to relax, and now that this experience of relaxation has been helpful, we are ready to enter into the "suggestions for change" part of the program. It is explained that these suggestions will be given to the patient by the clinician while the patient is in trance in the clinician's office. For the time being, the patient doesn't have to consciously listen to the suggestions, or try to repeat them during the daily practice of self-hypnosis.

We tell the patient:

> Your unconscious will hear everything that I am saying without your having to listen. The very nature of your relaxation experience automatically reinforces those things that I say to you when you and I are working together.

Note the phrase "when you and I are working together." This implies in and out of trance. These suggestions can be very powerful and liberating and can often prevent any distortion of the suggestions given by the clinician. They give the patient permission to stop worrying about making mistakes or unknowingly saying the wrong things. They also help the patient who is somewhat obsessive to avoid obsessing about the language used to bring about change.

We also give a very powerful reframing suggestion during the trance state that reduces or eliminates the patient's concerns that "because previous attempts to change may not have worked, why should this approach work?" When the patient is in a satisfactory trance state, the following may be said:

> This deep and comfortable level of relaxation that you are experiencing now is called the neutral state or the healing state. This is when the doorway to the unconscious opens and the unconscious can accept suggestions for change. But we can't go directly from negative to positive. That is too much of a leap. That is why you may not have been as successful before. In order to make the transition, we need to go from negative to neutral. When in neutral, everything is in balance. There is no wasted energy on stress or distress. All of the energy of mind and body is in balance, and available to the mind–body system to be used as an energy resource, for change, and to build a memory of deep relaxation that you can borrow every time you do your own relaxation, your own self-hypnosis. This allows the movement from negative, to neutral, and then to positive.

This approach fosters a collaborative team effort between the clinician and the patient. While the patient is learning self-hypnosis skills, the clinician, at first, takes the role of "director of change" and "administrator of suggestions." This approach allows the patient to focus on a single achievable goal. The patient's skill in "shifting into neutral" also adds to a growing self-confidence that encourages him or her to continue practicing self-hypnosis and learning more skills for change. This has strong ego-building and ego-strengthening characteristics (Frederick & McNeal, 1999; Hartland, 1965, 1971).

Patient-Administered Suggestions

By the time the patient becomes proficient and comfortable practicing self-hypnosis without self-talk, many of the presenting complaints and dysfunctional feelings and behaviors will have been reduced in intensity, or eliminated entirely. This may be the result of several interacting factors.

Marked alterations in the relative balance between sympathetic and parasympathetic nervous system activation and dominance appear to be associated with specific physical and psychological symptoms of pathology (Humphreys & Eagan, 1999), including the perpetuation of anxiety, depressive, and chronic pain disorders (Eimer, 1988, 1989; Eimer & Freeman, 1998; Melzack, 1999; Turk & Flor, 1999). Proficiency in practicing self-relaxation and self-hypnosis apparently leads to increased control over the autonomic nervous system and decreased sympathetic dysregulation and hyperarousal (Benson, Arns, & Hoffman, 1981; De Pascalis, 1999; Edmonston, 1981; Humphreys & Eagan, 1999).

Relaxation is the opposite of stress, pain, anxiety, rage and depressive states. A person cannot be relaxed and feel distressed at the same time. Learning self-relaxation and self-hypnosis is associated with increased thoughts and feelings of self-efficacy and self-control and the feeling of being "in charge" of oneself. Self-efficacy has been shown to account for a significant portion of the main treatment effects variance in psychophysiological treatment studies (Bandura et al., 1987; Blanchard et al., 1993; Eimer & Freeman, 1998; Gatchel & Blanchard, 1993).

The experience of symptom exacerbation as a consequence of "emotional overlay," which is partly associated with autonomic imbalance and dysregulation, is a real one to which clinicians ought to pay more attention. By doing so, the negative elements left are much easier to deal with. In the same way that positive suggestions sequentially attached to real experiences imply the reality of those suggestions, multiple negative symptoms attached to each other suggest that negatives are the only feelings and behaviors to expect. As the negatives are reduced or eliminated, this previous belief system is easily changed to positive expectations. The next natural step is for the patient to self-administer these positive suggestions.

Positive suggestions for specific disorders will be covered in detail in the following chapters that cover dysfunctional psychological and medical problems. However, at this point, we emphasize several considerations. One is the importance of frequently evaluating the patient's progress and reestablishing treatment goals. This will lead to giving the patient specific suggestions to be verbalized prior to his or her self-hypnosis sessions. These suggestions should be verbalized as positive rather than negative. They should be worded to suggest positive outcomes rather than to suggest not doing or not experiencing something.

For example, you would avoid having the patient self-administer the suggestion

I will not feel pain in my shoulder.

It would be more effective to have the patient say

I will enjoy feeling more comfort in my shoulder.

We avoid suggesting to the patient to not do something. This is because the harder we try not to do something, the more difficult it becomes not to do it!

Remember Coué's (1922) Law of Reversed Effect—for instance, try not to think of a pink elephant. Or try not to notice, or try not to scratch that itch on your nose, or try not to blink your eyes as you read this.

Self-Suggestions Before Entering Self-Hypnosis

When patients are ready to give themselves self-suggestions during their practice of self-hypnosis, they should be instructed to do so before they self-induce the hypnotic trance state. Help the patient write down specific suggestions that relate to the realization of the patient's specific change goals, or to a specific dimension of the patient's experience that the patient wants to modify. Then instruct the patient to read these suggestions before entering self-hypnosis. For example, before self-inducing hypnosis, the patient could read from an index card,

> I control my anger [or I will (or can) control my anger] and stay calm and in charge when my wife criticizes me. My shoulder feels really comfortable when I rest it and when I move it.

By reading pertinent, goal-oriented suggestions three or four times before entering self-hypnosis, as opposed to doing self-talk during self-hypnosis, the patient's unconscious is freed to do its "work" during and after the practice of self-hypnosis. This uncomplicates the utilization of self-hypnosis for change purposes. It provides a simpler way for the patient to communicate with his or her own unconscious mind.

GENERAL GUIDELINES

An experienced clinician may have his or her own favorite trance induction methods. That is okay. As long as the clinician follows the following general guidelines that were established for the practice of brief cognitive hypnosis, almost any induction procedure can be effective. In summary:

1. Use short uncomplicated induction procedures.
2. Do not teach self-hypnosis for single-session procedures, such as smoking cessation or simple habit extinction (covered in Part Three).
3. Use the initial learning of self-hypnosis for relaxation only.
4. Initially, do not add any self-talk or self-suggestion to the self-relaxation/ self-hypnosis procedure. In some cases, you may decide that self-suggestions are not necessary.
5. Pay attention to, match, and use the patient's individual language and sensory systems.
6. Choose a hypnotic induction procedure that is either internally or externally directed, based on your assessment of the patient's presenting problem and needs.

7. Be sure that the patient can give you feedback about the comfort of the chosen induction procedure and experience.
8. Encourage patients to practice their self-hypnosis regularly. We usually recommend 10 to 15 minutes twice a day, once in the morning, before breakfast, and once in the late afternoon, or early evening, before supper. It is better to practice self-hypnosis on an empty stomach. If the patient regularly exercises at a fixed time during the day, it is better to do a self-relaxation before rather than after exercising. After exercise, the process of adrenaline pumping is still going on, which makes self-relaxation more difficult to achieve.

THE USE OF TAPES

Many clinicians who teach self-hypnosis make tapes of sessions that they give to patients to use at home. They may feel that this is a valid vehicle for patients to use to enter into hypnosis. Those who use tapes often describe that their value lies in having a patient listen to the clinician's voice giving the specific suggestions for change that were given during the office session. Clinicians may even make new tapes during subsequent sessions that are then given to patients to replace the previous ones, or as part of a history (or record) of each progressive session. In our view, this may be giving too much information to patients that may cause too much obsessing and intellectual evaluation of the process of treatment, and not allow the unconscious to do its work.

Other clinicians encourage the use of selected commercial tapes that are geared primarily for relaxation, and that have some special sounds or music in the background. They usually are selected to meet the unconscious needs of the clinician, especially when there is a musical background that the clinician finds relaxing. Most clinicians have their personal favorite music and sounds. There probably are as many different individual favorites as there are clinicians. The patient may not have the same favorites.

Why We Rarely Use Tapes

We rarely use tapes in our practices. When we do, we do not use music. Music may or may not help relax the patient, depending on the patient's own musical tastes and auditory propensities. Also, music is not always available when it is important for the patient to practice self-hypnosis in a setting other than a quiet home. Our reasons for rarely using tapes are the following:

1. *Patients change, tapes do not.* Each time the patient initiates self-relaxation or self-hypnosis, some subtle or significant change takes place. Suggestions, which may have been valid when given in the office by the clinician, may no longer be valid the next day. Continued use of a tape containing sugges-

tions given during the first induction and self-hypnosis training session in the office may prevent change by regressing the patient back, during each subsequent use of the tape, to when the patient was in trouble. This can produce a cycle of progress–regress. This is also why we often start with no self-talk during the patient's self-relaxation/self-hypnosis practice.

2. *Tapes require special equipment and supplies and special settings.* If the patient uses tapes, the patient does not learn to do self-hypnosis as a self-contained, self-initiated independent process, but becomes dependent on the clinician's voice and the equipment to transmit it. This means that the patient's own power of imagination is limited to the words of the clinician on the tape, and this establishes further dependency on the clinician. Use of the tape recorder also limits where the patient can practice self-hypnosis without attracting unwanted attention.

3. *Commercial tapes are not individualized.* Generic commercial tapes are intended to be all things to all people. They are not individualized to meet the unique needs of the patient in terms of sensory system learning and change language that will be easily accepted by the patient's unconscious mind. Furthermore, they are often too long and too repetitive. Commercial tapes need to be of a certain length, usually a half hour on each side, to warrant charging a premium price for each tape. Such length requires frequent repetition of trance induction and therapeutic suggestions. This may cause the message to become redundant after more than a few minutes. Such redundancy paradoxically can negate the acceptance of the suggestions by the patient's unconscious.

4. *Patients loan out tapes.* Our experience has been that patients who have experienced clinician-made tapes as helpful often lend these tapes to others who may or may not have asked to borrow them. Unfortunately, they may do harm to others who borrow them, because the tapes were made specifically for the patient, not for anyone else. Therefore, if you do make tapes, instruct your patients not to lend them to others.

Special Circumstances

We may use tapes for special circumstances. For example, if an anxious patient has an impending trip and must travel before we can complete anxiety control training, we may give the patient a specialized relaxation tape that we make for the patient, but it is not taped during a therapy session. This tape can be used while traveling. If the patient is taking a difficult examination away from home, for example, or participating in an anxiety-producing work situation away from home, we may produce a special tape for use before the examination or meeting. This could be used the evening before and/or shortly before the event.

The tapes we produce specifically for a limited group of individual patients are for a time-limited purpose. They are individualized. Even so, we believe we must add suggestions that allow the patient to change, and allow the suggestions contained on the tape to be reinterpreted based on these unconscious changes. To achieve this, we add certain suggestion phrases at the end of the tape. The following is one example:

As you continue to grow and change, the meaning of my words and suggestions that you hear on this tape will also change. Although the words may be the same, the meaning of those words will be different. They will continuously change and be interpreted by your unconscious to meet your changing needs.

6

Common Factors in Dysfunctional Behavior and the Creation of Double Binds

Most patients who present for psychotherapy and hypnosis feel significant loss of control. Consciously, the patient may be aware that a particular behavior or symptom is dysfunctional, self-defeating, distressing or harmful, but he or she feels helpless or powerless to change it. The dysfunctional behavior or feeling originally may have been imprinted in the unconscious as the result of some traumatic experience and, through repetition, further imprinted. The unconscious continues to repeat the dysfunctional behavior or feeling, and it becomes a habit, because the unconscious does not have enough information to judge the behavior as no longer necessary, or as invalid.

If the patient consciously knows that the behavior or symptom is undesirable (i.e., egodystonic), but the patient's unconscious does not have the data or information to invalidate it, then this results in an incongruity between the conscious mind and the unconscious mind that controls the behavior or symptom. The conscious mind "knows" that the behavior or symptom is undesirable, but the unconscious mind does not know this.

Such an incongruity can produce a pathological double bind that manifests as psychological conflict and causes further dysfunctional thoughts, feelings, and behavior. The patient becomes "frozen" in the dysfunctional way of thinking, feeling, and acting because of a conviction of being trapped. The underlying belief is that there are no choices, that the patient is dammed if he does, dammed if he doesn't. Here the proverbial "being caught between a rock and a hard place" also applies.

In a pathological double bind, the uncomfortable, debilitating symptom behavior continues because the patient is trapped into believing that this behavior, which is a negative coping mechanism, is unchangeable. However, it is the only choice the patient has because of his or her belief that there are no other choices.

From our perspective, all "bad," dangerous, or self-destructive behaviors, most psychosomatic symptoms and all dysfunctional behaviors are precipitated and maintained by pathological double binds. These double binds are essentially internal miscommunication systems.

The conscious mind is aware that something is wrong but can't help it. The unconscious mind is unaware that something is wrong, so continues to perpetuate it. In fact, the unconscious mind may be maintaining the problem feelings and behaviors in the belief that the dysfunctional behavior is an appropriate coping behavior. Remember that all behaviors are both a form of communication and a way of coping.

At first, the coping behavior may have been temporarily appropriate. However, as it was repeated for its palliative value, it changed and evolved by repetition into a less palliative dysfunctional behavior. The original precipitating cause of this choice of coping behavior is no longer occurring, but the behavior has taken on a life of its own. It has now become imprinted as the behavior of choice because the unconscious mind is unable to reevaluate it and thus discard it. The dysfunctional behavior has been transformed into a habit. Habits are created by repetition, and the unconscious does not judge whether they are good or bad, or their appropriateness, except if they are life threatening.

ORIGINAL DOUBLE BIND THEORY

The double bind theory was introduced by Bateson et al. (1956) to describe the paradox established by certain unresolvable sequences of experiences confronting an individual in that individual's family interactions or primary interpersonal context (Sluzki & Ransom, 1976; Walrond-Skinner, 1986). The concept was further elaborated by Watzlawick, Beavin, and Jackson (1967). These clinical researchers proposed that these situations were "schizophrenogenic" because they placed the individual in a no-win situation in which whatever that individual did in response to the authority figure's communications and injunctions was defined as "bad." As Laing (1965) stated, the individual, which he described as a "divided self," was "mystified," and this "mystification" led the conflicted individual to develop unconventional communication habits that were appropriate or adaptive in that "crazy-making" context.

Thus, schizophrenia was not seen as an intrapsychic disturbance primarily caused by a biochemical imbalance or genetic factors. It was seen to be interpersonally induced primarily through a dysfunctional socialization process in which a person was bombarded by continuous, manipulative, and mixed communication messages by family authority figures.

In other words, the schizotypal behavior was posited to develop as an appropriate personal coping response for dealing with the conflict generated by ongoing, incongruent communications. Such a paradoxical assault on the developing individual's psyche could only be handled if the individual constructed a separate reality. This separate reality then gives rise to accompanying coping behaviors, which, in that original impossibly conflicted context, were life saving for the recipient of the discordant and "crazy-making" manipulations.

Beyond Schizophrenia

We recognize that this concept can be extended to understand the origins of most dysfunctional, fixed behaviors and beliefs. The experience of being trapped in dysfunctional feelings and behaviors is associated with the belief that there are no other viable choices. This belief structure perpetuates those feelings and behaviors. It also creates a closed feedback system of internal miscommunications that fixes in place rigid beliefs that give rise to the patient's distorted worldview and internal reality.

In his seminal work *The Psychology of Personal Constructs*, George Kelly (1955) posited that all behavior represents a test of the validity of a person's personal construct system. According to Kelly, a person's personal constructs (what we would call concepts or beliefs) are the "lenses" or "dimensions" or "channels" through which the individual sees or understands "reality," and anticipates and makes predictions about events. This conceptualization was further extended in the work of Powers (1973), who proposed a cybernetic feedback model in which behavior serves to control perception (and personal beliefs).

According to this compelling model, particular beliefs lead to specific behaviors that are unconsciously chosen to confirm those beliefs. In turn, a person's perceptions and feelings are seen to be determined by his or her beliefs and experiences in the world acting on those beliefs. When the predicted outcomes of particular behaviors do not occur, the discrepancy between the construing person's beliefs and predictions and the actual outcomes can create cognitive dissonance (Festinger, 1957). People are intrinsically motivated to resolve or avoid such dissonance because it is unsettling and uncomfortable. One way that it is often avoided is by reinterpreting the outcomes to fit the original beliefs and predictions. It is usually harder to change the beliefs themselves. However, it is often necessary, and hence adaptive, to do so, when "reality" does not turn out as anticipated or predicted. This is why the technique of reframing is so useful and important.

In our view, most of the choices people make are not conscious but unconscious. These unconscious choices lead us either to cope well and feel relatively good or to cope poorly and feel bad. We conceptualize all behavior and symptoms as an expression of the attempt to cope.

Beliefs, feelings, and coping behaviors, dysfunctional or otherwise, are imprinted in the unconscious through the processes of repetition or trauma. Dysfunctional beliefs, feelings, and behaviors (i.e., symptoms) can be changed through the appropriate application of waking state reframing, and these therapeutic changes can be fixed in place through hypnotic trance work.

THE ILLUSION OF ALTERNATIVES

Beliefs can be changed. That is what reframing is all about. Reframing involves changing beliefs that are discordant thinking processes. In addition to reframing, pathological double binds can be changed by establishing therapeutic double binds, which are also reframes. Therapeutic double binds maneuver the patient into a situation and new belief system in which the patient cannot lose. Instead of feeling "dammed if he does, dammed if he doesn't", the patient is helped to experience the belief that he wins no matter which choice he makes. In a therapeutic double bind, a patient is changed if he or she does what the clinician suggests or directs, and changed if he or she does not. This is called the *illusion of alternatives*, an integral part of the therapeutic approach of Milton Erickson (Haley, 1986). The illusion of alternatives was a part of many of Erickson's hypnotic trance inductions (Erickson, 1980a; Erickson, Rossi, & Rossi, 1976; Havens, 1992). For example, he often gave patients the choice of going into trance now, or going into trance later.

Case Study: Double Bind

Recall the preadolescent boy described in chapter 1 who could not speak above a whisper. This is an interesting case that demonstrates the two sides of the pathological double bind. His problem of not being able to talk above a whisper created a double bind for his parents, his siblings, his teachers and his friends. They were forced either to ignore him or to pay attention and move closer to him to hear what he was saying. Because he was such a nice, polite young man, they felt sorry for him and gave him even more leeway. They were responding to his unspoken directive that they pay attention to him. They had only two choices to deal with the double bind into which his behavior forced them. They could be unkind, and feel guilty, or they could give him the attention he required. Most chose to give him attention as a way out of this trap. However, this perpetuated the problem.

Once the boy established this power over others, he could not give up his whispering behavior and speak normally without exposing himself as a fake, and thus lose face. He was equally trapped in a "dammed if I do, dammed if I don't" double bind situation. Not recognizing that he had any other choices, he continued the controlling whispering behavior.

The therapeutic work with him accomplished two things. First, it allowed him to relinquish control and speak normally when playing fantasy pinball games during trance sessions. At first, he could allow this to happen only during trance, not in the waking state. However, that opened a small "crack" in the trap, which allowed him to acknowledge to himself and the therapist that under special circumstances, he could speak normally and still save face. The hypnosis did it, he didn't. This further helped him to unconsciously look for a more complete face-saving way out of the trap. Second, when it was suggested that the surgeon operating on his hand would be able to fix everything, he accepted that possibility as another appropriate choice. With the surgeon's help, saying that everything would be fixed, during his anesthetized altered state in surgery, the boy could allow himself to speak normally without losing face after awakening following the successful surgery.

RULES FOR CONSTRUCTING THERAPEUTIC DOUBLE BINDS

Some basic rules apply to the construction and use of therapeutic double binds. They have to do with (1) the choice of appropriate language and trance induction methods, (2) the effective utilization of the illusion of alternatives to limit the patient's number of choices to a few therapeutic ones, (3) the appropriate use of the reframe "You are trapped only if you believe that you have no choices," (4) the appropriate use of the reframe,; We only pay attention to events. We don't pay attention to nonevents," and (5) the appropriate reframing of the illusion of absolutes.

Choice of Language and Methods of Induction

Most trance induction language contains the makings of a series of small double binds that nudge the patient into the trance state. Each suggestion contains double-level requests that tell the patient not to do something, while at the same time implying that something will happen even while the patient tries not to make it happen. For example, the patient is asked to voluntarily look at an object and involuntarily experience eyelid fluttering and heaviness. The patient is asked to "pay attention to your breathing, but try not to change your breathing," and the breathing changes involuntarily. Then the patient is asked to be aware of the changed breathing that occurred automatically. This attention to a change in behavior that was not supposed to be consciously willed by the patient ratifies that the altered state labeled "trance" actually exists and is occurring.

We often say to the patient "I am not doing this to you. You are doing this to yourself. I'm just a guide, teaching you how." So the patient is being told not to try to relax, and that the patient, not the clinician, is bringing about the relaxation. This paradoxical statement, "Don't try, but you will do it anyway," is a therapeutic double bind that is a part of all hypnotic trance induction procedures and well-constructed trance language suggestions.

Remember the example "Try *not* to think of a pink elephant"? The harder you try not to do so, the more you become preoccupied with thinking of a pink elephant. If a patient is being instructed to relax, and there appears to be eye fluttering but no eye closure, an appropriate request might be,

That's very good. Now, try not to close your eyes; let them close all by themselves.

Limit the Choices (The Illusion of Alternatives)

As parents, those of us who feel we have been fairly successful in child rearing discovered or were taught that, in order to keep our children safe and happy, it works best to limit their choices when we offer them suggestions for learning or tell them what they should do. The more choices there are, the more difficult it is to make a decision.

For example, when a child is encouraged to go to bed but doesn't want to go, the parent may say, "Okay, then I am going to let you decide. You can go to bed now, but you don't have to go to sleep right away, or you can go to bed in 15 minutes and go right to sleep. You choose." Or the parent may say, "Do you want to go to bed at a quarter to eight or eight o'clock?" Usually, the child makes a choice. Either choice is acceptable to the parent, but the child believes that he or she made the decision. In fact, the child did make the choice, but because the choices were limited to only two alternatives, and they were both acceptable, this was a win-win situation for both the parent and the child.

Reframe: "You Are Trapped Only as Long as You Believe You Have No Choices"

Many of us were brought up believing that determination and willpower can solve most if not all problems. Many of us were taught that if we are determined to solve a problem, or accomplish a goal, we should keep at it and eventually we will succeed. Thus, the adage "If at first you don't succeed, try, try again" applies. However, if something isn't working, continuing to repeat what isn't working, to "try, try again," isn't going to make it work any better. Therefore, it would be better if we are taught "If at first you don't succeed, try something different." This principle requires the recognition that there are choices. By making a new choice, we are no longer trapped.

Patients usually come to us feeling trapped. Their prior choices that didn't work helped maintain their trap. The therapeutic choices that didn't work further fixed the trapped feelings and beliefs in place. Often you, as the current clinician, may be the patient's latest and last therapeutic choice. Therefore, it is important for you to have as much information as possible about what the patient's previous unsuccessful choices were and what actions were taken that did not work.

It is your job to help the patient realize that it is time to try something different. You do this by helping the patient understand that those previous choices didn't work as well as he or she would have liked. Now the patient has made another choice—to see you. You need to help the patient realize that he or she still has the power of choice, and that you will help the patient to be aware of other choices, and to make new choices, and, by doing so, to find a way out of the trap.

Reframe: "We Only Pay Attention to Events. We Don't Pay Attention to Nonevents."

We usually only pay attention to something when it is happening. For example, we pay attention to when we are smoking, biting our nails, pulling our hair, getting angry, or experiencing pain. We usually pay no attention when these and other negative habits, or dysfunctional feelings and behaviors, are not occurring. This normal process of "selective attention" can be adaptive, but it also gives rise to "selective memory." That is, if we have a problem, such as with handling anger constructively, selective attention can lead us to focus solely on and remember only when we had blow-ups or experienced temper tantrums, and not notice or remember those occasions when we did not. We are deprived of the positive reinforcement and validation that comes from "catching" ourselves being good.

To address this issue therapeutically, another type of double bind can be established, which we call a *perceptual contrast*. We help the patient become aware of the fact that the patient has been paying attention to the problem or symptom only when it has been happening, not when it has not been happening. Often, it is not happening more often than it is happening. For example, most smokers (addressed in Part Three) spend more time each day not smoking than they do smoking.

Similarly, many chronic pain patients present with the absolute belief that their persistent pain is constant (Ewin, 1992a). However, in most chronic pain states, the nature and quality of the pain frequently changes (Eimer, 2000a; Eimer & Freeman, 1998). It either comes and goes or goes up and down in intensity. Understandably, most patients coping with chronic pain pay attention to their pain when it is present and strong. Therefore, as one part of the therapeutic process of helping them manage their pain better, we draw their attention to the less painful intervals between the more painful intervals, using waking state reframing and trance state imprinting.

We can imprint the suggestion through hypnosis that the patient's less painful or more comfortable times will be extended, and that the painful episodes will shrink or diminish in duration and/or intensity (hypnotic time distortion and sensory alteration; see Brown & Fromm, 1987; Eimer, 2000a; Erickson, 1980b; Hilgard & Hilgard, 1994). These hypnotic strategies represent the imprinting of a perceptual contrast in the patient's unconscious. These and other therapeutic strategies for pain management are covered in detail in Chapter 11.

Redirecting the patient's attention to such perceptual contrasts can create a paradoxical message that can be a very powerful reframe. After all, the patient doesn't always do or experience these dysfunctional feelings and behaviors. By being aware of when they are happening and not being aware of when they are not happening, an illusion of absolutes is created, which needs to be altered in order for positive change to take place and continue.

The Illusion of Absolutes

Often, patients verbalize such things as "I *always* feel pain," or "I *never* get any sleep," or "I'm *always* feeling hungry," or "We are *always* fighting," or "I'm *never* happy," or "I can *never* relax," or "I *always* have a cigarette in my mouth," or "This has been going on *forever*." Notice the use of unconditional absolutes in each of these statements. They are the words *always*, *never*, and *forever*.

The illusion of absolutes is the ultimate pathological double bind. Yet *the only absolute is that there are no absolutes*." This is a powerful reframe that, when combined with the reframe *"We only pay attention to events"* is an excellent "double whammy" that can positively affect the patient's belief system about being trapped.

Case Study: Nail-Biting Reframing

A patient was referred to me (JIZ) by the patient's wife's physician to "help him stop his long-standing behavior of nail biting." This was a 53–year-old male who had retired early from his work and moved to Florida with sufficient money to live very comfortably. During the intake evaluation, it was discovered that the patient's mother and younger brother also bit their nails. He said, "I've bit my nails for as long as I can remember." When asked, "Can you remember if there was ever a time when you did not bite your nails?" (question containing embedded suggestion), he suddenly remembered that 15 years ago he had gone to see a therapist for hypnosis to stop smoking and that he hadn't smoked since. However, he had not remembered until just that moment in the interview that he had also stopped biting his nails for a whole year, even though he did not remember the therapist's making specific reference to his nail-biting behavior.

This positive recovered memory opened the door for the two reframes "There are no absolutes" and "We only pay attention to events; we do not pay attention to nonevents" after I further asked the patient, "Can you remember other times when *you are not biting* your nails?" Note the use of present tense (you are not) that was used as an embedded suggestion. The reframe "We only pay attention to events; we do not pay attention to nonevents" was delivered to the patient by asking questions such as "Do you bite your nails while you are asleep?," "Do you bite your nails while you are taking a shower?," and "Do you bite your nails while you are cooking dinner?" The patient answered with either "I don't think so" or *"No."* This further reframed the illusion of absolutes to an agreement that he bit his nails often but not always.

It was then explained to the patient that, without realizing it, the patient had told us that he had a memory in place, that was working and operational, that indicated that "there are times throughout the day and night when I do not bite my nails." It was then explained that his nail biting was an "empty" habit that was only hanging around by habit, not because of need. The patient was told that it would be easy to remove it without having to replace it with something else.

The details of the induction procedure and the change language employed during trance are described in detail in chapters 3 and 4. In this case study, the patient did not continue to bite his nails after the conclusion of the trance experience. The waking state reframing process that took place prior to the trance induction and trance experience was essential to helping the patient recognize that he no longer had to be trapped in his pathological double bind. There were other choices, and making a choice worked for him.

PATIENT TRUST

Why should the patient believe that choosing you and your therapeutic approach will work any better than what the patient has done before?

The answer is that every step along the way, the patient is offered suggestions and demonstrations that progressively reframe beliefs and experiences and provide credibility that your approach makes sense and offers hope. Under these conditions, a positive patient–clinician relationship is established. This relationship is the foundation for the development of trust, and trust is a key ingredient in efficient brief therapy.

Every interaction and communication between you and the patient must be recognized consciously by you as being therapeutic. Everything said is important. There is no such thing as casual conversation. This is what we mean by the clinician's "conscious use of self." Every question that is asked by you, even if it seems innocuous, has meaning and significance in the patient's conscious and unconscious search for solutions and trust. Likewise, every question asked by the patient has meaning and significance to you.

Case Study: Relaxation

In chapter 3, we described a patient of Dr. Jones who had been referred "to learn how to relax." At first, she did not respond to the procedures offered by the therapist. She was unable to allow herself to experience a relaxed state. When questioned further as to what Dr. Jones said when making the referral, she explained that Dr. Jones told her that it was "impossible" for her to relax, so he was sending her to this therapist "to learn how to relax." That iatrogenic, physician-induced, powerful suggestion was a paradoxical communication that forced the patient into a double bind. She couldn't relax because Dr. Jones said it was impossible for her to do so. At the same time, she was told that she would relax by visiting me (JIZ).

This contradiction, in effect, froze her in place. However, once we reexamined Dr. Jones's true intent, and after the patient accepted my reinterpretation (reframing), the patient had a new choice and was no longer trapped by the pathological double bind. Relaxation was now seen to be both acceptable and possible. The ensuing process of hypnotic trance induction and deep relaxation, and learning of self-hypnosis, did occur, and it validated her new belief and trust in me and in the real intent of Dr. Jones, her referring physician.

THE POWER OF DYSFUNCTIONAL LABELS

Another equally important common factor in dysfunctional behavior has to do with the compulsive need that many mental health professionals have to label each dysfunctional behavior as unique and different. Although this does allow us to establish formal diagnostic categories, as compiled in the American Psychiatric Association's *Diagnostic and Statistical Manual of Mental Disorders*, or DSM-IV (4th ed., APA, 1994), and it often legitimizes insurance coverage of psychotherapy, it also has its downside. It leads clinicians to employ diagnostic labels that can become dysfunctional.

Different dysfunctional behaviors are often labeled and categorized as different and distinct illnesses having specific behavioral characteristics, along with subcategories (labels) with added characteristics. In our view, this often unnecessarily complicates and obfuscates the diagnostic and treatment planning process. This can happen in several ways.

The clinician or therapist feels that it is necessary to place a diagnostic label on the patient that may not be therapeutic, or may in fact be antitherapeutic, that is, dysfunctional. Many of these labels (e.g., "borderline and narcissistic personality disorders," "addictive disorders," "dissociative disorders") are associated with the expectation that the patient cannot be helped to change, or that for change to occur, extensive personality restructuring is required that can only be accomplished with expensive long-term psychotherapy.

Such diagnostic labels often have negative or pejorative connotations that

NYACK COLLEGE MANHATTAN

can lead a patient to develop rationalizations for not changing, because he or she has, or is, a "borderline personality," or an "addictive personality," and so on. Thus, such labels are often a source of demoralization for patients and therapists. After all, why bother working at changing if one cannot? Why bother with expensive therapy that will make little difference in the end?

Patients who buy into such labels have excuses for not changing, for staying the way they are. Therapists who treat patients who are labeled as such often become burned out because their expectations are that therapy will be long, complicated, and difficult, and, in the end, little if any change is expected.

This type of dysfunctional diagnostic labeling sets up the need to require specific, ritualized, mechanistic treatment protocols for each major diagnostic category of dysfunctional behavior. For example, phobias require ritualized systematic desensitization procedures (e.g., see Hope & Heimberg, 1993; Wolpe, 1982). Borderline personality disorders require long-term, intensive, insight-oriented, dynamic psychotherapy incorporating ritualized treatment procedures (e.g., see Clarkin, Yeomans, & Kernberg, 1999), or long-term, intensive, cognitive-behavioral psychotherapy incorporating complicated treatment protocols (e.g., see Linehan, 1993).

In addition, many dysfunctional ritualized behaviors are treated by setting up and substituting other ritualized behaviors. Sometimes these mechanistic treatment protocols are as complex as the labeled and categorized dysfunctional behaviors. For example, obsessive-compulsive disorders require more intense rituals for controlling thinking and actions, such as these contained in specific step-by-step thought stopping, exposure, flooding, and response prevention protocols (e.g., see Kozak & Foa, 1999; Steketee, 1996).

EVOLVED NEGATIVE COPING MECHANISMS

One of the main theoretical constructs of brief cognitive hypnosis is that many complex dysfunctional behaviors involving compulsivity and avoidance are basically negative coping behaviors that have evolved over an extended period of time from simpler, less complex attempts to cope. This evolution into increasingly complex and more debilitating symptoms may have been driven by frequency of repetition, generalization, emotional intensification and developmental maturation.

In many cases, these evolved, complex, matured complaints may have been further exaggerated by futile attempts to apply complex, ritualized, mechanistic treatment protocols to change them. The reframe "The harder you try, the more difficult it becomes" might therefore be rephrased as "The more complex the treatment, the less likely the outcome will be successful."

Walter Cannon's Concept of the Fight or Flight Mechanism

Walter B. Cannon, the famous Harvard physiologist (Cannon, 1929) offered the "fight or flight" model to explain the automatic survival mechanism that is a programmed part of all of us. According to Cannon, our nervous systems are biologically "hard-wired" to respond to anything perceived as a danger or threat, with an automatic response that prepares us to either fight to protect ourselves or flee to escape from the source of the perceived threat. This physical-chemical-mental response to a stressor is called the fight or flight mechanism.

We recognize that the biochemical infusion of adrenaline following an interpreted signal of danger creates an anxiety-driven reaction that mobilizes the organism to either fight or escape (flee), to protect the organism. Thus, a response of anger to a perceived stressor can be interpreted as the "fight" part of the fight or flight mechanism and a response of fear-based avoidance can be interpreted as the "flight" part.

Hans Selye (1974, 1976) developed the concept of the "general adaptation syndrome (GAS). This theoretical model described the stages of any living creature's adjustive responses to a stressor. According to Selye, the GAS consists of three stages: (1) the initial "alarm reaction," (2) the intermediate "stage of resistance," and (3) the final "stage of exhaustion."

The Alarm Stage

The initial alarm reaction is a call to mobilize the body's defenses (i.e., the autonomic nervous system and the immune system). It is triggered automatically when an organism first encounters a stimulus strong enough to demand adaptation and change. This is what is meant by a "stressor." For example, when a person goes out into a cold, snowy day, the first reaction to the biting cold, which is a stressor, is an alarm reaction. Other examples of stressors would be when a person is yelled at, or verbally or physically assaulted or threatened.

The Stage of Resistance

Gradually, the human body adjusts to the cold stressor and produces its own heat to bring about adaptation, maintain homeostasis, and create comfort. This is the resistance stage. If the individual does not stay in motion or move out of the cold, by donning a warm coat, building a fire, or going inside where it is warmer, then the body cannot continue to produce enough heat to offset the body heat lost to the cold air. If the person has to continue to "resist" the cold, as would be the case if the person were stranded in the wilderness with insufficiently warm clothing, the inability to build or keep a fire going, or the lack of available shelter, the person would eventually succumb to the cold stressor and freeze to death. However, before this happened, the body and the mind would eventually reach the stage of exhaustion.

The Stage of Exhaustion

The person's body could continue automatically to try and produce the necessary amount of body heat for survival by shivering, but eventually the mind and body would exhaust their available supply of energy.

In the muscles, the wastes from each cell would begin to accumulate, resulting in tiredness, then numbness, and the body would eventually start to shut down. This is the third stage, the stage of exhaustion. Taking this example to its inevitable conclusion, the person would eventually freeze to death.

Similarly, the stressors of being repeatedly or continually verbally assaulted, yelled at, harshly reprimanded, or criticized would initially mobilize a person's bodily defenses (i.e., the sympathetic branch of the autonomic nervous system and the immune system) and alarm reaction. The assailed person tries to fend off the aggressor or hostile opponent. However, gradually, over time, if the person cannot satisfactorily fend off or resist the aggressor, or if the person has to continue to fight repeatedly, continually, or indefinitely, keeping the person in a prolonged stage of resistance, then, the stage of exhaustion is likely to set in. The repeated mobilization of the "fight or flight reaction" will, in all likelihood, take its toll physically and mentally. This too may then lead into the third "stage of exhaustion."

Most physical and mental stressors, over a limited period, only lead to changes of the first- and second-stage type. Initially, we may become upset about feeling alarmed and needing to adjust, but we eventually accept the stressful stimuli, adapt to them by changing our responses in some way, and become less stressed. This adaptation, when repeated often enough, over an extended period of time, becomes learned behavior. It is imprinted in our unconscious as our unique stress reaction or way of responding to and coping with stress.

Almost any stimulus that is interpreted as threatening, whether mild or extreme, evokes some level of anxious feelings. Even when these anxious feelings are interpreted as not life threatening on a conscious level, this anxiousness still evokes an automatic response to escape from the perceived threat and seek relief from the fear. This is a natural adaptive response mechanism in that it leads the organism to select a coping behavior that temporarily reduces the anxiety. This could be as simple as thumb sucking or as complex as agoraphobia.

This selection of a way of coping is largely an unconscious process. It is influenced by various factors, such as unconscious role modeling and observational learning (Bandura, 1976), selective positive and negative reinforcement contingencies (Bower & Hilgard, 1981), innate temperament (Chess & Alexander, 1996), developmental maturation and learning, and cognitive adaptational processes of assimilation and accommodation (Piaget & Inhelder, 2000).

ANXIETY-BASED BEHAVIORS

We have categorized anxiety-based coping responses into six progressively more complex systems of behavioral response.

Mild or Low-Level Feelings of Anxiousness

When mild or low-level feelings of anxiousness are spontaneously evoked during childhood, they can lead to the unconscious choice of a coping behavior, such as nail chewing or thumb sucking, that is further imprinted by repetition. Eventually, the behavior of unconscious choice may become a simple or empty habit, as referred to earlier.

In adolescence and adulthood, when continued unabated, low-level anxiety is experienced and no temporarily effective anxiety ameliorating coping behavior is initiated, the individual may experience a continuing anxious feeling whose cause is unknown. This may lead to a generalized feeling of uneasiness, diffuse emotional and/or physical discomfort, mild depression and feelings of impending negative expectations.

Generalized Anxiety

When mild or low-level feelings of anxiousness lead to obsessive worrying as the coping behavior of unconscious choice, more intense and longer duration feelings of anxiety may result. A generalized anxiety disorder involves intense, continual, or repeated feelings of anxiety associated with the misinterpretation of a wide range of situations and circumstances as potentially threatening and dangerous and repeated predictions of future harm. This creates a vicious, unending cycle of worrying, negative anticipation and predictions, apprehension, feelings of impending doom, helplessness and perceived vulnerability to many perceived threats, resulting in hypervigilance and physiological hyperarousal.

Unlike with the next category, phobic behavior, generalized anxiety does not typically lead to extreme behavioral avoidance. Rather, the individual with generalized anxiety disorder continues to physically move through the world repeatedly encountering situations that he or she predicts to be dangerous. That individual then continues to "control his or her perceptions" (Powers, 1973) by "proving" his or her predictions to be true through endless worrying.

Phobic Behavior

This is the anxiety behavior that we identify as evoking actions such as running away or taking extreme measures to avoid stimuli or settings that have been identified as dangerous or threatening. If not treated, *phobic avoidance behavior* can generalize into agoraphobia, which is a phobic reaction to everything outside of one's close "zone of comfort." However, the end result is that one's comfort zone progressively becomes more and more narrowed and confining, and the increasingly distressed individual eventually refuses to leave the confines and illusory safety of his or her own home.

Panic Attacks

A panic attack is a highly distressing and severely negative emotional response to an extremely negative or catastrophic interpretation of the bodily sensations of the fight or flight mechanism. For example, the afflicted individual develops the fear and conviction that he or she is dying of a heart attack or is completely losing control. This is often accompanied by difficulty breathing, accelerated heart rate (tachycardia), pressure in the chest, stomach pain, weakness in the legs, fear of passing out, sweating, dizziness, tremulousness, shaking and other physical symptoms.

In a panic attack, the body's fight or flight mechanism" is triggered unconsciously. The individual may be aware that the first or last time he or she had a panic attack, it occurred in a particular setting. This may then lead to future avoidance of that situation. However, the fear typically generalizes to other settings and stimuli, and the person may remain unaware of what sets off the panic.

Most individuals attribute their panic attacks to there being something wrong with them physically. This leads to repeated visits to hospital emergency rooms, family doctors, general practitioners and cardiologists that usually reveal that there is nothing physically wrong. However, the condition is perpetuated by a negative feedback loop. This cybernetic "Bermuda triangle" is driven by the individual's continued belief that there really is something physically wrong, and that he or she really is going to die or lose control. Consequently, overwhelming fight or flight reactions are triggered repeatedly and unexpectedly, and they are repeatedly misinterpreted as evidence confirming the sufferer's worst predictions. The repetitions of this extremely dysfunctional cyclical process imprints it into the unconscious.

Obsessive Thinking

This category of anxiety-evoked thought behavior can be experienced as mild to extreme. It can be as common as having difficulty getting a song or musical phrase out of one's head or as disruptive as having to repeat certain verbal phrases over and over again. It also can be as intrusive and anxiety-provoking as having repeated thoughts of doom and gloom about individuals or about situations that have already occurred or may possibly occur. Once again, by repetition, these thought patterns are imprinted in the unconscious and become habits.

Obsessive-Compulsive Behavior and Obsessive-Compulsive Disorder

This category covers extreme, repeated behavior that may be singular, such as repeated hand washing, or more complex, such as making sure that everything is shut off and all the doors are locked before leaving the house, then going back to check again and again and again before leaving. There may be only a few repetitions to reduce anxiety or many repetitions, even repeated rituals, to ward off or prevent feared catastrophic consequences. By repetition, the reoccurring thoughts and the behavioral responses aimed at reducing the anxiety associated with the thoughts, are imprinted in the unconscious. This reinforces the dysfunctional habit patterns and strengthens their compulsive aspects.

Each of the above examples has as its core component the experience of anxiety which is interpreted in different ways and to which is attributed differing degrees of danger. As we have mentioned before, we believe that the more extreme anxiety-related behaviors typically evolve from the less extreme anxiety-evoked behaviors.

Our treatment approach is to initially avoid treating the mature, evolved, extreme forms of the dysfunctional behavior. To begin and simplify treatment, we first go back and treat the original or originating behavior, what we call the "foundation behavior." In our view, the foundation behavior is simple anxiety, which is much simpler to address effectively than its more evolved manifestations. We begin to address it during waking state reframing, when we tell the patient that something may have happened a long time ago that produced discomfort or anxiety, but that whatever happened then, is no longer happening now (if this is true, which we determine in the intake evaluation).

The process is almost like doing a therapeutic waking state regression without formally regressing the patient. We believe that regression actually does take place during this reframing process as the patient remembers past sequences of events and spontaneously enters a hypnoticlike state (Cheek, 1994; Erickson, 1961, 1985; Grinder & Bandler, 1981). However, we do not identify it as such. Part Two of this book describes clinical applications in detail.

7

Dysfunctional and Therapeutic Rituals

RITUALS

The word *ritual* is derived from the Latin word *ritus*, meaning "rite." The term refers to a "formal pattern of behavior, culturally prescribed for use in specific circumstances. The term includes the social, religious and cultural practices which symbolically convey meaning about an event and those who are participating in it" (Walrond-Skinner, 1986, pp. 300–301).

For our purposes, rituals are conceptualized as a series of sequential acts or behaviors or procedures that are part of a prescription that must be followed, without interruption, to accomplish a set result. Religious rituals are excellent examples of this. Ritual behavior essentially is designed to establish a repeatable predictable order that creates an expectation and feeling of security because of a belief in knowing what is going to happen next. Rituals allow us to predict the future. The ability to predict the future builds a strong feeling of security.

Individuals, families, social groups, business organizations, religions, ethnic groups, political organizations, government organizations, societies and countries all establish "normal" ritual systems to maintain order and organizational integrity. Knowing what the structure is and knowing the appropriate procedures to follow make for a smoother and more orderly system.

The first introduction to ritual behavior that we experience is within the family system. The family constellation first establishes the rules of behavior that may include rigid time frames to establish order and harmony, with each family member assigned a role. Roles and rituals evolve as the family constellation changes. Most of us are taught from infancy that ritual and order are necessary and good.

Dramatic and powerful rituals are seen in organized religious ceremonies, ancient celebrations and worship routines, and ceremonial healing rites and "rites of passage." Most often these organized social order rituals are positive and do contribute to enriching the lives of individuals and families. On a personal level, many of the things that we normally do from the time we arise in the morning to the time we go to sleep at night are ritualized to best serve our need to take care of ourselves.

The Origin of Dysfunctional Rituals

Unfortunately, we all encounter crises at times, individually, as a family, within our greater extended family and in our general environment. Those living in Florida, for example, have their normal rituals interrupted by pending threats of hurricanes. In California, it is the threat of earthquakes. These crisis situations force us to interrupt normal everyday patterns of behavior. This disruption causes us to change predictable future activities and requires more or less drastic adjustments to deal with the crisis. At the same time, a crisis imprints a powerful emotional response in the unconscious and evokes some type of emergency behavior. A dysfunctional crisis ritual may then be established as a way of coping with the extraordinarily stressful occurrence, even though that ritual may not appear dysfunctional at the time the crisis is occurring.

The coping ritual established to deal with the crisis might be appropriate at the time and in the situation in which it is required. Eventually, however, the crisis passes, and then a more normal daily ritual is needed to attain stability. If the individual and family are generally well adjusted, this transition back to a more normal pattern of activity may be relatively comfortable and occur without leaving much negative residue in the wake of the crisis situation. However, if there are other dysfunctional forces at work prior to the crisis, the crisis response may be fixed in place and continued long after it is needed. Thus, it may become a dysfunctional ritual. As with most negative behavior that is repetitious, this too can evolve into more complex and disruptive behavior patterns.

Dysfunctional rituals that at first may seem appropriate, may later become uncomfortable, because the ritual no longer satisfies its original purpose. Although the dysfunctional ritual may be uncomfortable and may be recognized by the patient as dysfunctional, it may still meet a fundamental need. Often you may hear a patient say something like, "I know that this behavior is bad, but at least I know what to expect. If I get rid of it, what might happen next? Things could be worse!" Many smokers are afraid to give up their smoking ritual for fear of the possible discomfort of withdrawal behavior. This fear of the problem getting worse, combined with fear of the unknown and intolerance for uncertainty, may help maintain the dysfunctional ritualistic behavior. However, the behavior is also strengthened and maintained by repetition. Trauma initially imprints a coping behavior, and repetition further imprints the behavior. Imprinted behavior that is repeated often and long enough can then generalize and evolve.

Visible Rituals

Obsessive-compulsive behavior and extreme phobic behavior are familiar examples of major and extreme dysfunctional rituals that are presented to many clinicians by patients asking for help. These are the kinds of dysfunctional ritualistic behaviors that are most often referred and seen in clinical settings. They are dysfunctional and extreme enough to force some search for help. They are very visible both to the patient and to others. For example, the hand-washing ritual is a cleansing ceremony and is very visible. Recalling the past reference to "we only pay attention to events," visible ritual behavior is "event behavior."

Invisible and Covert Rituals

There are also many unrecognized ritual behaviors that go on for years, that are not identified as such, and that permeate almost all of the other more frequent problems that are presented to most clinicians. Some of these invisible rituals are treatment or health focused. That is, they evolve in order to help the individual cope with a problem that may or may not be ongoing. Other rituals are associated with the enactment of certain social roles in particular social contexts and occur without much notice in certain social situations. For example, many dating behaviors and sexual or mating behaviors are ritualistic. Other examples have to do with eating behaviors and social etiquette and role expectations at social events, when eating out, when going to worship and so on.

Many of these "invisible" rituals may actually be visible, but they may remain unrecognized or covert because they have become "the norm." They continue to exist as a part of the expectations attached to many everyday experiences. Their establishment as "normal" rituals may become "nonevents," which makes them invisible.

Medical Rituals

There are also many medical rituals that, by definition, are the behavioral manifestations of certain medical treatment protocols. Each disease or illness has prescribed its own treatment ritual. The administration of medication, radiation, chemotherapy, surgery, physical therapy, spinal manipulation and alternative therapies all establish their own rituals designed to help the patient feel better. Some rituals can be identified as very powerful placebos. That is a good thing.

Placebos capitalize on the power of positive expectancies (Evans, 1974; Kirsch, 1990, 1999a, 1999b).

Rehabilitation programs for people who abuse drugs and alcohol also establish treatment rituals that often serve to rationalize long expensive inpatient care and after-care. Often, when the treatment ritual is "completed" (after the insurance runs out), the patient is removed from the controlled ritual environment (the hospital or clinic) and sent back home, and the problem reoccurs. A new adaptive readjustment ritual takes time to establish and may often not be a formal part of the discharge program. However, many medical rituals, both visible and invisible, serve positive therapeutic purposes.

There are also a number of medically oriented social rituals that also serve to imprint beliefs and evoke social support. A significant one that quickly comes to mind is the Alcoholics Anonymous 12–step program. This ritual form has become so culturally popular that it has been adopted for a wide range of other compulsivity problems, such as drug addiction, pathological gambling, sexual compulsivity, overeating and many other difficult-to-change behaviors. Other medically oriented social rituals include the formation and evolution of various support groups for almost every significantly dysfunctional behavior or illness, from anxiety to cancer.

Consider many of the DSM-IV diagnostic categories. When examined closely, many of these include behavioral criteria, which are defined by extended ritualistic behaviors that may in fact be given little or no attention by the patient. Also, note the many ritualized treatment protocols that have been created to treat many of these carefully delineated DSM-IV diagnoses.

We are not suggesting that all of the above are negative approaches that harm patients. We are suggesting, however, that some social support and medical-psychiatric treatment rituals further develop obsessive thinking and obsessive behavior in some patients, and thus may become iatrogenic in some cases.

For example, many patients suffering from anxiety should not be in an anxiety support group. This is because such groups usually are made up of individuals who have not succeeded in freeing themselves from anxiety. The regular meetings, or "get-togethers," may certainly help many patients recognize that they are not alone, but they may also further reinforce their mental preoccupation with the problem, and the feeling of being trapped, because most members of the group may not have gotten much better. The same could be said for such programs as Overeaters Anonymous.

It is our opinion that all persons who have been diagnosed as having cancer should not automatically be referred to a cancer support group, because it may not be within each patient's best interests. Nevertheless, almost all of them are. Some would do better living life more normally while undergoing medical treatment for the disease. When the disease is established as terminal, a support group, directed by a health care professional, can be valuable.

THE USE OF RITUALS FOR THERAPEUTIC PURPOSES

Rituals are widely used for various therapeutic purposes in varied psychological treatment settings (Haley, 1984; Imber-Black, Roberts, & Whiting, 1989; Van Der Hart, 1982). They can lend structure and order to the therapeutic encounter and set the context and frame for the treatment (Frank, 1974; Langs, 1995). Therapeutic rituals also can confirm both the treatment provider's and the patient's expectations about what will take place. This serves to reduce uncertainty and anxiety. It also socializes the patient to the therapy (Eimer & Freeman, 1998; Freeman et al., 1990) and can facilitate patient compliance (Meichenbaum & Turk, 1987). Rituals in psychotherapy also can assist in creating new corrective emotional experiences, as has been discussed by psychoanalytically oriented psychotherapists such as Alexander and French (1946).

"Exchanging new rituals for old, dysfunctional ones forms a major therapeutic ingredient of social skills training, problem-solving interventions and *coping skills learning* and new rituals for engaging in more productive interpersonal relationships are consciously taught in sex therapy, marital therapy, and family therapy" (Walrond-Skinner, 1986, p. 301). Palazzoli et al. (1995) describe the use of rituals in the context of changing severely dysfunctional family systems of interaction. They define a *therapeutic ritual* as "an action or series of actions usually accompanied by verbal formulae or expressions which are to be carried out by all members of the family" (as quoted by Walrond-Skinner, 1986, p. 301). They are sometimes referred to as "homework assignments."

Eimer and Freeman (1998) describe a number of interventions that are incorporated in the practice of pain management psychotherapy that fit the above definitions of rituals. In pain management psychotherapy, these rituals serve various purposes, which include helping patients dealing with chronic pain build greater tolerance for pain, increase self-control and develop improved problem-solving and coping skills.

Hypnotic Inductions as Rituals

The hypnotic induction process has been aptly described by some experts as a formal "ceremony" or ritual (Spiegel & Spiegel, 1987). Spiegel and Spiegel state that "trance phenomena may occur spontaneously, or in response to a myriad of *ceremonies* of induction . . ." (p. 35). They define a ceremony as "an action usually performed with some formality but lacking in deep significance. If the subject interprets the cues properly and conforms to what is expected, the trance ensues" (p. 35). Their major thesis is that hypnotizability is the capacity to experience trance that manifests as a stable trait and that should be measured by a standardized "formal ceremony," such as their hypnotic induction profile (HIP). They also make the point that for highly hypnotizable individuals, a myriad of induction *rituals* or *ceremonies* can serve to induce hypnotic trance.

Relatedly, Spiegel and Spiegel redefine *deepening techniques* as procedures for "clarifying the context" and "clarifying the patient's motivation or the relevance of hypnosis in the first place; correcting misunderstandings or aesthetic preferences of the patient; altering expectations of the patient, the therapist or both" (p. 36). Finally, their HIP procedure is "regarded as another ceremony" and also as "a measurement of hypnotizability in which a systematized sequence of instructions, responses and observations are recorded with a uniform momentum in a standardized way, as the subject shifts into trance to the extent of his ability, maintains it and exits in a prescribed manner" (p. 36).

Thus, hypnotic trance induction ceremonies can be seen as fitting the definition of a ritual in that they are a series of sequential acts or behaviors or procedures (a formal pattern of behavior) that are part of a prescription that must be followed (in certain specific clinical circumstances) without interruption, to accomplish a set result (i.e., the induction or evocation of the hypnotic trance state).

Other Ways to Use Rituals Therapeutically

The use of rituals for therapeutic purposes does not necessarily involve the prescription of new rituals designed to be therapeutic. Often, what we do in the practice of brief cognitive hypnosis is add therapeutic elements to existing normal rituals. In this way, we can take advantage of and capitalize on the "piggyback effect" of potentiating normal, everyday, healthy coping behaviors with additional therapeutic behaviors. One such example is incorporating the practice of self-hypnosis into daily ritual activities.

Case Study: Treatment Ritual

This may be an appropriate place to make a personal statement regarding rituals. I (JIZ) was diagnosed with prostate cancer some years ago. In consultation with an oncologist, a number of treatment options were offered to me, including joining a cancer support group as an adjunct to my medical treatment. I explained to the cancer specialist that I wanted to choose the most aggressive, least intrusive approach that would allow me to continue my normal daily schedule and allow me to travel to San Diego to teach, in 3 months, as scheduled. I declined the support group option and chose 26 weeks, 5 days a week, of radiation therapy, that would also allow me to interrupt treatment for my teaching trip.

I added to my regular daily activities stopping at the hospital on my way to my office for the 15-minute radiation treatment. For years, I have been practicing self-hypnosis twice a day. I added to this regular daily ritual, suggestions for healing. (These will be discussed in detail in chapter 11.) The outcome was that I had no side effects from the radiation treatment and the treatment process became normalized as part of my everyday activity.

I live in a condominium community, and no one there knew I had cancer. When I went to California to teach, none of my colleagues or workshop participants knew I had cancer. I didn't look like a cancer patient, feel like a cancer patient or act like a cancer patient. I saw the oncologist every 3 months after the completion of the radiation therapy, then every 6 months for a blood work-up and now continue to see him only once a year. I have had no further symptoms or return of the cancer. What I did was attach to my normal daily rituals the additional cancer treatment and the self-healing power of my self-hypnosis practice, which served as my personalized adjunct to the traditional medical cancer treatment ritual.

In sum, societies have established culturally based therapeutic rituals that then become the custom and establish predictability and order. Marriage ceremonies, funeral rituals, bar and bat mitzvahs and confirmations are but a few examples of therapeutic social rituals. Given the times, with the increase of broken marriages, we can add the ritual of divorce as therapeutic in many cases.

When we mentioned medical rituals, both visible and invisible, we were implying that many of these serve a positive therapeutic role also. In the psychotherapy context, there exist a variety of rituals that lend structure to the psychotherapy process and that are employed by both the therapist and the patient, some consciously, some unconsciously.

REPLACING DYSFUNCTIONAL RITUALS WITH THERAPEUTIC RITUALS?

When considering the concept of therapeutic rituals, we are talking about two separate processes. Both of these processes are important, and often integral, to the success of the treatment.

Visible Rituals

One process involves the removal of dysfunctional rituals and the establishment of therapeutic rituals to replace them. This initially requires an examination of the visible rituals that constitute the presenting problems. These should be uncovered, understood, demystified and reframed during the waking state reframing process. This is when we establish the concept that the presenting problem and its accompanying rituals are an evolved exaggeration of an original attempt to cope with an earlier event that was once interpreted as threatening. That earlier event is no longer happening. Therefore, the original attempt to cope and the current exaggerated behavior are no longer needed.

Invisible Rituals

The second process involves the invisible rituals associated with previous unsuccessful attempts by the patient to cope with previous treatment failures. These too need to be uncovered, understood and reframed. This will help in the reframing process, when the patient wants to know why previous attempts to get relief from symptoms, or to cope, did not work. Uncovering these invisible rituals may also help you to avoid repeating things that did not work before and in establishing a treatment plan that is likely to work now.

Problem Interruption, Not Ritual Substitution

When deciding on a treatment plan, you need to be aware of how ritualized the plan is. You then need to simplify the treatment ritual so that it is not interpreted by the patient as a substitution for the undesirable and problematic presenting ritual. You do not want to suggest to patients that you are going to give them a better, more functional ritual as a replacement. Recall that we suggested that the current symptom is an exaggerated evolved outcome of a coping response. By suggesting a substitute ritual, the patient could postulate consciously and unconsciously that the new ritual could negatively evolve.

In brief cognitive hypnosis, the description of the treatment, such as learning and practicing relaxation, is presented as a way to interrupt the dysfunctional ritual by treating the original preevolved attempt to cope. For example, we say to patients whose presenting problems involve anxiety, "You can't be anxious when you are relaxed. They are physical and emotional opposites of each other."

Single therapeutic prescriptions are not considered rituals. However, they can become ritualistic when they are repeated and attached to other repeated behaviors. For example, teaching a patient self-relaxation, then suggesting that the patient practice self-relaxation or self-hypnosis, is a process of posttrance imprinting. The suggestions are consciously evoked by the patient and thus are visible. Other therapeutic behaviors can gradually be attached to the practice of daily relaxation, such as feelings of energy following the relaxation, then exercise, because of the increased feelings of revitalization and energy. When these additional therapeutic behaviors are added to the regular daily schedule of the patient, they become incorporated into the patient's daily rituals.

Note that the heading of this section, "Replacing Dysfunctional Rituals with Therapeutic Rituals?," ended with a question mark. All treatment programs and protocols are, of course, assumed to be therapeutic. Very often, they are also ritualistic. However, the more regimented they are, the more rigid they tend to become; the more rigid they become, the less therapeutic they tend to be.

Complex therapeutic rituals are designed to give order to the work of the patient and to enhance compliance. However, our experience has been that they often create more stress and further the patient's feelings of confusion, of being trapped and of being preoccupied with the problem. The intended purpose of ritual behaviors, which is to help the patient to predict the future, to know what is coming next, is valuable only if it can be experienced as comfortable and eventually become invisible and hence unconscious.

For this reason, we prefer to attach our therapeutic prescriptions to existing, normal and comfortable everyday rituals. If those daily rituals include dysfunctional aspects, we help the patient to remove those parts of the rituals that are uncomfortable. We do this by adjusting the order of the activities or changing the time frame of the activities or slightly altering or adding to the activities. We suggest other choices and new ways of thinking about what is being experienced. For example, let us examine the ritual of eating that caused a patient to seek help because of weight gain and preoccupation with food.

Case Study: Adding to an Established Ritual

Session 1

A 52-year-old, divorced, successful, professional woman was referred to me (JIZ) by her physician because she complained of being preoccupied with thoughts of food and could not lose 20 pounds that she had gained in the past year. She was 5 foot 3 inches tall and weighed 143 pounds. She worked as a financial planner and experienced a great deal of job stress.

During the intake evaluation, she reported that she had breakfast between 8:00 and 8:30 A.M., which generally consisted of a half cup of juice with vitamins and a boiled egg, or plain oatmeal with boiling water, or cottage cheese and fruit. Sometimes, she had cheese sticks between breakfast and lunch. Lunch was eaten at about noon and she usually had a lunch salad with dressing or meatballs without pasta with a house salad and part of a roll. Her liquid intake with her lunch consisted of a glass of water with a wedge of lemon. Between lunch and dinner, she had some nutrition bars. Dinner was taken between 6:00 and 8:00 P.M. and was usually made up of leftovers, such as salads, soup, a barley drink or water with lemon. She ate at home most evenings. She said that she did not snack in the evening and went to bed between midnight and 1:00 A.M. What was reported so far appeared very positive.

When asked, she answered that she did eat fast. She stated that she would become so hungry that it would make her feel weak. She had also just started a "Sugar Busters" diet that involved eating no sugar, if at all possible.

When questioned further about her feeling so hungry, she said that she felt a pressure in her stomach and heard stomach noises that told her that she was hungry. She had been on hormone replacement pills but had stopped them because she gained weight while on them. When asked at what times of the day she felt most hungry, she answered that it was usually late in the afternoon. Her office always had cakes, cookies and candy available, so she ate what was there.

This led to her commenting that she had a "sweet tooth." Note the new negative feeling and eating behavior that was elicited by further questioning.

Something just didn't add up, so she was questioned further regarding how often she thought she was hungry because of stomach pressure and noise and how often she thought about food and eating. She admitted that she felt "hungry" much of the time and that she thought of food most of the time. She stated that her "strong will" kept her from eating more often. Then she said that maybe she snacked more than she admitted to, even to herself.

In terms of exercise, she rollerbladed for 40 minutes every morning before she went to work and walked for an hour or more on the sand at the beach near her home after work. This, of course, was considered positive and healthy.

On initial examination, it seemed that she basically ate right and she did exercise regularly. She appeared to have control. However, she did have a problem properly interpreting the messages of her body, some snacking behavior had been invisible to her, she was preoccupied with the fight over food and she was exaggerating her weight problem.

Further examination of the data obtained suggested that many of her "visible" eating rituals were in fact healthy. However, there were some "invisible" rituals that were not healthy. She did have a problem with her kinesthetic awareness of her body's messages. In her case, as in many cases of "weight problems" that present to clinicians who use hypnosis, fluid retention may have been more of a problem when she was on hormone therapy than body fat. She ate too fast. She also had a problem with sugar and it was hypothesized that she may have been hypoglycemic, as indicated by her late afternoon hunger, which is often caused by a drop in blood sugar level. She also carried an unrecognized low level of anxiety related to the pressure of her work and her limited social life, so she ate when stressed.

The issues that needed to be addressed were (1) her low level of continual anxiety, (2) her stress eating, (3) her habit of eating too fast, (4) her misinterpretations of body messages, (5) her fluid retention, (6) her "sweet tooth," and (7) her possible hypoglycemia. These were discussed with her during the waking state reframing portion of the first visit. I told her:

> "There are a number of patterns and feelings that need to be dealt with in order to help you feel and look better. My approach will not be to help you lose weight, so you are not to weigh yourself while we are working together. I will help you change your behavior, and you will notice that your clothes fit more comfortably. You will be aware that you are loosing inches. You will be taught a form of self-relaxation to remove the anxiety feelings. Those anxiety feelings, which you may not have even been aware of, are your reaction to the many things that you identify as stressful. You said that you eat when you feel stressed. By practicing relaxation for about 10 minutes once or twice a day, you will no longer feel stressed, so you will no longer feel like eating. When you are relaxed, you can't feel stressed because they are physical and emotional opposites of each other.

You will be helped to eat very slowly. The stomach fills up on a time frame, not a volume frame. So the slower you eat, the less volume you will consume when your own individual "full time" is reached.

You will be helped to ignore body messages that you thought meant that you were hungry, and to better recognize the true messages of your body.

You will be helped to reduce your fluid retention that makes you feel heavy, by drinking more of the water with lemon that you already enjoy doing.

You will be able to avoid sweet, sugary foods easily and reduce any hypoglycemic reaction, which occurs in the late afternoon and which makes you snack. You will also be aware that sweet foods no longer taste as good as they did. This will make it easy for you to start your "Sugar Busters" program. By the way, it is better to call it a "program" and not a "diet". This will make it easier to follow.

All of this will happen as you add daily relaxation exercises to your normal daily routine. We will need up to five sessions after this evaluation session. If we can accomplish your goals in less than five, fine. How does that sound to you? Good. Then, let's set up an appointment for you. During the next session, I will explain about the two parts of the mind that control your behavior and teach you self-relaxation to start the change process.

Session 2

The second session included the waking state reframing material about the conscious and unconscious mind and the explanation about hypnosis and relaxation. The patient stated that she was already eating better after the last session and that she looked forward to learning self-relaxation.

She was taught to enter trance (relaxation) using an eye fixation with attention to breathing induction procedure. This was chosen because she would be taught instant relaxation using three slow, deep breaths during the second session. This induction also helped in reframing her body's messages. Redirecting her attention to her breathing helped to make the sounds and other feelings she interpreted as hunger invisible.

During trance, she was asked to be aware of how good this relaxation experience felt and that she could experience it on her own by doing at home what we did in the office, without my help. Before the induction, we had agreed that the best time for her to practice was in the morning, before her exercise activity and in the afternoon, right after she got home from work and before her walk on the beach. It is better to practice self-hypnosis before as opposed to after physical exercise.

The following suggestions were also given during this trance experience in the office:

You will be eating very slowly and filling up very quickly in a comfortable way, and eating less and enjoying it more.

When you think you are feeling hungry, pay attention to your breathing without trying to change your breathing, and the feelings that brought the thoughts of hunger will disappear.

You will drink your water with lemon between breakfast and lunch and in the afternoon and evening, in addition to water with your meals. This will help you eliminate more of your body fluid retention and your feeling of bloating.

Do not give these suggestions to yourself. You are to do no self-talk while doing your own self-relaxation. Every time you do your own relaxation, you will automatically reinforce the things that I say to you when we work together.

Session 3

At the third session, a week later, the patient reported a 5-pound weight loss and felt that her clothes were fitting better. I asked her how she knew that she had lost 5 pounds. She said that she had "cheated" and had weighed herself that morning, the day of her appointment, but not before. I told her that it was okay to weigh herself once a week on the day she was to come in to see me. She further reported that she was feeling much more relaxed, thinking about food hardly at all and drinking more water instead of snacking. She enjoyed the relaxation time and said it gave her more energy for her exercise.

She was surprised that she did not feel hungry. I asked her if she found herself occasionally paying attention to her breathing. She answered yes, but hadn't remembered until I asked if she had been doing so. It had become invisible and unconscious as it became comfortable.

We usually are aware of invisible change only in retrospect. In order to know about changes that have been suggested but that are not described by the patient, we ask the patient if they are aware of such changes. That is because changes that become invisible become "nonevents." They become a part of "normal" behavior.

I asked the patient to put herself into relaxation the way she was doing at home and to signal me by lifting one of her hands to let me know when she was ready to have me take her deeper. The hand lifting is not an ideomotor signal. It is a simple acknowledgment in answer to my request to be informed when she was ready. I could have, as I often do, just as easily asked her to nod her head. Some therapists might use ideomotor signaling here, we think unnecessarily. Our approach is to keep things as simple as possible. I then explained the following:

> I am going to take you deeper into relaxation by my counting slowly from 20 down to 1. I use the word *deeper* because I don't have a better one. I am really talking about improving the quality of your relaxation experience rather than the distance traveled. With each number that I count, you will find yourself feeling more and more comfortable, and more and more relaxed. Just listen to the numbers and let yourself go, and enjoy the feeling of going deeper into relaxation.

When I reached number 1, my observation of the patient's posture, breathing, facial coloring and eyelid flutter indicated to me that she was much more relaxed than when she had signaled me earlier. I then said:

> That's very good. You are much more relaxed after my countdown from 20 to 1. From now on, when you do your own relaxation, when you are about as relaxed as when you signaled me, start your own silent countdown to yourself from 20 to 1. By the time you reach the number 1, you will be much more relaxed. That deeper feeling of relaxation is the deeper level of relaxation that you will be able to reach every time you do your own self-relaxation. That is the level of relaxation that allows all of the changes you have made and all of the changes that you will make to be imprinted in your unconscious mind. They become new memories of success and change that are repeatable and enjoyable. So all of your successes now become a part of your normal everyday life, continued and improved as each day goes by.

Session 4

We scheduled a fourth session for a week later to make sure that the routine was established and that the changes were in place. The patient reported further weight loss, feelings of greater confidence, less stress, and being very much in charge. The patient was asked to relax herself. I reinforced her personal success and decided that this could be her last regular session with me. She was told that I was as close as the telephone. She could call me if she had a question or if there was some additional help that she thought she could benefit from. I congratulated her on her success and told her that I very much enjoyed working with her. Her parting words were, "Thank you. I have a lot of friends that I am going to send to you."

"NORMAL" IS "INVISIBLE"

A colleague once told us that calling this kind of process a "therapeutic ritual" was "a stretch." I (JIZ) explained that, in order for any change behavior to become effective, it had to become normal behavior and almost invisible. I further explained that behavior modification rituals and progressive relaxation rituals were not long lasting because they could not be incorporated into normal everyday activity. They stood out as attempts to change behavior rather than becoming a part of normal everyday behavior. That is why we prefer the label rituals that are therapeutic rather than *therapeutic rituals*.

The chapters that follow in Part Two will be descriptions of the clinical application to specific dysfunctional problems of what we do and why we do it that way. The seven chapters that have been presented as a foundation for learning will make the clinical applications to follow very easy and natural to learn and apply.

Part Two

Clinical Applications

8

Irritating Habits as Dysfunctional, Outdated Coping Skills

Dr. Knight Dunlap, then professor of experimental psychology at Johns Hopkins University, wrote in his 1932 book *Habits: Their Making and Unmaking* that "If we limit the term 'learn' somewhat narrowly, we can truthfully say that a definite process of learning is the formation of *a habit*; and conversely, a habit is a process of living that has been learned" (p. 8).

From the brief cognitive hypnosis perspective, irritating habits are dysfunctional and outdated behaviors that have been imprinted (learned) and fixed in place by repetition. They are automatic, often autonomous behavior patterns that are performed with little conscious control. Habits are a process of living that has been learned. They often represent shortcuts to valuable behaviors that serve a very constructive purpose. Habits make living easier by selectively responding to daily needs in an automatic way. These behaviors, called dysfunctional, may have started as ways of coping with long ago negative stimuli and were imprinted by repetition. They may have have been valid attempts at coping behaviors, but may no longer be valid or useful. The precipitating situation that started them is no longer present. The behavior continues out of habit. These behaviors are now simple or empty negative habits.

Although it is important to recognize that we identify simple negative habits as those behaviors that no longer have purpose or validity and are not complex in nature, they are not multifaceted. They are not made up of a series of behaviors. They are not ritualistic. They are many kinds of different individual behaviors that are presented as expressions of a loss of control by the patient that have become learned and established as a habit by repetition. They are specific and direct. However, like some behaviors of compulsivity that are anxiety based, problematic repetitions without resolution can lead to more generalization.

Generalization means becoming more intense, more widespread, and more visible and thus more dysfunctional. This will be discussed in more detail when reference is made to nail biting. Nail biting is an empty habit that can extend to cuticle biting and picking, as well as finger scratching and itching, with further dermatological complications.

A BASIS IN ANXIETY

All irritating habits, which we call simple or empty habits, have an initial foundation of being anxiety based. Something occurs in an individual's life, usually at an earlier age, although it can happen later, evoking a fight or flight reaction. This is experienced as a sense of anxiety, fear, or discomfort, requiring some immediate response to become more comfortable. The organism seeks a solution in a behavioral response. The individual experiences anxiety, not identified as such, that is noted as feeling very uncomfortable. This evokes a coping response. This response could be thumb sucking, hair pulling or any of a number of other behaviors that for the moment relieves the discomfort. The temporary comfort is imprinted lightly in the unconscious. When similar uncomfortable happenings occur, the chosen palliative is repeated. By repetition, this behavior is further imprinted and becomes a habit. It continues not because it is needed, but because of the habit function.

Because the habit that develops is simple and the initiating behavior is no longer present, its continuation is called an empty habit. It is empty of meaning and is no longer needed. It serves no continuing purpose. Some behavioral examples of these simple, empty habits are summarized below.

THUMB SUCKING

This is a common childhood habit that, in the early years, is a developmentally appropriate behavior that satisfies the infant's sucking needs. As the child grows older, the habitual use of thumb sucking gives pleasure, relief from anxiety and a feeling of safety. Sometimes a child may give up thumb sucking for the security offered by a teddy bear or a favorite blanket. These are usually given up as the child matures and feels more secure in the family environment. However, thumb sucking may reoccur later during a stressful situation, as a way of coping with that stress. If other family members, such as older siblings, suck their thumbs, this may act as a model for the behavioral choice. This is often identified as a behavioral regression to an earlier oral mode of coping.

Continued thumb sucking beyond adolescence is not common. This kind of problem usually will be seen in referrals of preadolescent or adolescent patients. Often these referrals are made, or initiated, by dentists who are preparing to straighten the patient's teeth.

Nail Biting

The onset of nail biting most often occurs in the grade school years. It is often accentuated by anxiety. This is one of the dysfunctional habits that does not extinguish itself as the individual matures. "Treatment" usually consists of home remedies such as bitter liquid applications, gloves, nail hardeners, nagging and punishment. None of these work effectively, and the behavior may continue into adulthood on a continual basis or during extreme stress. This, too, is often a coping behavior of choice because it has been observed as taking place with other family members.

Nail biting behavior may become more generalized to include cuticle biting or picking and finger and hand scratching. It can even extend to scratching the palm of the hand or fingers. It then can cause significant dermatological problems.

Neurodermatitis

Itching, along with the temporary relief brought about by scratching, is another common dysfunctional habit that is difficult to control. This can start as a result of a real dermatological problem or it can be initiated by a neurologically based itching response to anxiety.

The repeated scratching abrades and irritates the skin and often causes a rash and skin lesions. These lesions frequently become infected, leading to further treatment attempts with lotions, medications, surface coverings even tranquilizers. There also can be an allergic etiology involved in this problem.

Failure to remediate the problem through repeated medical treatment may lead to social embarrassment as more and more attention is focused on it and it becomes more visible. This may become a strong motivating factor for the patient to seek a new, more effective approach to treatment.

TRICHOTILLOMANIA (HAIR PULLING)

Repeated hair pulling may involve pulling out hair from the scalp, eyebrows or eyelashes. It sometimes includes eating or chewing the hair that has been pulled out. It is often exacerbated by apparent anxiety and may be a sign of a deeper emotional problem. The patient may be taking medication prescribed by a physician or psychiatrist and may be under treatment by a hair or dermatology specialist. If there is a suspicion of deeper emotional involvement, such as self-punishment and anger issues, direct symptom removal is not recommended. The possible medical causes, concomitants and consequences of chronic hair pulling (e.g., skin and scalp irritation, trichophagia [eating the hair] and its associated gastrointestinal complications, alopecia areata and mucinosa, balding and hair loss, lupus erythematosus, and folliculitis) warrant appropriate medical evaluation and consultation prior to behavioral, psychological or hypnotic treatment.

Interestingly, this particular dysfunctional habit has been identified in the DSM-IV as an impulse-control disorder (APA, 1994). Although they are not so identified, many of the simple habits described in this chapter are problems of impulse control to some degree. Trichotillomania may actually be dealt with as a simple habit or as a complex habit, depending on its complexity and ramifications. Complex habits are discussed in chapter 9.

Some simple habits evolve into more complex automatic behavior patterns, as the original behaviors generalize to a wider range of situations that present more demands for psychic gratification. The evolved symptoms and behaviors begin to provide "secondary gains." This means that the original coping demands that initiated the habit may or may not be present, but the habit behavior begins to provide a way of controlling the current external environment. The individual may begin to feel trapped in the behavior as the behavior becomes the unconscious coping mechanism of choice in a wider and wider range of situations (generalization). The need to "save face" may necessitate the continuation of the behavior. Recall the case example in chapter 1 of the adolescent who could only speak in a whisper.

There are a number of other habit behaviors that may have physiological expressions or be associated with medical or dental problems that may respond to the simple or "empty" habit approaches to treatment, such as snoring, bruxism and other irritating oral behaviors.

Our approach to eliminating simple irritating habits, when medical and psychiatric complications have already been ruled out, is a rather direct one that usually is accomplished in one office visit. This visit takes from 45 minutes to an hour. However, there are some cases where more than one visit and the teaching of self-hypnosis are required. Both types of cases will be addressed in this chapter. Below is a general treatment plan schema that you can follow.

Referral and Preintake

If a patient who has been referred by a physician or dentist calls you, obtain the patient's permission, during the initial telephone conversation, to speak with the referral source before conducting the initial intake in the office. If a patient calls about a problem that could have medical or dental ramifications and has not been referred by a physician or dentist, suggest to the patient that he or she be seen by the appropriate medical or dental professional before you see the patient for hypnosis or brief therapy.

When a patient calls, ask the patient to tell you exactly what the referring person said to him or her when making the referral. If the patient found you through a Yellow Pages or other advertisement, ask what it was about the ad that attracted him or her. The answers provide information about the patient's expectations and response set.

Intake Evaluation

Refer to chapter 1 for a full description of the process of intake evaluation. Once you have established that the presenting problem is indeed a simple habit, you can then move into the next phase of the process, which is waking state reframing.

Waking State Reframing

First, describe to the patient the two parts of the mind, what hypnosis is, what to expect and what the planned outcome of treatment will be. Then, begin to reframe the patient's ideas about the reasons for the habit's continuation.

You can do this by explaining that there are behaviors that were established, some time ago, that served as appropriate coping behaviors at the time that they first started. You don't have to know what precipitated the problem behavior or exactly when it occurred. You do know, however, that the precipitating event is no longer happening. That is, what started the behavior happened a long time ago but it is not happening now. The behavior continued and was repeated. This repetition imprinted the behavior in the unconscious mind; thus, the behavioral response was learned and became a habit.

Once it became a habit, it continued because it was now controlled unconsciously and became automatic. This automatic aspect was initiated without conscious thought. When the behavior came to consciousness, it was recognized as an event and became uncomfortable on a conscious level. Although the patient could interrupt it, this produced more anxiousness and discomfort that caused the behavior to increase in intensity. Trying to stop the behavior made it worse. Tell the patient that "the harder you try to stop the behavior, the more difficult it becomes."

Because the original cause is no longer present, the behavior is no longer necessary. Explain to the patient that you will help him or her into hypnosis, during which time he or she will feel very relaxed and comfortable. During this relaxation experience, ask the patient to give permission to his or her own unconscious to remove this behavior that is no longer necessary and no longer needed.

TRANCE INDUCTION AND TRANCE LANGUAGE

The trance induction for simple habits is one that would usually not include the teaching of self-hypnosis. It is important to repeat the rationale for this here.

A simple habit usually can be eliminated in one session. Once the behavior has been removed without a symptom or behavior substitution, it is no longer an issue that needs to be addressed. Therefore, it should be allowed to disappear from current conscious awareness. The regular practice of self-hypnosis suggests that the patient needs to do something, frequently and regularly, to avoid the return of the problem. Yet the problem no longer exists. Therefore, the directive to practice a regular activity for something that is no longer a problem keeps the thought of the problem conscious and worrisome. Such a directive is not necessary.

There are exceptions to this that may require two, three or four visits and the teaching of self-hypnosis, when there are continuing reminders of the negative dysfunctional behavior or stressors that are internalized by the patient. However, these continuing stressors may not be related to the original onset of the problem. They may have arisen from more current problems that are being dealt with in an outdated way. In these cases, as will be seen later in this chapter, self-hypnosis does need to be used.

By referring to chapter 3, you will find some trance induction procedures that do not include teaching self-hypnosis and that are appropriate for producing the trance state in dealing with simple habits. Any short direct induction will do. We tend to use the eye fixation attention to breathing induction because it includes visual and kinesthetic elements that allow for externalizing the start of the induction and internalizing the control of obsessive thinking, while helping the patient to go deeper into relaxation.

Nail Biting Script

A typical induction and following trance state suggestions for the simple habit problem of nail biting would go something like this.

> Sit comfortably in the chair with your feet flat on the floor and your arms resting on the arms of the chair. Look at the hands of the Buddha in the picture on the wall in front of you (it can be any object small enough to concentrate on). As you continue to visually concentrate on the hands of the Buddha, you will be aware that your eyes begin to blink more frequently than they usually do. Your body will begin to relax, and your breathing will begin to change all by itself. You will be aware that, as your eyelids blink more rapidly, they become very heavy. When you close your eyes, leave them closed until I ask you to open them, and don't squeeze them tight. Just let them be loose and comfortable and relaxed.
>
> Now that your eyes are closed, concentrate on your breathing, but don't try to change your breathing, and allow yourself to go deeper and deeper into relaxation and hypnosis. You will notice that your breathing becomes deeper and more regular, and then more shallow and more regular, as you relax even more.
>
> If your mind wanders, the moment you realize that you are thinking of something different, bring your thoughts back to concentrating on your breathing. By

concentrating on your breathing, you will have control of your thoughts and go still deeper into relaxation.

You will go deeper with each breath that you take, deeper with each word that I say, regardless of the meaning of those words. As you continue to feel more relaxed, the doorway to your unconscious opens. With your permission, I can talk to your unconscious to give it information it can use to change the behavior that you want to change, namely, to no longer bite your nails.

Some time ago, and we don't have to know when, something happened that made you feel very uncomfortable, or afraid, or nervous. You started biting your nails at that time, and for the moment it helped you to feel more comfortable. Because, a part of you felt more comfortable by biting your nails, you did it again at another time when something upset you or bothered you. You did it again at still another time when you felt upset, and so on. By repeating the nail biting, you learned that it helped when you were upset. Therefore, you continued to do it until it became a habit.

We may not know exactly what happened way back then, but we do know that it is not happening now. Because it is no longer happening, you no longer need to continue to bite your nails. You can give yourself permission to keep your hands away from your mouth so your nails can grow back normally. By doing this, you will feel even better than you did before, because the nail biting behavior will be no more, and you can enjoy their gradual growth and return to health. If it is okay to give yourself permission to no longer bite your nails, just nod your head for me, so I will know that it is okay. Thank you.

Now that you have given yourself permission to no longer bite your nails, you will immediately begin to feel better about yourself. You can take pride in treating yourself with more care, with more dignity, and with more self-respect and with more self-love. Because you now feel so much better and so much more in charge, others will be aware of how much better you look and feel.

Sometimes the habit of your hand moving toward your face that may have led to biting your nails may occur. Most often it will not. If it does, you will realize that once your hand begins to make the move, it stops part way up and does not reach your face. You will be pleasantly surprised that it doesn't do so, and you will immediately be comfortable with the knowledge that the habit is gone.

Now I am going to help you become more alert, more awake yet comfortably relaxed at the same time, by my counting slowly from 1 to 5. With each number that I count, you will be more and more alert. At the count of 5, your eyes will open, and you'll feel great.

Okay. Ready. 1—2—3—4—5. Eyes open, wide awake.

Case Study: Nail Biting

A 15-year-old 10th grader, who lived with her mother and father, presented to me (JIZ) for treatment with hypnosis for nail biting. She did well in school and had a comfortable relationship with her friends and peers. She wanted to be a teacher. Information gathering during the intake revealed that she did not consciously experience anxiety and did not experience any phobic behavior. She didn't remember when she first started biting her nails, and she was usually unaware that she was biting her nails except when she was experiencing tension, such as durng an exam. She and her father were both stubborn and argued a lot. She commented that she was aware that her father bit his nails.

I explained the concept of the conscious and unconscious parts of her mind. Then I proceeded to tell her the following: I told her that we didn't have to know what started the habit or when it started. Something happened when she was younger that made her uncomfortable. Without being consciously aware of it, her unconscious mind had searched for something that she could do to help her feel better. This unconscious part of her mind was aware that when her father was upset, he chewed on his nails. Not knowing what else to do, her unconscious took the example of her father's behavior and transferred it to her because she was aware that this is what he did when upset. The nail biting did make her feel better. Whenever something else occurred that made her feel uncomfortable, she again bit her nails. By repetition, nail biting became the pacifier of choice and became a habit.

I proceeded to explain that, as she got older, the behavior of unconscious choice became uncomfortable because it embarrassed her, so she tried to stop it. Unfortunately, her unconscious mind did not know that she wanted to stop because she didn't know how to communicate with her unconscious. The harder she tried to stop, the more uncomfortable she felt, because the behavior continued. This discomfort made her bite her nails even more.

I explained that this was an empty habit that was no longer needed, because what originally happened was no longer happening. I said that we could remove the behavior without substituting another behavior. I described what to expect with hypnosis and told her that she would feel relaxed but always be aware of everything that was going on.

I then helped her into a hypnotic trance using the eye fixation with attention to breathing induction. I then administered trance state suggestions using trance language similar to the above script. Following the delivery of these suggestions, while she was still in trance, I told her:

> If you become aware that you are a little uncomfortable about anything in the future, and you can recognize this by some pressure in your chest, shoulders, or neck, just take a few very slow deep breaths. Slowly breathe in relaxation through your nose and breathe out tension through your mouth, to melt away the discomfort. You are sitting in the chair, already relaxed. Take a few very slow, deep breaths now and be aware of how much more relaxed you feel. You did feel more relaxed, didn't you? If you did, just nod your head for me. Thank you.

She was then awakened and we discussed her experience. I further emphasized the availability of the deep breaths for any kind of discomfort, such as school tests. Follow-up over the next few months indicated that she continued to be free of her nail-biting behavior.

A year later, the patient transferred to a new and more and more demanding school and was having trouble adjusting. She did not return to nail biting although she was going through a difficult adjustment. She came back for some help and I taught her self-hypnosis to deal with her fears and anxiety regarding the new school, the increased challenges and the need to develop new friendships.

Cuticle Chewing or Picking

The same sample script used for nail biting above with the exception of changing the label nail biting to Cuticle Chewing and Picking will bring the same successful result. If this behavior accompanies Nail Biting, added suggestions might include:

> No longer biting your nails also means no longer chewing or picking on your cuticles. It will be really great to stop the ugliness and the bleeding that have been so uncomfortable for you.

Thus, no longer chewing or picking the cuticles is tied to or linked with no longer biting the nails.

Hair Pulling and Chewing (Trichotillomania)

Hair pulling and chewing, when evaluated as such, are other empty habits that often respond to this same approach. There is often greater frustration on the part of the patient because of the visible loss of hair and the greater length of time it takes for the hair to grow back.

If, during the evaluation, it is determined that this presenting behavior is more complex because of the presence of deeper anxiety levels, it may be necessary to deal with this in more than one session.

Bruxism

Bruxism, or teeth grinding, is a dysfunctional habit that most often presents as occurring at night while the patient is asleep (nocturnal bruxism). Like all habits, it is controlled by the unconscious mind and the patient usually is unaware that he or she is doing it. Through repetition, the behavior is further imprinted in the patient's unconscious. It is responsive to hypnotic approaches that emphasize simple relaxation, reframing of the problem and imprinting suggestions for the control of the problem by the unconscious mind (Clarke & Reynolds, 1991; LaCrosse, 1994).

Patients exhibiting bruxism are often aware of awakening in the morning with gum, tooth, jaw and facial pain, neck pain and headaches. When a patient reports being aware of bruxing during the day, the patient is also likely to say that he or she is only aware of it when consciously paying attention. The patient is usually aware of having a tightly clenched jaw and may report that he or she "is under," and "holds onto," a lot of tension. Others may remark to the patient that he or she often looks angry or tense, frustrated or anxious.

Continual clenching or bruxing has serious medical and dental ramifications. It puts heavy wear and tear on the muscles of the face, head, and neck, on the gums and teeth and on the temporal-mandibular joints (TMJ). This dysfunctional habit often causes or is associated with TMJ and other oral-facial and dental disorders. In serious cases of bruxism, the patient's teeth may be severely ground down, resulting in undue chronic strain on the patient's bite, TMJ, and jaw muscles.

Most bruxism referrals are made by dentists and physicians. These health care professionals often are treating the patient's medical or dental problems that are made worse by the bruxism or that are a consequence of the problem. Often, the patient's bruxism and clenching have been undoing or undermining what the physician or dentist has been trying to accomplish. The typical goal of such referrals is to help the patient eliminate the behavior, or at least control it better.

Frequently, the patient has a dental appliance, such as a night guard or bite guard, but has not been compliant with wearing it. In such cases, the referring agent's goal may be to help improve the patient's compliance with the treatment regimen. Referral sources also are also typically aware that such patients have trouble relaxing and that the bruxism and clenching are a way of releasing tension in a dysfunctional way. They therefore may be referring a patient to learn to relax. They may view our input as a "court of last resort," as is often the case with patients dealing with chronic pain (see chapter 11).

Occasionally, bruxism patients are self-referred or referred by word of mouth (no pun intended). In such cases, it is important to make certain that the patient is receiving appropriate medical or dental consultation and care before beginning treatments. Otherwise, you will be wasting the patient's time and money and your time, given the medical and dental complications of the problem.

Essential Suggestions and Treatment Strategy

Bruxism sometimes can be treated as a simple habit, that is, in a single session. However, if the imprint has become intensified by nonsuccess in treatment from other sources, such as with a dentist or in a pain clinic (often prescribed for the treatment of complicated bruxism), the behavior persists and can evolve into a complex habit. When it evolves into a complex habit, it becomes an ongoing way to handle current persistent anxiety. It may be necessary to teach the patient self-hypnosis and have the patient practice self-hypnosis on a regular basis. The goals of self-hypnosis that are suggested in session are to produce control, to feel more comfortable, to reduce the need to grind the teeth and clench the jaws and to interrupt the iatrogenic imprinting that has resulted from repetition of the dysfunctional behavior or failure in the treatment process. Most importantly, it is to reduce and control anxiety.

You can determine if the patient's bruxism is a simple habit or a more complex condition by exploring what attempts have been made in the past to treat the bruxism and by evaluating how persistent it is despite multiple treatment attempts. You also need to evaluate whether it involves a number of other medical problems or problems that are the result of responses to stress.

If bruxism is isolated, has not been going on for a long period of time and isn't complicated by other issues, it usually can be dealt with as a simple habit. However, if it's been going on for a long period of time, has become quite complicated in terms of destruction of gums and teeth and requires the use of various dental appliances, then it is no longer considered a simple habit but is a complex habit.

Waking State Reframing

The following sample script shows one approach to reframing.

There are a number of issues involved in grinding your teeth and chewing on your gums. One of the ways that you have dealt with discomfort, anxiety, fear, or anger been to grind your teeth. Grinding your teeth can often be an expression of internalizing anger of holding it in. "Gritting your teeth" is the term that we often encounter when someone talks about the anger that they are experiencing. For example, someone may say, "I grit my teeth and hold it in." So, very often, what happens is that, when they start to feel uncomfortable, they get slightly angry, and in order to not express the anger or blow up, they grit their teeth. That leads to the grinding experience, the tightening, the clenching, even chewing on the gums, the cheek, and the tongue. So the anger is dealt with by oral irritation, by oral means.

If you determine that the bruxing problem is a simple habit, you can go on to say:

"Sometime ago, when you got angry, you started to grit or grind your teeth, and you found that that helped you feel a little better because you were able to hold in the anger. So, the next time you were feeling upset or angry about something, you tended to repeat the gritting or grinding of your teeth. Whenever you had the slightest sense of discomfort, this repetition of the teeth grinding imprinted that behavior into your unconscious mind as a simple habit.

Whatever was happening then is no longer happening now. Therefore, the grinding habit is no longer needed now. Because you no longer need to do it, perhaps you can give yourself permission to no longer grind your teeth.

When you relax, you can't be angry, because relaxation and anger are physical & emotional opposites. Because you haven't been doing the grinding for so long that it's caused major dental problems (if this is true), we may be able to help you to eliminate this behavior by teaching you some simple relaxation skills that you can use "on the fly" when you start to feel upset or a little angry or uncomfortable.

You can then go on to do a simple induction. Using trance language, help the patient give himself or herself permission to let go of the teeth-grinding habit for good.

The basic treatment strategy for eliminating bruxism is to teach the patient simple relaxation.

Nocturnal Bruxism

It really doesn't matter whether the grinding is done during the daytime or at night. The approach is essentially the same, with the exception that several suggestions are added to address the fact that, at night, the person is not conscious of grinding his or her teeth. For nocturnal bruxism suggest that the behavior of chewing or grinding the teeth no longer has to continue during the sleep period because it is no longer needed and no longer has current value.

Case Study: Bruxism

A 46–year-old, married bank president was referred to me (JIZ) by her dentist for treatment of bruxism. Most of her teeth grinding took place at night while she was sleeping. Because of her job responsibilities, she led a very stressful life. She had headaches almost constantly. She also had a professional trainer and worked out regularly. When she worked out, she had fewer headaches. During the day, she did not grind her teeth, but she did clench her jaws and she kept them tightly clenched much of the time. This gave the outward impression that she was an uptight and angry person. She knew that, in her position, this was not a good way to appear.

The patient had a root canal a few months before seeing me. She still had pain, and she believed that the dental surgeon "botched the job." She woke up several times during the night from tooth pain and she realized that her clenching and teeth grinding worsened the pain and soreness. Because of this, she labeled herself a "restless sleeper." Her family dentist, she stated, believed that the pain was secondary to her bruxism. However, the patient would not accept a nocturnal bite guard because she felt that it caused more mouth pain.

This patient was rather intense and described herself as either "on" or "off" in her intensity. Mostly she was "on." We discussed her appearance of anger and I explained that she was internalizing her anger and expressing her tension through teeth grinding and jaw clenching. She did relieve some of the anger during workouts. However, that was only a temporary solution because of the continuing pressure from her job. Given the multiple factors maintaining the presenting problem, this case required more than one visit and the teaching of self-hypnosis.

As part of the initial waking state reframing, before doing a trance induction, I explained that she needed another way of freeing herself from the anger buildup and a better way of coping with the work pressures she was experiencing. The following transcript includes the explanation of trance, some of the waking state reframing, the trance induction, the teaching of self-hypnosis and trance state suggestions for change.

> The fact that you have been unable to reduce the demands on yourself at the bank is based on two things. First, when professionals are good at what they do, they are often asked to do more. Second, because of your drive and intensity, you strive to be the best you can be, and that leads to your sometimes taking on more than may be necessary.
>
> Both of these are admirable characteristics. You do, however, require a new way of coping with your drive and responsibilities. Currently, you are hurting yourself, physically and emotionally, and creating an image of an angry person to your peers and staff. There is a better way to cope. In addition to the physical activity that helps some and is good for you, you can learn to dissipate the anger instead of internalizing it.
>
> So far, the only way you know to relax is to exert yourself physically. I am going to teach you how to experience relaxation by being in repose. When you are physically and emotionally relaxed, you can't be tense, stressed, or angry, because these feelings are physical and emotional opposites of relaxation. The teeth grinding and jaw clenching are learned behaviors. I will help you to learn a better way.

I explained about the two parts of the mind, conscious and unconscious, and about what to expect during hypnosis, as described in chapter 2. Usually with internalized anger, I would use a marble induction. However, in this case, I chose an eye fixation and attention to breathing induction because there was a sleep problem component. When using a form of self-hypnosis to assist in sleep, the marble induction is not appropriate.

Trance Induction

I initiated the eye fixation and attention to breathing induction. When I felt that the patient was relaxed, I continued as follows.

> This deeper level of relaxation is called the "neutral place" or the "healing place." We can't go directly from negative to positive. It's too big a leap. We can go from negative to neutral, however. Then we can go from neutral to positive. The neutral place and the healing place are the same. This is when all of the resources of mind and body are in balance during deep relaxation. There is no wasted energy on anger or pain or discomfort. All of that energy is now available for positive healing and growth and change.

Recognizing how comfortable you now feel allows you to also recognize that you can, in fact, feel comfortable. This means that you are no longer trapped in discomfort. Because you are very relaxed and in the neutral healing place, you can now move beyond the discomfort into positive, comfortable feelings while relaxed during hypnosis and when not in hypnosis.

The memory of this comfort will imprint itself in your unconscious mind and will be available to you when awake, and while sleeping, and will be strengthened and reinforced every time you do self-hypnosis.

I am going to teach you now how to do this by yourself. Set your alarm a half hour earlier in the morning. After you have awakened and done your usual toilet activities, gotten dressed, and before you have had your breakfast, find a comfortable chair to sit in, and start relaxing yourself the way we did here in the office today.

Look at some object not too far away and be aware of your eyelids fluttering and your breathing beginning to change all by itself. When your eyelids get very heavy, gently close your eyes and continue to concentrate on your breathing without trying to change your breathing. If your mind wanders, as it may, bring your attention back to your breathing. These occasional wandering thoughts and your growing ability to control them will take you much deeper into relaxation.

Self-talk during your own self-relaxation is not necessary. Every time you relax yourself this way, you will automatically reenforce the things that I say to you when we work together. Stay in this continuing deepening experience of relaxation for a while, until you are ready to awaken yourself. I use the word awaken as a convenience. You are not asleep. You are experiencing deep relaxation as part of the current hypnosis and future self-hypnosis experiences. When you are ready to awaken, count slowly from 1 to 5, as I will be doing with you very shortly. With each number that you count, you will become more and more awake. At the count of 5, you will then open your eyes and be wide awake, and continue to feel very relaxed and comfortable for some time into the day as you go about your business.

In fact, you will find that you experience much less pressure at work and when you are at home. Later in the day, after work, before you start your exercise program, take 10 or 15 minutes to do your relaxing self-hypnosis again. You will be able to melt away any lingering stress and give yourself more energy for your exercise activity.

One other important thing. When you are ready to go to sleep at night, be aware that your jaws no longer feel tight. Lie down in your most comfortable sleep position. Gently and softly close your eyes. Take two or three very slow, deep breaths. Then concentrate on your already changing breathing and allow yourself to gently drop off to sleep. You will sleep more peacefully, without jaw tension or grinding, and awake refreshed and comfortable in the morning.

During the day, every once in a while, take those same three very slow, deep breaths, as you are sitting at your desk or going from one place to another, to melt away any tension before it starts.

Now, I am going to count slowly from 1 to 5, as you will be doing silently to yourself, to help you awaken from this deep relaxation refreshed, energized, and very comfortable.

1—2—3—4—5. Eyes open and wide awake.

I saw the patient 2 weeks later for a second visit. She said that there had been no more grinding at night and no more jaw clenching during the day. She spent about 5 minutes at bedtime lying in her most comfortable position and concentrating on her breathing. She fell asleep and did not awaken until morning, and she recognized that she did not feel tense or experience pain in her jaws. One night she decided to test herself by not doing the bed-time attention to breathing, and she had a bad night. This was during the first week after her first visit. The next night she did pay attention to her breathing, as instructed and she slept fine.

During this second visit, I had her relax herself in my office, as she had been doing at home. I reinforced her successes by repeating the original suggestions. I also added suggestions about continuing her success, by saying,

> You have taken charge of the way you feel and have changed the way you feel. So now you are in charge of you.

I gave her the suggestion in trance that she could give herself permission to change the behavior. I also suggested that her unconscious would from now on be automatically aware of when she either ground her teeth or clenched her jaws while sleeping, and it would automatically have her change her position to a more comfortable one, and unclench and stop grinding. The principle behind this suggestion is that, if the unconscious detects the clenching and changes the person's sleep position to a more comfortable one, the grinding or clenching will stop.

We scheduled an appointment for 2 weeks later, with the provision that she could cancel at the last minute if all was well. She called 2 weeks later and told me that she was doing fine and decided not to come in. She did call about 3 months later to thank me and say that the presenting problems had gone away. Her dentist also called with congratulations on the successful treatment.

Case Study: Rubbing and Sucking on Tongue and Biting Gums

This case involved a 60-year-old married woman who was referred to me (JIZ) by her dentist and a consulting oral surgeon. They had found that there were many lesions on her tongue and in her mouth and a number of white pimples that had developed on her lower gum facing her lower lip and elsewhere in her mouth. She had a burning tongue, and, in an attempt to find relief, sucked her tongue and rubbed it all over her mouth, teeth and gums. Neither dental specialist could find a medical cause for her problems. She also clenched her jaws tightly to try to sleep at night and was given a mouth guard to wear at night to prevent this.

During the intake evaluation, the following facts were elicited that I felt were important. The patient had had a hysterectomy 3 years before. About that time, her husband had decided to retire, and they began to plan a move from their home in another state to Florida. She had a large circle of friends and networks that she would lose in the move. Shortly before the planned move, she developed what she called an "irregular heartbeat," but her doctor could not find a problem and told her not to worry.

The couple moved to a country club community, where her husband could spend every day playing golf. She found it difficult at first to make friends. She related that she experienced "loud heart palpitations" that occurred every afternoon when she was alone at home and sometimes in the evening as well. She also stated that there were times when she felt lightheaded, with a "rushing" feeling to her head, without dizziness. She had discussed none of these uncomfortable feelings with her dentist.

She worked out in a gym with a personal trainer two mornings a week and did stretching and swimming pool aerobics the other three mornings. She also played golf with a group of women or with her husband two afternoons a week. (Note the frequent activities that pump adrenaline.)

She used a lot of visual language and described much of her experience in visual terms. When asked to more fully describe how her mouth felt or how her heart palpitations felt, she was unable to be very descriptive kinesthetically.

I explained to the patient that, based on my evaluation, a number of issues had to be addressed:

1. She was very visual and was unable to accurately interpret the messages of her body.
2. She was probably experiencing a continuing feeling of anxiety that she interpreted as heart palpitations and head rushes.
3. These symptoms started after her hysterectomy and while the plans to move were being worked out.
4. Anxiety can cause dry mouth, which started her using her tongue to increase the flow of saliva.
5. Once the move was made, her anxiety increased. It was further exacerbated by her loneliness and increased physical activity, which pumped adrenaline and increased the experience of heart palpitations and tongue movement and biting. This was especially evident in the afternoon and evening, after exercising, when she was alone and attempting to relax. This caused further and more frequent repetition of tongue and mouth activity and imprinted that behavior as a habit. Even though she had now made friends and adjust to the move and the new home, the uncomfortable behavior continued and was now an empty habit, and therefore no longer needed.
6. She was still feeling problems of separation (depression) from her old home and friends. Although she was adjusting better, she was still not fully accepting of the move.

Session 1

During this first visit, using the process of waking state reframing, I explained about the conscious mind and the unconscious mind and about what to expect during hypnosis. I told her that we would give information to the unconscious that would allow her to give up the uncomfortable habit and allow her mouth to heal normally. I also explained that I would be teaching her a form of self-hypnosis that could help her experience deep relaxation. This would reduce her anxiety and help her to feel more comfortable with the move and her new environment.

I answered her questions, and we then scheduled a second visit for later in the week, to start the treatment process. Note the list of five issues that were discussed with the patient. These helped to establish the goals of treatment and the treatment plan.

Session 2

At the start of the second visit, she told me that she was already feeling somewhat better and was looking forward to the hypnosis experience. She was asked to pick any marble she wanted from my large jar of marbles that was on a side table near her chair. She chose a very large translucent marble with yellow spirals, because it was very "ethereal looking" and she liked its heaviness. (This kinesthetic comment could be used as an opening to help her become more aware of inner feelings and to externalize some of her discomforts, as will be seen later.)

Before we started the trance induction, we explored her daily schedule to determine when to fit in her twice-daily self-hypnosis sessions. She arose at 7:10 A.M. each day, 5 days a week and skipped breakfast. She was at the gym from 8:15 to 11:00 A.M. For 2 to 3 hours, she did stretching and aerobics in the pool. Two days a week she worked out with a personal trainer.

It was suggested that she plan to get up 15 minutes earlier and do her self-hypnosis before she went to the gym, which was only five minutes away. By doing self-hypnosis before exercising, she would have more energy and more stamina. Two days a week she played golf, at around 2:00 P.M., then relaxed in the clubhouse and had a drink with her friends. She usually returned home by 5:30 P.M. We decided that she would do her second self-hypnosis session after she returned home at about 5:30 P.M. every day. These self-relaxation times would fit easily into her already well-planned schedule without changing the rest of her daily rituals.

She was instructed to sit comfortably in the chair and to hold her marble between her thumb and index finger. I told her to look at it, to feel it and to notice the smile that appeared on her face as a result of her instant regression to a happy time in her childhood. While she was doing this in the office, a smile did appear on her face as she told me about when she used to play marbles with her brother and always win. We continued with the marble induction.

As you roll the marble between your finger and thumb, you notice how much warmer it is getting. That warmth is moving right from your hand and fingers into the marble, in the same way that you will soon be able to move discomfort from your body and mouth into the marble. The weight of the marble seems to increase slightly, bringing your hand down to your lap [using what I observed was already occurring]. Notice that your eyes are blinking more rapidly, and your eyelids want to close [leading from what I observed to be happening to a reasonable outcome that I wanted to happen next]. That happens when someone begins to experience relaxation. When your eyes close, let them close gently without squeezing them tight, until I ask you to open them. Close your hand around the marble and concentrate on the marble in your hand. Picture it fully, and begin to feel it getting even warmer. Pay attention to its weight, its roundness, and how comfortable it helps you feel. As you do this, you will relax more and more, deeper and deeper.

If you find your mind wandering, the moment you are aware that you are thinking of something other than the marble, bring your thoughts back to fully concentrating on the marble in your hand. This will help your mind to wander less and less, until it hardly wanders at all.

You know that you are deeply relaxed and continuing to go deeper still because your breathing has become more shallow and more regular, and you hear and feel your heart beating softly and regularly and normally. This recognition of a regular, steady heartbeat adds to your experience of comfort and deepening relaxation.

By now you have reached that deep level of relaxation that we call the neutral place, the healing place. It is very difficult to go directly from negative to positive, because it is too big a leap. But you can go from negative to neutral. This neutral place is where the healing and change begin. This is when your body and your mind are in balance. There is no wasted energy on stress or distress. So all of the energy of your mind–body system can be used for healing, for change, as an energy resource, and as a way of building a memory of deep relaxation that you can borrow back when you do your own self-relaxation, your own self-hypnosis. Now you can begin to see and feel yourself moving to positive.

During deep relaxation, your body creates more saliva, so your mouth feels better and your tonguing behavior can stop. This also allows your mouth to heal and your jaws to remain relaxed and comfortable. What you are really doing is giving yourself permission to let behaviors that are no longer needed leave your mind and body and travel down your arm and hand into the marble, where they can dissipate into the air and be gone. You can almost see, and you can certainly feel, the pain, tension and discomfort moving down to the marble, turning into smoke, and disappearing harmlessly into the air.

Starting tomorrow, you will relax yourself at home, as we did here today in my office. Each morning before you exercise, and each afternoon after golf or other activities, at home, you will use the marble to help yourself into deep relaxation, the way we did today. By carrying the marble in your purse or pocket, you can also hold it in your hand from time to time and feel it helping you be more relaxed without even closing your eyes. During your own self-hypnosis sessions, you do not need to talk to yourself or attempt to repeat what I say to you when we work together. In other words, no self-talk. The reason you do not need to talk to yourself is that, every time you do your own self-relaxation, you automatically reinforce the things I say to you when we work together here in my office. You will also be aware that you are enjoying and appreciating your home and your friends and your sunny environment much more than you have been.

Now, I am going to awaken you from this deep relaxation. I use the word awaken because I don't have a better one. You are not asleep, just experiencing the deep relaxation of hypnosis. I am going to count slowly from 1 to 5. With each number I count, you will feel more and more aware and alert, and still feel relaxed at the same time. This sense of relaxation will continue for some time after you awaken, even while you function fully and alertly. This slowly counting up is the same way you will help yourself to "awaken" when you do your own self-hypnosis each day.

1—2—3—4—5. Eyes open. Fully aware now. That was great. You really appeared very relaxed. How was that?

We then discussed what her trance experience had been like, and how she now felt. Her report was very positive. I then asked her to put herself back into self-relaxation using the marble, the way she would be doing at home. I told her that I would not assist her. She was to do this by herself while I observed. Having the patient repeat an induction directly after awakening from the trance state is a powerful reinforcer of the trance experience. It ratifies the patient's ability to do it to himself or herself.

The patient spent about 10 minutes in relaxation. Then, after opening her eyes, she smiled brightly and exclaimed, "That felt great". She was scheduled for a third appointment a week later and encouraged to practice self-hypnosis regularly twice a day, as agreed, to continue the healing and change process by herself. She had an appointment with her dentist for the day before she was to see me again and I suggested that she tell her dentist about what we were doing and how she was feeling.

Session 3

When the patient came in for her third visit a week later, she said that she had experienced no heart palpitations or head rushes all week. Her mouth was much better and her dentist agreed that there was much improvement. Her tongue was quiet most of the time and she could recognize that her mouth was healing. The patient had practiced self-hypnosis regularly twice a day. She said that her mind had wandered a lot but she was able to bring herself back to concentrating on the marble. She stated, "It is kind of nice to be able to do that." The patient was more aware of how her body felt and could easily make herself feel relaxed.

She further commented that she had more energy at the end of the day. "Yesterday was my best day," she said. "I can often 'feel' the marble in my hand and experience relaxation even when it is not there."

I asked her to put herself into self-hypnosis with the marble and to say "okay" when she felt relaxed enough for me to take over and to help her to go much deeper into relaxation. When she said "Okay," I said:

> Thank you. I am now going to help you go much deeper into relaxation by counting slowly from 20 to 1. With each number I count, you will recognize that you are going deeper and deeper into relaxation. Just listen to the numbers and let yourself go and enjoy the experience. 20—19—18—17—16—15—14—13—12—11—10—9—8—7—6—5—4—3—2—1. Deep, deep, very deep relaxation.
>
> From now on, when you relax yourself, you will add this countdown from 20 to 1 to your own self-hypnosis procedure to reach this same deeper level of relaxation. This deeper level of relaxation will increase the successes that you have already achieved and increase the process of healing that is already taking place. This deeper neutral place, healing place, will also help you recognize how important it is to treat yourself better. Every time you relax yourself, you are treating yourself with more care, with more dignity, and with more self-respect. You are taking better care of you.
>
> Now, I am going to back off and leave you in relaxation. Stay there for a while and let the things I have said to you imprint themselves deeply into your unconscious mind. When you are ready, you can awaken yourself and feel really great, relaxed and alert at the same time.

Session 4

The patient was scheduled for a planned last visit in 2 weeks. At that time, she reported a quiet tongue and no nocturnal jaw tension. Her dentist allowed her to remove the night guard. Her mouth sores had mostly healed and the few pimples that remained were very small and not a problem.

The patient told me that when she practiced her twice daily self-hypnosis, she saw colors that were bright, changing and very soothing. She was asked to do self-hypnosis in the office, and to say "okay" when she finished her deepening countdown. I then emphasized her very deep relaxation in the healing place and suggested that the healing would continue in her mouth. I told her that continuing to practice self-hypnosis on a regular daily basis and using the marble, as needed, for almost instant stress control, would assist her unconscious to help her deal more effectively with any future problems, increase her comfort with her new environment and new friends, and continue to take better care of herself. She was told to awaken herself when she was ready. Upon doing so, the patient exclaimed that she saw the colors again and could picture the future as being very bright. I explained that I was always available should she need me again.

Three weeks later, her dentist called to thank me, stating that the patient was free of mouth lesions, and jaw tension and that her tongue had healed.

The same general procedures can be used in a one- to four-visit treatment program for thumb sucking (rarely seen in adults, but often present in children, teens, and sometimes young adults), hair pulling, nail biting, skin picking, and other similar simple habits.

"Simple" and "Problem" Snoring

A somewhat different approach can often be helpful for snoring. Some 45% of normal adults snore at least occasionally, and 25% are habitual snorers. Problem snoring is more frequent in males and overweight persons, and it usually grows worse with age (American Academy of Otolaryngology—Head and Neck Surgery [AAO-HHS], 2000). Snoring is caused by a physical obstruction of the free flow of air through the passages at the back of the mouth and nose and throat while the person is sleeping. In the back of the mouth, this area is the collapsible portion of the airway where the back of the tongue and upper throat meet the soft palate and uvula. This physical obstruction occurs when the muscles of the palate, the uvula and sometimes the tonsils relax during sleep and come into contact with each other. These structures then act as vibrating noisemakers when the air moves across them during breathing, usually during inspiration.

Snoring can be the result of a number of medically diagnosable physical-anatomical conditions (AAO-HHS, 2000). These include poor muscle tone in the throat and tongue, excessive bulkiness of throat tissue, a long soft palate and/or uvula, nasal or nasal septum deformities and/or nasal airway obstruction. Severe snoring can also be one symptom of obstructive or central sleep apnea, both of which are serious medical conditions requiring medical treatment, that involve frequent episodes during the night of totally obstructed breathing.

Behavioral Issues

Understandably, snoring can be a problem for both the snorer and the person he or she sleeps with. It can disturb both the snorer's and the snorer's bed partner's sleep patterns, and thus lead to sleep deprivation for one or both individuals.

We have had a number of requests over the years to help people control their snoring behaviorally and with hypnosis. These requests usually came from former patients, seen successfully for other problems, or from family members or friends of former patients. Physicians and dentists have also made referrals for behavioral and hypnotic treatment of snoring.

When considering the use of hypnosis, it is important to acknowledge that snoring is an automatic physiological behavior that is controlled by the unconscious part of the mind. Therefore, when a person is sleeping, that person does not have conscious control over the snoring behavior. Because it is controlled by the unconscious, this part of the mind needs to be addressed to modify the unconscious behavior. We use the hypnosis tool to give the unconscious the information it needs to solve the problem.

As stated by author Anthony Burgess (quoted in Moore-Ede & LeVert, 1998), "Laugh and the world laughs with you. Snore, and you sleep alone." This is an eloquent and somewhat humorous statement about a not so funny problem that has destroyed many a marriage bed. The fact is, many snorers are only aware of their snoring as a problem because their spouse or sleeping partner is kept awake by the sound of snoring. These individuals are rarely awakened as a result of their snoring. Although there may be a minor nasal obstruction present, due to nasal allergies or sinus conditions, it may not cause significant discomfort to the individual and may not be associated with any significant airway obstruction, or apnea. These cases usually can be handled in a single session. We label this problem as *simple snoring*.

In many cases, we have had success in using hypnosis and suggestion to help patients experience a drying up of their postnasal dripping and to breathe more easily through their nose. However, these cases may require more than one visit. We label this problem as *complex* or *problem snoring*.

Suggestions for Simple Snoring

Our usual intake evaluation is done to determine if the snoring problem can be conceptualized as a simple habit that has been imprinted by repetition. If it is determined that this is indeed so, we proceed to treat the problem as a simple habit through the use of waking state reframing and direct trance state suggestion approaches.

Very often, we may hear from the patient, or the patient's sleep partner, that the sleep partner says, "When his/her snoring awakens me, I poke him/her and he/she moves into another position and stops snoring for a while. Then it happens again. Then I poke him/her again." In such cases, it is suggested that the patient give the unconscious mind permission to be aware of when the snoring starts. It is then suggested that the unconscious mind will cause the sleeper to change his or her body position to interrupt the snoring behavior, without disrupting the sleep pattern. Suggestions may include closing the mouth and breathing more easily through the nose.

Specific suggestions, such as the following, are verbalized:

> The approach I am suggesting is very simple, and it works. It works in the same way that, if you're in bed sleeping and you're snoring, and your wife kicks you or hits you, or says something to you, somehow you change your position, and you stop snoring. So, from now on, when you are snoring during your sleep, a part of

your own mind will become aware of it, without your awakening. And that part of your mind will slightly change your breathing and move your body and head just a little. This will immediately interrupt your snoring. Any time during the night when you are asleep, if you should start to snore again, the same response will occur.

Choice of Induction

Waking state reframing is used first, as described previously, to explain the conscious and unconscious parts of the mind. The snoring problem is then reframed as being only a simple habit that is no longer needed. Hypnosis is then explained, and an appropriate hypnotic induction is chosen.

When choosing the induction for this problem, some important considerations must be explored. First, we must decide whether or not to teach the patient self-hypnosis. If we plan on using the single-session simple habit protocol, we do not teach self-hypnosis. However, if we conceptualize the problem as being more complex and we plan to see the patient for several sessions, then we teach self-hypnosis.

The method that we usually use is the eye fixation attention to breathing induction. However, breathing is usually a problem for snorers. If the breathing is too labored, we avoid suggesting attention to breathing. If the breathing is not labored, or not too labored, this induction is good because it can include suggestions for awareness of improved breathing during the experience of relaxation. This actually can help to eliminate the snoring problem. The patient is asked to be aware of the relationship between the experience of relaxation and the improvement of breathing during the induction process and to acknowledge this awareness with a simple head nod.

Suggestions can be given that the sleep experience is also one of the ways that we experience relaxation. It is suggested that, during sleep, the patient can breathe better, the way he or she did in the office while relaxing in hypnosis.

Sample Induction and Suggestions for Snoring

The following is an example of the induction and suggestions to deal with a case of simple snoring.

> Sit comfortably in the chair and look at something in front of you. How about the hands of the Buddha in the large picture on the wall, or the large crystal ball on the windowsill? Which would you like to look at? The crystal ball is an excellent choice. Keep looking at the crystal ball, and notice that you are beginning to blink more frequently than usual. That increased blinking happens during the beginning of a more relaxed feeling and is an indication that hypnosis is starting to occur. Notice how much heavier your eyelids have become.

Now, gently close your eyes without squeezing them tight, and leave them closed until I ask you to open them. You will notice that your eyelids are fluttering rapidly. That tells us that you are in fact going into hypnosis. After a while, you will no longer pay attention to your eyelids as you direct your attention to your breathing. As you continue to relax even deeper, your breathing will become deeper and more regular, then shallow and more regular. Concentrate on your breathing and notice how much easier it is for you to breathe. Nod your head for me so I will know that you are aware of that. Thank you. The improved breathing is a direct result of your growing feeling of relaxation.

Continue to concentrate on your breathing, and go deeper and deeper into relaxation—deeper with each breath that you take and deeper with each word that I say, regardless of the meaning of my words. If your mind wanders, the moment you realize that you are thinking of something other than your breathing, bring your attention back to concentrating on your breathing and allow yourself to continue to go still deeper into relaxation, deeper with each breath and deeper with each word.

This deeper level of relaxation also relaxes your breathing, and you breathe so much better and so much easier. You are more aware of your easier breathing, aren't you? Just nod your head so I will know that you are. Thank you.

This deep relaxation is when the doorway to the unconscious opens. With your permission, I can give information to your unconscious to help you eliminate the snoring behavior. Remember we talked about the snoring as only a simple habit, imprinted by repetition? Well, now, during this deep relaxation, this deep hypnosis experience, you can give yourself permission to no longer snore. As you breathe better during sleep, which is one of the ways that we all relax deeply, you will sleep better and more restfully.

Recall that your unconscious mind controls all of your automatic bodily functions such as your breathing and your sleeping. It also controls all of your habits, including the snoring. So, when you are sleeping, your unconscious mind is immediately aware when you first start to snore. Therefore, from now on, when you first start to snore, your unconscious, which is immediately aware of this, will automatically move your body into a more comfortable position and interrupt the need to snore. This will happen throughout the night. By automatically being aware of the beginning of a snore, and by moving your body into a more comfortable position, snoring will be interrupted and no longer occur. You will sleep better, be more rested, and wake up feeling more refreshed and relaxed. After a while, by removing the need to snore, the natural sleep experience will be free of snoring. So you need not snore again.

Now, I am going to awaken you from this deep relaxation by my counting from 1 to 5 slowly. With each number that I count, you will be more and more awake. With the number 5, you will be wide awake and feeling great, just the way you will feel when you awaken from a restful, peaceful sleep.

After the patient emerges from the trance state, we discuss the patient's relaxation experience, the improved breathing and we reinforce the belief that the snoring behavior is gone.

Problem Snoring

When the patient presents significant blockage in the nasal passages due to extensive mucus buildup and postnasal dripping, suggestions are given that the experience of deep relaxation changes breathing so that tightness is reduced and drying up of the nasal passages can almost immediately take place. We also add the following suggestions to the previous simple snoring script.

> As you enjoy a deeper feeling of relaxation, notice how much better your breathing is. Also, be aware of less constriction in your nose and throat. In fact, this comfortable relaxation experience allows greater comfort to take place in your nose and throat. The reduction of stress allows your immune system to use its available energy to quickly dry up the postnasal drip and blockage. That healing will continue. You will find that your unconscious mind will recognize this and further reduce the snoring behavior.

Posttrance Imprinting

Directly after exiting trance, the patient is still very susceptible to suggestion. Therefore, we reinforce the suggestions for change that were given earlier during the waking state reframing and during the trance state. Here, we carry on a casual conversation with the patient, commenting on how great the patient did and how relaxed he or she appeared to be. We ask the patient to describe how much the experience of relaxation was enjoyed, and how good it felt to be so relaxed.

Falling Asleep during Trance

The topic of treating the problem of snoring brings up an interesting and not too uncommon issue for clinicians who use hypnosis. That is, what should you do when a patient appears to fall asleep during trance work? The way we handle this apparent problem is based on our belief that patients don't usually fall asleep during trance work (although some therapists may fall asleep).

Sometimes, although rarely, patients do indeed fall asleep. You should suspect that a patient has fallen asleep if the patient is sitting there with his or her mouth open and begins to snore. If this happens, simply say to the patient in a authoritative manner:

> Please close your mouth.

That almost always brings the patient right back into the trance state without interrupting the flow of the process, and without in any way drawing the patient's attention to the possibility that the patient was sleeping.

SUMMARY

Most simple habits respond to the procedure described above. The key is to assess the presenting problem during the intake evaluation to be certain it is really a simple habit. Then, use a short hypnotic trance induction and employ the trance language demonstrated above, inserting the name of the habit behavior. The trance script is modified as necessary.

9

More Complex Habits as Ways of Dealing with Anxiety and Stress

Complex habits are repetitive behavior patterns that are motivated by multiple factors and often underlying psychodynamic issues. These issues create anxiety that seeks resolution by invoking some behavioral response more powerful than what occurs in cases of simple habit responses. The forcefulness of the invoked response often produces additional emotional and behavioral responses in the person and others. The initial imprinting may occur as a result of some major emotionally charged event that initiates the chosen response, or results from it. The problem coping behavior is further imprinted by repetition.

It evolves into a more complex habit when it initiates a chain of events that present additional coping demands. These invoke additional emotional and behavioral responses. As the habit pattern occurs in a wider range of situations, response generalization take place. That means that the habit response becomes attached to more and more stimuli. Different situations invoke the same or similar responses, and through the process of repetition, the habit pattern is further imprinted. Thus, stimuli that are far removed in time, distance, form and psychological and physical characteristics from the original initiating stimuli can come to invoke similar responses (i.e., habit patterns).

The habit pattern serves the individual as a way of coping with, and to some extent, reducing anxiety, so it is repeated and strengthened. Under stress, which exacerbates anxiety, the frequency, duration, or intensity of the negative habit behavior tends to increase.

PROBLEM EATING

Overeating, or "problem eating," is a complex habit that is usually initiated and maintained by multiple factors (physiological, psychological, and interpersonal-social) (Brown & Fromm, 1987; Cochrane, 1987, 1992; Russ, 1987; Vanderlinden & Vandereycken, 1994). It can be an anxiety-based coping behavior that tends to occur frequently and repetitively, with or without much conscious control. The individual may overeat in many different situations without realizing it until after the fact. This automatic behavior is usually associated with a misinterpretation of the messages being received from the body. The behavior is immediately reinforced or gratified because it feels good, or satisfies the need to make sense of the body's message that is being misinterpreted. However, the behavior may also trigger negative feelings, such as guilt, further anxiety or shame. It is a behavior that is recognized as typically having negative health consequences.

Effective brief hypnotic treatment of overeating or compulsive eating typically requires more sessions than does the brief hypnotic treatment of most simple habits. This is because this behavior generally occurs in response to a variety of anxiety-provoking situations that require resolution. Although you can stop some behaviors completely, you can't stop eating. The behavior must be changed and controlled, not stopped. Furthermore, issues of self-esteem, body image and physical health often have to be addressed as part of the reframing process (Brown & Fromm, 1987; Bryan, 1980; Cochrane, 1987, 1992; Reaney, 1987; Russ, 1987).

Many patients who present for hypnosis for weight control have a history of going on and off various diets (Cochrane, 1987, 1992; Levitt, 1993). For the majority of these patients, these diets have not been successful at keeping the weight off for the longterm. Many weight patients experience some success on some diets initially, then, at some point, begin to have difficulty continuing to adhere to the particular dietary regimen. Initial weight losses that aren't maintained are often followed by larger weight gains, or "weight rebound." These dieting failures often lead to greater and greater demoralization and depression associated with negative coping behaviors.

Many patients with weight and food problems show patterns of overzealous food deprivation, resulting in severe reductions of caloric and nutrient intake that can result in serious medical complications (Russ, 1987). Overweight patients who are severely deconditioned and out of shape present significant health risks when they start physical exercise and conditioning programs without medical supervision. In addition to the above considerations, marked losses or gains in appetite and unhealthy eating habits can be caused by a variety of medical or psychiatric conditions that should be ruled out through appropriate initial medical and/or psychiatric consultation.

Given the variety of medical complications that can be associated with food and weight issues, it is unwise to begin hypnotic treatment for problem eating without first checking that the patient is receiving competent ongoing medical care. Our treatment protocols described below assume that the patient has been properly medically evaluated (Hunter, 1987). We never want to use hypnosis to treat a patient's symptoms that are due to an untreated medical problem.

PROBLEM DRINKING

"Problem drinking" is another complex habit pattern that responds well to the brief cognitive hypnosis model. This problem behavior requires extensive reframing of such popular belief systems as the alcohol disease model and the belief that everyone with a drinking problem is an "alcoholic." Further reframing is required about the issue of total abstinence versus controlled drinking (Brown & Fromm, 1987; Sobell, 1978). Here again, however, patients with drinking problems should not be treated psychologically or with hypnosis until they have been adequately worked up medically, given the myriad of serious medical consequences of alcohol abuse.

Our conceptual and treatment model is also effective with other complex habits, such as performance, examination, learning, and concentration anxiety. The brief cognitive hypnosis treatment approach that is applicable to all of these types of problems will be addressed with case examples in this chapter.

OVEREATING

There are many reasons why a person may eat too much or too often. On a conscious level, a person may answer the question "Why?" with responses such as "I love sweets," "I enjoy it," "I can't help myself," and "I like to indulge myself." These are all conscious rationalizations that do not address what is really going on. The overeating may produce a sense of inner comfort and reduce feelings of anxiety. It may be a response to biochemical imbalances. It may be related to family patterns, as when a person is influenced by repetitive pressure of a parent to "finish what is on your plate." It may even be related to the time of day that the person eats, the place (e.g., eating at home or at a restaurant), or a host of other environmental and emotional factors.

Dabney Ewin, MD, a physician who specializes in the use of clinical hypnosis, stated in an e-mail communication (May 2000) that "Hans Selye demonstrated long ago that when he stressed animals with heat, cold, physical exhaustion or psychologically, they all ultimately developed functional hypoglycemia as a result of chronic stress. Under chronic stress, when the nervous system is not getting enough glucose, it reacts the same way it does when it's not getting enough oxygen. This produces anxiety, dizziness, palpitations, and other panic type experiences." The drop in blood sugar level that takes place with the manufacture of insulin motivates a person to eat sugary foods. This calms the anxiety and removes the uncomfortable symptoms of hypoglycemia. Even though the person may be upset about weight gain or weight maintenance, the repetition and imprinting of the pattern of being calmed by food is often more powerful than the embarrassment, shame or discomfort of being too heavy or overweight.

A suggestion of blood sugar problems may require further questioning during the intake about the possibility of a family history of diabetes and hypoglycemia.

Developing a thorough initial understanding the patient's eating patterns is essential to establishing a treatment plan for the utilization of waking state reframing and Trance Language with this problem (Brown & Fromm, 1987; Russ, 1987; Zarren, 1996a). People who are successful at changing and controlling problem eating behavior and losing weight "reframe their relationship with food and with formerly problematic food-social situations" (Cochrane, 1992, p. 114). For example, people who overeat often have the following kinds of problems:

1. They have difficulty recognizing the messages of their own body. They interpret every sound, every gurgle and every momentary twitch in their body as a sign of hunger.
2. They usually eat very fast. The stomach fills up using time cues, not volume cues. The faster one eats, the more volume one consumes before the stomach informs the brain that it is full (Raloff, 1996).
3. They avoid eating breakfast because they are "not hungry in the morning," and thus do not start the process of digestion early. This leads to starting the day without sufficient energy and a lethargic metabolic process.
4. These same individuals often have a very late, large, heavy dinner. They then spend the rest of the evening passively, not burning off body fat and going to bed with a full undigested stomach. They often snack in the evening.

When discussing points 3 and 4 with patients who present this pattern, we may use a metaphor to explain what is happening, such as the following:

Imagine that your body is a mountain cabin heated only by a fireplace. By the time you wake up in the morning, the fire is out, so it is cold. You don't start a fire. That is, you don't have breakfast. By not having breakfast, you don't start a fire to heat up your body and to give it energy for the day and start the process of burning off body fat.

By noon, you realize that it is cold, so you start a small fire. You have a small lunch. But you have used only a few small logs, so by 4:00 in the afternoon, as the sun is setting, it is cold again. This is when there is a normal drop in blood sugar, making you hungry for a snack, so you throw another small log on the fire, by having some sweet snack food. You are warming up the cabin only a little bit. You keep throwing a few twigs on the fire as you continue to snack.

Then the sun goes down, the wind picks up, and between 7:00 and 9:00 P.M., the cabin is very cold. You throw a number of logs on the fire to start it roaring to produce more warmth. You have a large dinner. You keep throwing logs on the fire. You keep snacking. By the time you are ready to go to bed, the fire is roaring to keep you warm through the night. You go to bed having had a lot of food, building body fat while you are sleeping. You have had no exercise, no activity, no way of burning off the fat. During the night the fire dies down, the cabin gets cold;

you wake up in the morning cold, with no breakfast and start the process over again. You are not giving yourself enough energy to burn up body fat during the day. You are taking in too much food at night, when you don't need the energy, not exercising and going to sleep to build more body fat.

5. Frequently, there is a problem relating to taste. Overeaters usually prefer sweet foods to foods emphasizing other tastes. They may have a blood sugar problem. Often, people who overeat prefer "comfort foods" that taste like those they were fed while growing up. Frequently, foods falling into this category were given to them when they were feeling "low" by overzealous mothers who encouraged overeating. On the other hand, some foods are avoided because the taste is not considered enjoyable or desirable. This information can be used to suggest taste changes to other healthier foods to make them more desirable. By asking questions about taste, you can force a patient to pay more attention to tastes that produce feelings that encourage overeating and those that can become satisfying without being associated with the need to eat too much.

6. Many people eat to reduce feelings of stress. They are not "stress eaters." Well, not exactly. They eat to reduce feelings of anxiety that may or may not be related to current stress. These feelings of anxiety, however, are not recognized as such. The individual who eats to reduce feelings of stress and anxiety may only be aware of being uncomfortable and of the fact that eating food helps him or her to feel more comfortable. Anxiety can be low level, continuous, and invisible to people who, as suggested in point 1, have difficulty recognizing the messages of their own body. The use of food to change these uncomfortable feelings is imprinted by repetition and fixed in place as a habit. Although the behavior may no longer needed, it is continued unnecessarily.

7. Some women, even some men, unconsciously may overeat to be unattractive to members of the opposite sex. Maintaining excess weight can function as an insulator that helps the overweight person avoid being attractive and prevent unwanted sexual advances. It also can serve as a way to avoid intimate relationships. There may be a history of sexual abuse or family trauma that established this defense. If an overweight woman is married, being overweight can sometimes be the result of subtle encouragement by her husband to keep her unattractive to other men. Your experience and professional instinct will give direction as to how to deal with this issue.

LIMITING THE FOCUS OF BRIEF COGNITIVE HYPNOSIS

We limit the focus of therapy to goals for change that are attainable and that usually can be realized within several sessions. Neither of us treats sexual abuse problems. If this issue stands out as an important one during the evaluation, we offer to make a referral to a competent therapist who does treat these problems, or we negotiate a compromise goal with the patient. The compromise may include two issues:

1. If the patient wants to change his or her appearance enough to feel more confident and comfortable with himself or herself, we may establish a verbal contract to continue within established parameters that are agreed to between us.
2. Often the control of anxiety that influences dysfunctional behavior can be taught to a patient without having to uncover and deal with the deeper fearful issues. This is done by addressing the current symptoms while helping the patient remain insulated from past traumas. This approach may be considered controversial and should only be considered by an experienced clinician who is comfortable with it. We both have had some success with this approach in our own practices.

One of the keys to success in this type of situation is to be very clear about the goals of the therapy and to make sure that the therapeutic contract is acceptable to the patient. It is also essential to agree to work within a fixed number of sessions, then to evaluate what has been accomplished and what remains to be accomplished after those sessions have occurred.

It is also important to structure each therapy session adequately. The degree of structure is dictated by your intuition regarding how much direction versus permissiveness the patient needs and can tolerate. However, it is important to Not allow the sessions to go off on tangents that may be precipitated if the patient is distractible, hysterical, emotional or has marked character pathology. The degree to which each session addresses whatever comes up is directly proportional to the degree of open-endedness and duration of the therapy.

PROBLEM EATING REFRAMES

The following eight reframes usually are delivered when we are doing brief cognitive hypnosis for overeating or problem eating. They focus the patient's conscious and unconscious mind on important concepts that need to be accepted consciously and imprinted in the unconscious mind to start the process of behavior change when it comes to eating. These reframes are presented both in the waking state and during the trance state. When they are delivered in the trance state, they are presented in a simpler, more direct and less wordy form.

Reframe 1: We Will Not Be Watching How Many Pounds You Lose

We are not interested in monitoring pounds lost, by frequently weighing yourself on a scale. In any given day, you may be up or down 3 or more pounds based on how much fluid you retain. Usually about 4:00 P.M. you will weigh more than you did at 9:00 A.M. because of fluid retention. We are more interested in how much more comfortable your clothes fit than in how many pounds you lose.

Reframe 2: The Stomach Does Not Inform You It Is Full Based on How Much Food You Eat

The stomach does not signal the brain that it is full based on how much food you have eaten. It is really a time frame system. Time spent eating is more important than volume of food consumed. After a certain period of time, which varies with each person, a signal will go to the brain that says your stomach is full, no matter how much you have eaten. It will be helpful to teach you how to eat very slowly, to eat less and enjoy it more. That way you consume less food.

Reframe 3: You May Have Difficulty Recognizing the Messages of Your Body

Very often people with weight and eating problems have difficulty recognizing the messages of their body. They often misinterpret body signals as meaning that they are hungry, even if they are not. Stomach growling may be interpreted by you as a signal that you are hungry. It may not be. What it may mean is that you have swallowed too much air and your body is dealing with that. There may be other internal sounds and feelings of a similar nature that you are not consciously aware of that create the same false impression of hunger. I will help you to correct those misunderstandings.

Reframe 4: Diets Don't Work

Some people do lose weight while dieting. Almost any change in food intake will accomplish that for a short while, regardless of the particular diet. That is why there are so many different diets for weight loss. Many of them contradict each other but still bring about some weight loss temporarily. But diets stop working after a while. They cause the dieter to become too preoccupied with thoughts of pounds gained or lost, grams ingested and choices of foods that are supposed to be helpful. This preoccupation becomes obsessive and increases anxiety and feelings of guilt when the diet rituals that are prescribed are not followed. Therefore, you will not be dieting. You will be changing the way you think about food, about how you deal with food. You will be changing your eating behavior.

Reframe 5: There Are "Weight Loss Plateaus"

Even though you will not be weighing yourself, your body will know when you have lost enough weight to stop for a while. When you have really lost 8 to 10 pounds, and not from fluid loss, you will reach a plateau at which you appear to stop losing weight for about a week to 10 days. You will continue to lose fluid during this time, so you may continue to find that your clothes fit better. This plateau is when your body makes whatever internal adjustments are needed to accommodate the change in weight. It is like going down a staircase and reaching a series of landings that create occasional resting places in the descent. As you continue to change, you will reach these resting places and recognize them as helpful stops rather than problems.

CASE STUDY: OVEREATING

Session 1

A 77-year-old, 5-foot-8 inch-tall man weighing 205 pounds was referred to me (JIZ) by his physician for help in losing weight. His doctor was concerned about the patient's blood pressure and did not believe he would follow a prescribed diet. The patient lived with his 72-year-old wife. Four years earlier, the patient had colon cancer. He was treated surgically followed by a year of chemotherapy. At the time of referral, he had no signs of cancer.

The man had been a restaurant owner before he retired. He played tennis avidly almost every day and stated that he liked to eat and drink. His occupation made this easy to do when he was working. He and his wife ate out three or four times a week, and he would have six or seven beers a week, usually when he ate out.

The patient typically ate a light breakfast and a very light lunch. About 4:30 P.M. he would start to get hungry and would begin to snack. Usually this included fruit or a cookie and milk. Dinner was usually eaten around 6:00 P.M. and was very large. It might consist of spaghetti and meatballs or baked chicken, with soup, salad, and bread, and constituted a large volume of food. After dinner, the patient continued to snack, and between 10:00 and 11:00 P.M. he usually had something more to eat to "fortify himself" before going to sleep.

As is typical, the patient ate very quickly, always filled up his plate, finished everything on the plate, then took another helping and finished that also.

The issues that had to be addressed and the behaviors that had to be changed were outlined using many of the reframes listed above and employing the mountain cabin metaphor given earlier in the chapter. The goals of treatment included imprinting the following new habits: (1) eating slowly, (2) eating less food, (3) eating three small meals, (4) not eating after dinner, (5) understanding the messages of his body to interrupt the belief that he was hungry, (6) exercising in the evening, and (7) reducing alcohol intake.

The intake evaluation took up the entire initial session. A second session was scheduled later in the week, so that we could get started sooner.

Session 2

During the second session, the concepts of the conscious and unconscious minds were explained, as were the issues of what to expect during hypnosis. The tasks and behavioral change goals of the therapy also were reviewed. Any questions the patient had were answered, so that he could understand what we would be doing in the office and what he would be doing at home. It was further explained that he would be learning self-hypnosis and that he would be relaxing himself twice a day for about 10 to 15 minutes each time. We explored the best times for him to do this and agreed on before playing tennis in the morning and shortly after 4:00 P.M. when he usually started his "eating behavior."

The eye fixation with attention to breathing induction was chosen because the patient was visually oriented and had difficulty identifying the internal messages of his body. After we had finished the initial induction, he appeared restless and not very relaxed, so a slow 20-to-1 countdown was added as a deepening procedure. By the number 1, he looked very relaxed and an explanation was then given as to how he could do this himself, when at home or anywhere else, without my help.

The patient was to do self-hypnosis in the morning, before he went out to play tennis, and in the afternoon, between 4:00 and 5:00. It was explained that while he was in deep relaxation, in hypnosis, here in the office, he would be given information that his unconscious could use to start the process of changing his behavior. He was instructed not to attempt to give these same suggestions to himself when he did self-hypnosis. He was not to talk to himself. His only responsibility was to concentrate on his breathing to maintain and deepen his own level of relaxation. If his mind wandered, he was to immediately bring his mind back to concentrating on his breathing. He was also told that every time he did self-hypnosis he would automatically reinforce everything that was said to him when we worked together here in my office. (Note that I said "everything" that was said to him. This implied everything I said, during both the waking state and the trance state, without my specifically saying so.)

The specific suggestions administered were as follows:

> You will find yourself eating very, very slowly, taking one small bite at a time and finishing what you have in your mouth before you take another bite. You will actually eat less and enjoy it more. You will find it unnecessary to finish what is on your plate and at first push your plate away unfinished, then place less on your plate and still push it away unfinished. When eating out, you will order smaller portions and sometimes realize that you put your fork down while finishing what is in your mouth. You will choose foods with less sugar and drink fewer beers with

your meals and after. After dinner you will experience no hunger and no need to snack or eat before you go to bed. You will sleep more deeply and more restfully and awaken feeling very good. Now, I am going to count from 1 to 5 to awaken you, as you will be doing to awaken yourself. With each number I count, you will feel more and more awake. With the number 5, you will open your eyes and be wide awake and feel really great. You will be relaxed and comfortable, yet wide awake at the same time. 1—2—3—4—5. Eyes open, wide awake.

After the patient opened his eyes, he was asked how he felt. He answered that he did not remember ever having been this relaxed before.

It was then suggested:

Now put yourself back into relaxation without my help. I will just sit here and watch, without saying a word. When you finish the 20-to-1 countdown, allow yourself to stay in relaxation for a while and enjoy the experience of having done this by yourself. Then you can awaken yourself when you are ready.

The patient's eyes closed very quickly, his breathing changed, and he remained in relaxation for about 8 minutes. After he opened his eyes, he stated that he felt as it he had a full night's sleep and was surprised and elated at how good he felt. He was reminded to practice this self-relaxation twice a day until he came back for a third appointment in a week.

Session 3

When he came in a week later for his third appointment, the patient reported, that he had lost 6 pounds. He stated that the previous day he had been in a drug store that had a free scale. Even though I had told him not to weigh himself, he did so anyway. He felt elated, and his wife told him that he looked great. He then said that he was very encouraged by the changes in his behavior and wanted to continue. He was eating slower, consuming less food and stopping himself from putting too much on the plate.

However, he still had a perception of having hunger pangs. I reframed his interpretation of certain physical messages as signs of hunger. I explained that frequent swallowing of air produces gurgling sounds that are not related to hunger. It was also suggested that he drink more water, a few sips at a time and that the frequent swallowing behavior would go away.

The patient was practicing his self-relaxation exercise twice a day for about 10 to 20 minutes and was amazed that he could relax himself so easily. He did not crave sweets and was not eating after dinner. He stated that he sometimes had a glass of juice. He reported that the other evening he had hard shell crabs and a pitcher of beer, indicating that this was the first beer he had since we had started our work together and that he believed he could have just that much and no more. We discussed this as a "testing process."

The patient was then asked to relax himself as he had been doing at home and to indicate when he finished his silent countdown. When he said "Okay," I directed his attention to concentrating on his breathing without trying to change his breathing. Through suggestion, I linked his breathing and my words to further deepening of his relaxation experience. I said:

> You will experience deeper levels of relaxation with each breath that you take and each word that I say, regardless of the meaning of my words.

The suggestions given before about eating slowly, filling up quickly, eating less and enjoying his food more were delivered again. I also repeated the suggestions that he would reject sweets and not eat after dinner, and I added the suggestion that he was already successful at controlling his eating behavior and therefore would find it easier to continue his control.

I also reinforced the reframe of interpreting the messages of his body correctly. The reframe was that body sensations usually did not indicate that he was hungry. I also repeated the suggestion that when he relaxed, he would not talk to himself. He would just enjoy the experience of deep relaxation so that his unconscious mind could automatically use what I said to him when we worked together to fix the new and positive behavior in place. I then asked him to awaken himself. After he opened his eyes, we talked about his trance experience, and scheduled a fourth appointment for 3 weeks later.

Session Four

Three weeks later, the patient returned, having lost another 12 pounds. He had stopped at the drug store to weigh himself on his way to the session. His clothes were very loose, and he was happy about his comfort with continued relaxation and the easy behavior change. He was told that he would probably plateau from time to time so that his body could adjust to the changes. These plateaus might last for a week to 10 days and were not an indication that there was a problem. It was further explained that, at some point, his body would stop the weight loss because it had reached a point of balance (i.e., a set point), but that he would be likely to continue to lose inches as his body contours changed. I suggested that, when his body was most comfortable, he would continue to maintain his improved weight and shape. When that happened, I stated, it would be important for him to continue his self-hypnosis at least once a day, to maintain his control over stressors and thus remain in charge of how he felt and what he did.

These same suggestions were repeated during his self-hypnosis trance experience during this final session. Everything I had said to him during previous trance experiences were summarized and repeated using slightly different words, adding that he would continue to enjoy being in charge of how he felt and what he did. After awakening, we discussed the fact that he no longer needed to see me and that should he have any future questions or problems, I was as close as the telephone. He called six months later to report that all was well, and to thank me.

Case Study: Preoccupying Thoughts of Food

A 50-year-old woman, who had been divorced for 17 years after having been married for only 2 years, was referred to me (JIZ) by a local psychologist because of her constant preoccupation with food. The referring psychologist was seeing her for relationship problems. The patient stated that she had never had a successful social life and was considering joining a singles dating club. Before doing so, however, she wanted to lose 15 to 20 pounds in order to feel comfortable about meeting new people. She was 5 feet 3 inches tall and wieghed 138 pounds. Her best weight was between 115 and 125 pounds. She was physically active, but she consumed a lot of sweets and ate out about half the time.

The patient had been to see a therapist a few years earlier who used hypnosis to help her lose weight. However, the patient did not like this therapist and felt that she had not been successful at losing weight because the therapist was not very good. I asked her why she thought she might do better with me, and she responded that I was highly recommended by the psychologist, whom she felt was helping her with her current relationship problems.

When the patient was 30 years old, she had gone to India. While there, she learned to meditate. She had been practicing meditation ever since, off and on, including visualization and breathing exercises. However, she had not been able to apply these practices to her goal of losing weight.

This patient thought about food constantly. However, she only ate breakfast when she woke up "starving." If she felt stressed, she would eat candy in the morning. Lunch was her "most important meal and was usually eaten out. She chose "light foods," such as a salad for lunch, but she would then "take several steps backward" by consuming a bag of pretzels. By 4:00 P.M., she felt starved. She would drink about a gallon of water every day, eat very fast, and consume much more when under stress. As in the previous case study, she interpreted almost every sound, twitch, and gurgle from her stomach as a hunger signal. Dinner was usually eaten late, between 8:30 and 9:00 P.M. Again, she ate dinner very fast and usually ordered large portions, or cooked much more than she could possibly eat. She would freeze all of her leftovers and, when eating dinner at home, mix them together, almost always reheating too much food.

Treatment Plan

This patient's *treatment plan* was outlined for her as follows.

1. To interrupt her continuous preoccupation with food.

2. To correct her belief that the body messages she was aware of meant she was hungry.
3. To teach her how to safely externalize her feelings of stress that had been influencing her frequent eating.
4. To change her eating patterns and behaviors.
5. To substitute self-hypnosis and relaxation for her meditation, which was not working.
6. To teach her to use a marble, either real or imagined, to do self-hypnosis and for instant thought interruption and control of momentary stressors.
7. To assist her in "ego strengthening" as an adjunct to her work with her psychologist.

Because the first visit allowed only time for evaluation and discussion of a treatment plan, another appointment was made for later in the week because the patient wanted to get started as soon as possible.

Session 2

During the second session, further waking state reframing included an explanation of the conscious and unconscious minds, the experience of hypnosis, how she would be using self-hypnosis, and when to practice it twice a day. The difference between her previous practice of meditation and the use of self-hypnosis was clarified.

> Meditation, as you already know, is practiced as a way to achieve a higher level of awareness and consciousness. In its purer form, it requires many hours of continuous practice. Relaxation is a side effect of meditation, not its essential purpose. Would you take medication for its side effect? Meditation also rejects the concept of the unconscious, and it does not encourage specific suggestions for behavior change.
>
> The kind of hypnosis and self-hypnosis that we will be using specifically employs relaxation as a way of assisting the doorway to the unconscious mind to open, and with your permission, enabling the unconscious mind to accept suggestions for change. You learn to relax, and the learned relaxation is imprinted in the unconscious. This allows you to borrow back a part of this relaxation to interrupt stress when it starts to affect you."

Because the patient tended to be somewhat compulsive, the times we chose for her twice-daily practice were designed to fit comfortably into her daily rituals, for example, before her exercise activities in the morning and right after leaving work before she started her early evening exercise and late dinner. She agreed that these two times would be easy for her to keep.

I clarified any questions she had regarding our goals, my responsibilities, and her responsibilities. Her responsibilities would include, with my help, eating a small breakfast, a small lunch, and an earlier small dinner. She was not to weigh herself on a daily basis, but could do so before her appointments with me. Ordinarily, the weekly weight check would not be permissible, but her compulsivity needed to be tempered by reduction of this activity rather than elimination. This would further demonstrate that she really had control over what she did. We talked about my giving her suggestions to eat slower and fill up more quickly and why this would be so.

We also discussed the necessity of reducing her sugar intake to diminish the insulin–sugar "seesaw effect." That is, I explained that too much sugar stimulated the repeated release of insulin to break down the sugar, which in turn caused an increased need to eat sweets.

I told her that I would give her another suggestion to possibly increase her metabolism. This would help her be more aware of increased body heat throughout the day and evening, as an indication that she was burning off body fat faster. She was a very active woman, and there is an increase in body heat when a person exercises. By helping her be more aware of this heat, we could increase her belief in the effectiveness of the treatment process. Belief leads to change. This would also be helpful in filtering out body messages that she had misinterpreted as hunger signals. I suggested that, as she continued to drink water, she would reduce not only fluid retention but also her thoughts of food.

I did the marble induction and gave her suggestions similar to the preceding case study, with the added elements indicated. After she "awakened," I asked her to relax herself again, without my help. She did so easily and with great satisfaction and enjoyment. An appointment for a third visit was then set for a week later.

Session 3

When the patient arrived for her third visit, she mentioned that she had lost 8 pounds and that her clothes felt loose, as if she had lost two sizes. She had easily added the self-relaxation routine to her daily activities, twice a day, and was enjoying doing it. She also noticed that she was experiencing greater warmth in her body during exercise and to a lesser degree during the day and evening. She was eating slower and less, and having dinner earlier. Her use of the marble was helpful in taking her thoughts away from thinking about food, but she still thought about it more than she wanted to.

She was asked to relax herself as she was doing at home and to say "okay" when she felt she was deeply enough relaxed for me to take her to a new and deeper level of relaxation. It took her about 5 minutes to say "okay." I then added the countdown from 20 to 1 to help her to experience a deeper level of relaxation. At the completion of the countdown, I congratulated her on doing so well and suggested that she would be able to continue her successes as she continued her own self-hypnosis, until the new behaviors and feelings became automatic and habitual. She would find that, as she drank water, each sip would help her feel comfortably full and leave her thoughts of food as part of the past. I also suggested that she could add the 20-to-1 countdown to her own self-hypnosis to achieve this deeper level of healing relaxation. I further gave her ego-strengthening suggestions:

> As you continue to practice your own self-hypnosis and enjoy the experience of healing and change, you will be treating yourself with more care, with more dignity, and with more self-respect. This will help you feel better about yourself and help others to feel better about you.

I repeated this suggestion three or four times before having her awaken herself. The word *remember* was added to the last two repetitions.

> Remember, as you continue to practice your own self-hypnosis and enjoy the experience of healing and of change, you will be treating yourself with more care, with more dignity and with more self-respect. This will help you feel better and better about yourself, and help others to feel better and better about you.

Note the repeat of *and better.*

Session 4

The patient was seen for a fourth and final visit 2 weeks later. She had lost 7 more pounds and had started to plateau, as I had discussed with her during the waking state reframing earlier. I told her that she would probably start losing more inches in a few days, then a few more pounds. I suggested that she was approaching her desired weight and that soon her body would begin to stabilize at its most comfortable weight level. By continuing her twice-daily self-hypnosis, she would be able to further imprint her most comfortable body metabolism and new way of feeling and behaving. She would have more energy and look and feel better than she had in years.

The patient told me that she had joined a singles group and was feeling increasingly confident in relating to the people in the group. In fact, she was planning on taking a trip with the group. I congratulated her on this, and said,

> It is time for you to begin to enjoy yourself. You deserve it. Now that you are in charge of how you feel and what you do, you can be less compulsive and more outgoing.

She was asked to relax herself and do a silent countdown to deepen her experience of relaxation. When she finished her countdown, she was to say "okay," so that I could give further suggestions to her unconscious mind. When she signaled me, I reviewed her successes, suggesting that she would be able to continue this success until it became automatic. By then, she would, if she chose, be able to do self-relaxation once or twice a day for the pure pleasure of it. This would keep her comfortable and confident and appropriately in charge.

I repeated the suggestions about enjoying herself in the trance state that I had given to her in the waking state. I then suggested that she could awaken herself, when she was ready, and feel great. She did so, and after talking about her experience, she told me that she felt so good about what had been accomplished that she didn't feel she had to come in anymore on a regular basis. She would call me if she needed any further help. She has called from time to time to say that she was doing great and to thank me.

Her psychologist called me a month after her last visit to tell me that she had done so well with the self-hypnosis and growing confidence that they had decided to discontinue her psychotherapy sessions.

PROBLEM DRINKING

We do not view all excessive alcohol intake as a "disease." Generally, we view it as another way of dealing with stress and anxiety. Sometimes it is learned by the behavior modeled from family members or other important persons. Sometimes it is the result of cultural, environmental, or severe stress influences. Usually, it is exacerbated by unrecognized blood sugar problems, such as hypoglycemia. Often, the problem drinker has comorbid medical problems that are already recognized and possibly being addressed by a physician.

Very often, problem drinkers come to us after extensive treatment in a residential or outpatient alcohol rehabilitation program that includes a twelve-step program and attendance at Alcoholics Anonymous meetings. They may stop drinking for a while, after treatment in these programs, then start again when under stress, or because of social or other external influences.

One of our patient selection criteria is the patient's previous ability to stop or control drinking behavior for a short or long period of time, without serious withdrawal problems. Another criterion is the patient's previous ability to refrain from drinking in specific situations, such as when driving a car or operating machinery. Relative to this second criterion, we have been successful in helping some problem drinkers to learn to control their drinking in specific situations where serious physical or legal consequences are associated with uncontrolled drinking, such as injury to self or others, loss of the right to drive, or possible jail time.

An extensive waking state reframing process is required with problem drinkers who are accepted as patients. This is necessary because of the very powerful societal beliefs and publicity regarding alcoholism as a disease that is forever and that requires total abstinence, and nothing short of this, to control it. Also, if the patient has been in other treatment programs or has made other attempts at control that have failed, extensive reframing is necessary to help the patient believe that control of the behavior is possible with our treatment modality.

CASE STUDY: PROBLEM DRINKING

Session 1

A patient who had been seen successfully 5 years earlier for smoking cessation called and wanted to see me (JIZ) about an "alcohol problem." She was now 35 years old and had married a farmer who drank heavily himself. She told me that she had a drinking problem since the age of 16 that she had mostly controlled until her marriage. Since her marriage, she had been drinking daily. She mostly drank wine. However, she typically consumed several glasses to a whole bottle every day, depending on the situation and the circumstances.

The more her husband drank, the more she drank. She also found herself drinking wine while cooking dinner, as well as during and after the meal. She and her husband ate out three or four times a week and could consume one or more bottles of wine together during and after the meal. She stated, "It's a habit and it is causing me some problems."

The patient's husband did not drink every day, but he did drink at least 5 days a week. He drank mostly red wine, from one glass to a whole bottle. Occasionally, he drank whiskey, from one to several glasses. He thought that she had a drinking problem and wanted her to do something about it. He verbalized that he needed to stop drinking also, but he did nothing about it, and actually continued to encourage her to drink when he was doing so. The patient's 10-year-old stepson also thought that she had a drinking problem. He spent more time with her because his father worked long hours on the farm. The boy did not comment on his father's drinking.

The patient stated that drinking made her feel happier, less inhibited and more open. I asked her, "Compared to what? If you don't drink, do you feel less happy, less open, and more inhibited?" She replied that she wasn't sure, but that this was the way she thought about alcohol and about drinking. She further stated that she kept a lot inside and that she didn't express her opinions because her husband didn't listen anyway. As a result, she didn't talk to her husband about the way she felt.

The patient reported that she was usually the one who tried to "fix things and make them right" between her and her husband when there was conflict. She and her husband had gone for marital counseling about 2 years before she came to me. At that time, they saw a marriage counselor, a man, for a year, every 2 weeks, then once a month. Her husband's father reportedly was a brutal man, and her husband was also reported to be brutal "sometimes" and to be very "rough around the edges." He certainly did have some very hard mannerisms. The patient insisted that they see a marriage counselor, and she felt that her husband had agreed to do so in order to keep the marriage intact. During the counseling process, she felt that it was she who was repeatedly expected to make changes, whereas her husband did not make any. She felt that the marriage counselor seemed to be more on her husband's side than on her side.

The patient believed that her drinking allowed her to talk to her husband sometimes. I asked if her drinking might also serve to reduce her fear of her husband, to protect her marriage. I said "What would happen if you changed your drinking behavior and your husband didn't?" She felt that these were important questions, and she admitted that she considered alcohol to be a form of "bottled courage." She said that she felt some sense of relief and of fear, having had this verbalized. However, she also admitted that she was not sure what would happen and that she would have to think about it.

Following this admission, she went on to say that her husband was verbally abusive and that he also was a "workaholic." She then admitted that she did have a lot of anxiety, that she was constantly fearful and that she never felt relaxed, except perhaps when she drank a lot.

The patient reported that she had an escalation of feelings of panic and anxiety before her monthly period and during menstruation. She admitted to being unhappy and to having not told her husband recently about the extent of her unhappiness. He would listen sometimes to her expressions of anxious feelings, but he would make no comments. She obsessively cleaned house, did the dishes immediately after finishing a meal, and took classes to improve her cooking ability. She stated that she did these things "to keep busy" and also to please her husband.

We discussed why she might be working so hard to please her husband, and she answered that she was aware of the problems in their marriage, but that she was more afraid of being alone. She didn't want to try counseling again because she didn't believe it would help change her husband. She decided that she needed to deal with herself more appropriately and improve her own life within the marriage, and she wanted to start with her drinking problem. Apparently, both she and her husband had strong reasons for keeping the marriage together. He needed her for housekeeping and child rearing, and she needed him so as not to be alone.

She called me because of the smoking cessation success we had 5 years before. She was surprised that, with all of her problems, she had not gone back to smoking. She felt comfortable talking to me and trusted me.

As part of the waking state reframing process, I postulated that she had reverted to the use of alcohol because, in the past, she had used it to deal with her fears and anxieties. I explained that alcohol is a central nervous system depressant, and that it temporarily reduces anxiety and fear. However, the anxiety and fear come back stronger later, so more alcohol is needed. I told her that she was using the alcohol to feel relaxed.

Next, I asked the patient if she would like to learn to be relaxed and not anxious or fearful without the use of alcohol. She replied that this was exactly what she needed. I then reviewed the information about the conscious and unconscious minds, and told her that this time I would be teaching her how to do self-hypnosis so that she would be able to change how she felt and what she did. Time was running out in this initial session, so we set up another appointment for early the following week.

Session 2

At the beginning of her second visit, we discussed what I would be teaching her and what her responsibilities would be. We outlined a treatment plan and the rationale for each goal. The goals of treatment were as follows:

1. To immediately teach her self-hypnosis for the purpose of twice daily self-relaxation to calm her anxiety and fear. This daily self-relaxation would also help her feel more in charge and more self-confident. It would be a way for her to begin to treat herself with more care, with more dignity and with more self-love.
2. To teach her to use an instant-relaxation tool to remain in charge of her anxiety and mood between the practice of relaxation. This would help her to continue feeling relaxed and in charge by using something to hold onto (a marble) as a bridge to the memory of her deep relaxation experience, here in the office and when she did it herself.
3. To begin the gradual reduction of alcohol intake. Her self-hypnosis relaxation and instant relaxation practice would reduce her need to use alcohol as a way of dealing with her anxiety and fear.
4. To change her responses to her husband's verbal abuse and his lack of attention to her needs. It was suggested that, by changing her behavior, her husband might learn to behave differently. As she responded differently to his "button pushing," he would naturally be forced to look for a more positive way to reach her. Our rationale was that the patient's husband desired her compliance with his wishes; to earn it, he would have to learn to behave in ways that were acceptable to her.

I used the marble induction (see chapter 4) because there was a need to externalize this patient's fear and anxiety, to teach her self-hypnosis, and to give her instant control over the many daily stressors that exacerbated her drinking behavior. This was accomplished as follows:

Choose a marble from the large jar near you that you will have as your own. Pick a color, design, texture, and size that feels most comfortable to you. Notice that, as you hold that marble in your hand, you are smiling. Marbles produce an instant regression to a good memory from childhood, when there were not so many problems.

Once the patient was in deep relaxation, I continued with the following:

This deep relaxation that you are feeling, we call the "neutral place", the "healing place." It is very difficult to go directly from negative to positive. It is too big a leap. But it is easy to go from negative to neutral, then to positive. That is what is happening to you right now. All the negatives are being neutralized so you can make room for positives, here today and in the future.

This is also when the doorway to your unconscious mind opens. With your permission, I can give information to your unconscious that it can use to help you to feel better and for you to be in charge of you. Part of your being in charge of you involves your practicing self-hypnosis and relaxing yourself twice a day, in the morning and in the late afternoon, for about 10 to 15 minutes each time. You won't even have to pay attention to the time. Your mind will know when it is time to awaken and will help you do so.

You will relax yourself the way we did here in the office today, without using words to talk to yourself. The words that I say to you when we work together will be in the background, helping you remember how to use the marble to relax. Following your morning self-hypnosis, you will continue to feel very good throughout the day. Following your afternoon self-hypnosis, you will continue to feel very good throughout the evening.

By keeping the marble handy, you will be able to interrupt those anxious or fearful feelings, should they start to occur, within seconds, without even closing your eyes. Just play with the marble, or hold it in your hand, or imagine it in your hand and those negative feelings will immediately leave your body and your mind.

Soon I will ask you to slowly open your eyes, then open your hand and look at the marble and feel wide awake, yet continue to feel comfortably relaxed at the same time. This is also how you will awaken yourself when you do your own self-hypnosis. Now, open your eyes and be wide awake.

We discussed how she felt and her experience of being relaxed and in hypnosis. She commented that this was very different from her memory of hypnosis when she came to see me for smoking cessation. I explained that it was different because there were many more things that needed to be dealt with than the single behavior of no longer smoking.

I then asked her to put herself back into hypnosis without my help, using the marble once again, as she would be doing at home. I reminded her not to talk to herself, but to concentrate on the marble as her full focus of attention. I also told her that she would be able to awaken herself, when she decided to do so, the way we had just done.

She went quickly into trance again, remained with her eyes closed for about 7 minutes, then awakened herself with a smile and said, "That was so great. It was so easy." A third visit was scheduled for 1 week later, with the suggestion that I was as close as the phone if she had any questions.

Session 3

There were no calls from the patient between visits. After she was seated comfortably in a chair, she told me that she had practiced her twice-daily relaxation, accept on Saturday. She did notice a real difference in how she felt.

She woke up feeling much better and was drinking less. She had one glass of wine with dinner, instead of a bottle, and was not drinking during the day. Her head was clearer, and what her husband was saying to her seemed to "roll right off my back." It seemed to have stopped bothering her. She said that because she was thinking more clearly, she was aware that their treatment of each other was absurd and had to be changed.

I asked her to describe what she had been doing to relax at home. As she was telling me what she did, her successful transfer of the self-hypnosis procedure used in the office to her home was verbally reinforced. It was then suggested that she replicate that success by doing the same thing here in the office, and to say "okay" when she felt relaxed enough for me to talk once again to her unconscious. She said "okay" after about 5 minutes. She was then directed to continue to concentrate on the marble as a way of continuing to go even deeper into relaxation, while I gave more information to her unconscious that it could use to continue the process of change and help her to be more in charge. I suggested:

> As you continue to concentrate on the marble and listen to the sound of my voice, you will continue to go much deeper into relaxation, reaching that neutral place, that healing place. This allows you to continue to mature and change and be in charge—to go from whatever negative is left, to neutral now, to positive from now on.
>
> You continue to gain greater control over your alcohol intake, as you recognize that alcohol is no longer needed to help you to relax and feel confident. You have better and more positive ways of doing that. You continue to find it easier and easier to deal with your husband's behavior and not internalize it as yours. Be more aware that, as you become more comfortable being more confident, your husband communicates with you differently, and more kindly. Because you no longer reward his gruffness by being upset, he will change how he behaves to you from negative, to neutral, to positive.
>
> Continue to relax and enjoy your relaxation. When you do this by yourself, what I have been saying to you now will automatically be reinforced then, without your having to talk to yourself. When you have relaxed long enough, you can awaken yourself and feel great, rested and still very relaxed and very much in charge.

I scheduled her for a fourth appointment in 3 weeks, and reminded her that she could call if she needed to talk to me.

Session 4

She did not call during the 3 weeks between visits. During the fourth visit, she said that she felt like a new person. She was hardly drinking at all and was getting interested in doing gardening and planting vegetables. She regularly practiced self-hypnosis and was feeling energized so she was exercising longer.

She commented that she had a new positive friend, the marble, and had pretty much absented herself from her old negative friend, alcohol.

She said that her husband had voluntarily acknowledged that he tended to try to control her and that this wasn't a good way to behave toward her. He seemed to be less aggressive, but she acknowledged that she needed to wait and see whether this slight softening he demonstrated would continue. She wanted to stop coming in on a regular basis because she felt so much better about herself and her personal power. She would call me if she needed any further reinforcement.

She was asked to relax herself, using the marble, and to again say "okay" when she was ready for me to talk to her. The experience of deeper relaxation was suggested, as above. The successful changes that she had accomplished were reinforced, and it was suggested that those successfully changed ways of feeling and behaving would continue to grow stronger and more automatic and effective long into the future, as she continued to regularly include self-hypnosis in her daily routine. Upon realerting herself, she thanked me for helping her so much and said that she would call if needed.

SUMMARY

By now, readers can no doubt recognize the common themes that are part of the brief cognitive hypnosis treatment plan, and how basic approaches are individually tailored to apply to each patient's needs and personalities. The single-session and limited-session protocols recorded here also have been applied successfully to the problems of procrastination, studying for exams, increasing concentration, performance anxiety, and skill enhancement. Essentially, removing the intense emotional overlay that is a part of these negative behaviors and helping the patient to experience a relaxed state can be very powerful in controlling most anxiety-based dysfunctional behavior, whether simple or complex.

10

Panic Disorders and Other Complex Anxiety-Based Behaviors

This chapter will deal with more complex anxiety-based dysfunctional behaviors, including severe generalized anxiety, phobias, panic attacks, performance anxiety, obsessive thinking, obsessive-compulsive and dysfunctional ritual behavior, impulse control and mood problems. With the exception of patients with simple habit anxiety-based behavior problems who are treated in a single session, patients with more complex anxiety-based dysfunctional behaviors are taught self-hypnosis and relaxation skills. These new coping tools serve as "interrupters" of negative experience, and help in managing and changing a wide range of dysfunctional behaviors and uncomfortable situations.

Anxiety is a central feature of most psychological disorders and psychiatric illnesses (Kaplan & Sadock, 1981). If the experience of anxiety is chronic, persistent, and constant, then, once medical causes are ruled out (see below), it is probably diagnosable as a generalized anxiety disorder (American Psychiatric Association, 1994; Kaplan & Sadock, 1981). If the experience of anxiety is chronic but episodic and very intense, it is probably diagnosable as a panic disorder (see below).

The form the anxiety takes and the individual's pattern of symptoms are determined by the nature of the unconscious and conscious inner and outer objects of the patient's fears, as well as the complexity of the interactions and conflicts between the original sources of fear and the individual's continuing or evolving attempts over time to cope with them. A patient's specific anxiety symptoms are affected by (1) the particular inner drives, impulses, thoughts, feelings, and experiences he or she fears and (2) the consequences he or she fears if those experiences are expressed, acted out, or continue to occur (Kaplan & Sadock, 1981).

Complicating Medical Problems

If, during the intake evaluation, it is determined that the numbers and kinds of medical problems expressed by the patient may be the primary cause of the presenting problem, a referral to the patient's physician or to a physician, should be made for further medical evaluation, before treatment continues.

If the referring agent is a physician, prior medical and psychiatric work-ups and treatment need to be discussed with the physician so that the clinician/ therapist is thoroughly informed about the patient's prior medical history.

PANIC DISORDER

Perhaps the epitomy of complex anxiety-based dysfunctional behavior is panic disorder. Panic disorder with and without agoraphobia is a debilitating condition whose essential features are recurrent, unexpected panic attacks and the tendency to be overly concerned about having attacks (Antony & Swinson, 2000): "These rushes of fear, which seem to occur out of the blue, are associated with a number of intense physical symptoms as well as a feeling of impending doom" (p. 11).

As defined by the DSM-IV (American Psychiatric Association, 1994), a *panic attack* is a discrete episode of very intense fear and/or discomfort that starts abruptly, reaches its peak within approximately 10 minutes, and is accompanied by at least 4 of the following 13 somatic and cognitive symptoms: shortness of breath, dizziness, heart palpitations, trembling, sweating, feeling of choking, nausea/abdominal distress, depersonalization, paresthesias (numbness and tingling), flushes/chills, chest pain, fear of dying and fear of going crazy or fear of doing something uncontrolled.

Many of these somatic symptoms are also present in the other anxiety disorders we will discuss in this chapter. The motivation to avoid or ward off these uncomfortable experiences forms the basis for many of the dysfunctional behaviors that characterize these disorders. The etiology of the particular complex anxiety-based disorder that develops is influenced by a host of factors that are based on a vulnerability-diathesis-stress relationship (Cohen, 1974; Haynes, 1992; Kraemer et al., 1997).

Diathesis is defined as the inborn or constitutional predisposition of the organism that makes it vulnerable to developing a particular pathological condition when exposed to particular environmental stressors or experiences. The diathesis may include genetic predisposition, biochemistry, medical disease, an injury, learning experiences, cognitive and behavioral factors, trauma, and previous failures to cope (Maxmen & Ward, 1995; Rosenbaum et al., 1997). The stressors and precipitating experiences can involve biochemistry, medical disease, injury, trauma, learning experiences, imprinting, repetition and cognitive and behavioral factors.

To be eligible for the diagnosis of panic disorder, according to the DSM-IV, an individual must experience at least two unexpected panic attacks followed by at least a month of apprehension about experiencing another one. The frequency of attacks varies, ranging from several per day to several per year.

Panic disorder is a chronic condition that waxes and wanes in severity and that can begin at any stage of life. Unfortunately, most people with this condition do not receive appropriate or effective treatment and the severity of the condition severely restricts quality of life. The condition is associated with feelings of poor physical and emotional health, impaired social and marital functioning, financial dependency, and increased use of health services and hospital emergency services.

Panic Disorder with Agoraphobia

Epidemiological data suggest that approximately one-third to one-half of persons who have panic disorder also develop agoraphobia (Antony & Swinson, 2000). However, it is believed that the majority of people with panic disorder who do seek treatment present with agoraphobia.

Agoraphobia is defined as the experience of anxiety in situations in which escape is considered difficult and/or help is considered unavailable in the event of a pain attack, such as when being alone. Common agoraphobic situations include closed-in spaces such as planes, buses, trains, cars, elevators and crowds, as well as open spaces such as malls and the outdoors. Because the fear of having a panic attack tends to generalize to a wider and wider range of situations, it can eventually become associated with every situation conceivable. The individual then tends to become psychologically and behaviorally "paralyzed" by fear and restricted to the relative safety of the home. The agoraphobic individual's confinement to the home makes it exceedingly difficult to obtain appropriate treatment. Therefore, estimates of the prevalence of agoraphobia may in fact be underestimates.

COMMON ELEMENTS AMONG ANXIETY DISORDERS

Anxiety, fear, panic and even anger are fight or flight mechanism evokers. The physiological and biochemical processes that are initiated involve excitation of the central nervous system and the hypothalamic-pituitary-adrenal axis, which produces a surge of adrenaline. This signals the basic survival instinct in the brain to respond by either escaping the perceived source of the threat or danger (flight) or attacking (fight) in defense of the organism. The arousal of the instinctive fight or flight reaction usually includes complex physiological reactions, such as changes in breathing, muscle tension, stomach upset, greater intestinal motility, bowel and bladder irritability, elevated heart rate, heart palpitations and in̄ ͤͅsed startle and perspiratory response. If these responses are severe, the person may believe a heart attack is occurring. Accompanying emotional responses may include panic reactions. If this is so, these reaction patterns can evolve into phobias, obsessive thinking, obsessive-compulsive behavior and other negative coping behaviors.

THE BRIEF COGNITIVE HYPNOSIS MODEL OF ANXIETY-BASED BEHAVIORS

Simply stated, in terms of the brief cognitive hypnosis model, these physiological and biochemical responses, along with their accompanying emotional overlay, are the physical and emotional opposites of deep relaxation. When a person is deeply relaxed, these physical responses and types of negative emotional thinking are not present. The system is in repose and in balance and is not responding to an interpretation of danger to the organism.

There is a naturally occurring continuum of evolving complexity in anxiety responses. This means that when the anxiety condition of unconscious choice goes untreated and makes the individual's quality of life more and more dysfunctional, there is a natural tendency for the current anxiety-based condition to become more complex. The condition becomes transformed as it evolves into an anxiety condition of a higher level of complexity.

As we will illustrate later in this chapter, the crux of our treatment approach is to go back to and address the anxiety-based origins of the condition, taking into account the individual patient's unique needs and belief system.

A SCHEMA FOR CATEGORIZING ANXIETY RESPONSES

Based on our model, we categorize the evolving gamut of anxiety responses as follows:

1. *Generalized anxiety.* The label *Generalized anxiety* involves uncomfortable feelings, continual and obsessive worrying, misinterpreting a wide range of situations and circumstances as potentially threatening or dangerous and predicting possible future harm. Generalized anxiety can evolve into phobic behavior. The most common descriptors for the feeling state are "anxious," "worried," "nervous," "jumpy," "uncomfortable" and "afraid."
2. *Phobic behavior.* Phobic behavior is a label for anxiety that leads to running away or extreme avoidance of a dreaded situation or fearful object. The unconscious choice of the feared situation or object is usually imprinted into the unconscious during the initiating fight or flight experience, which may or may not be associated with a trauma of one type or another. A reason for the fear is searched for, and the setting or object that was present at the time of onset is usually identified as the source. Phobics tend to

externalize their anxiety feelings onto someplace, something, or someone else as the cause of their discomfort, so that the object of anxiety must be avoided at all cost. Avoidance then leads to the emergence of another form of anxiety called *anticipatory anxiety*, which occurs before an action that is interpreted as frightening, dangerous, threatening, uncomfortable, even if the feared consequences have never happened to the individual. For example, having never flown, someone may nevertheless develop a fear of flying. The most common descriptors are "phobia" and "fear of."

3. *Performance anxiety.* Performance anxiety may include problems of public speaking, loss of concentration and freezing by professional performers, difficulty concentrating and learning related to test anxiety and generalized social anxiety, or "social phobia." This category also includes sports under-performance problems and slumps by amateur and professional athletes. The individual may have felt comfortable and skilled in the past, then later developed fear and avoidance or may have been uncomfortable or afraid as far back as he or she can remember.

4. *Panic attacks.* The term *panic attack* is both a professional and a colloquial label for an extreme emotional interpretation of the sensations of fight or flight that are essentially internal and physical in nature, for example, the fear of having a heart attack, in which no causative environmental or definitive medical factor is identified. What is distinctive about this condition is that panic attack sufferers tend to internalize their anxiety feelings and attribute the danger or threat to their own body or themselves. (Descriptors include "I can't breath," "I'm having a heart attack," and "I'm going to lose control and go crazy or get hurt or die.")

5. *Obsessive thinking.* Obsessive thinking is a label for severe anxiety that involves gloom-and-doom thoughts that the individual cannot shut off, about self, other individuals or situations that may have already occurred or may possibly occur. It may include music or words or thoughts that are repeated ritualistically to ward off the possibility of calamity. There is a relationship of this type of ritualistic thinking to obsessive-compulsive behavior. Obsessive thinkers often believe that they are losing control or "going crazy" because they can't stop thinking about things, or can't stop repeating the verbiage or sounds in their head. This is an intense internalization process in which the auditory system is the major sensory information processing system. The thought process in these cases is usually verbal in nature. The most common descriptive labels are "obsession," "obsessing," "trapped" and the misuse in these circumstances of the label *phobia*.

6. *Obsessive-compulsive behavior.* Obsessive-compulsive behavior is a label for extreme anxiety that forces the individual into ritualized behaviors that are repeatedly acted out to ward off anxiety. The individual's experience is that somehow repeating the rituals will make him or her feel safe, and that not doing so will cause catastrophic consequences. Obsessive-compulsive

sufferers must act out their insecurities over and over again in order to quiet their feelings of anxiety and fears of pending doom. This form of dysfunctional behavior is an exaggerated evolution of the attempt to cope with and control extreme manifestations of anxiety. Unfortunately, it can further evolve and become intensely ritualistic. Rituals are sequences of behaviors that must be performed in the same way every time. They may be substituted for simple repetition when the fear element is directed to fear of the future. As we noted earlier, being able to predict what will happen next creates some sense of security.

Note that there is much overlap of the kinds of feelings, thoughts and behaviors experienced by anxiety sufferers. There is also a great deal of change in the form of coping behavior favored by the patient's unconscious as a result of an evolving system of increasing generalization and complexity. The behavior can change from one form of dysfunctional anxiety coping mechanism to another.

IMPULSE CONTROL DISORDERS: EXTERNALIZED AND INTERNALIZED

Impulse control disorders stem from dysfunctional ways of coping with unresolved feelings of jealousy, generalized anger, rage and mood problems. They include explosive behavior and short-duration extreme mood swings. They may be acted out verbally or physically or both verbally and physically. They also may be internalized and exacerbate or initiate serious medical problems. This latter issue will be addressed in chapter 11.

Patients who present for treatment of extreme mood behaviors, especially anger disorders (to a large extent patients with DSM-IV-diagnosable Axis II personality pathology) frequently find themselves in situations they interpret as being emotionally threatening. Many of these patients tend to get angry when they do not identify any serious physical danger to their well-being, yet feel wronged or narcissistically injured. They tend to be strongly opinionated and to overreact to any suggestion that judgments or opinions other than their own (which are often unstable or highly rigid) are possible.

These individuals externalize the cause of their feelings to someone or something else. For example, statements such as "You made me angry" and "That product was designed by a moron; no wonder I became angry" can lead to acting out the anger or frustration. Personal responsibility for the feelings is depersonalized through the defense mechanism of projection. This protects the individual from having to examine his or her own responsibility or culpability.

When the individual internalizes, as many do, the individual tends to become depressed as a result of feeling unable to react in a manner that is appropriate.

The individual becomes angry, then turns that anger against the self. This internalized anger is experienced as situational depression and involves feelings of guilt.

The label *losing (one's) temper* is applied to anger externalized when there is no apparent physical danger involved. It is often described as "having a short fuse." The anger also serves to control those at whom it is directed or who are present when it happens. The repeated expressed anger establishes a flinch reaction in those in close proximity, usually family members, and their resulting automatic responses are imprinted by repetition. These predictable responding behaviors are perceived by the person expressing anger as a reward for the anger behavior and produce a secondary gain and a ritualized pattern that further fixes the expression of anger in place. The expression of anger becomes "button pushing" and the repeated predictable response reinforces it.

People who have impulse control problems that are externalized are inclined to interpret the fight or flight response as requiring a fight response. People who internalize their anger and experience situational depression interpret the fight or flight response as requiring a flight response.

Readers may have recognized that, in the brief cognitive hypnosis model, we view anger and depression as opposite sides of the same coin. One side externalizes, and the other side internalizes. Both are anxiety based.

We do not treat major depression in our practices. However, referrals are often made by knowledgeable physicians who have prescribed medication for such problems. Their referrals ask us to address the frustration, emotional, behavioral, ego and self-esteem components, as well as the social problems that are an integral part of the depressive experience. We address all of these as well as the cognitive underpinnings of the dysfunctional coping behavior.

ANXIETY AS THE COMMON INITIATING ELEMENT

All of the coping behaviors described above have a single common initiating element. They are a response to the perceived experience of anxiety. They differ in that the dysfunctional behaviors presented for treatment are variant end products of the exacerbation of differently evolved unconscious behavioral response choices. However, the evolved presenting problem in every case is still anxiety based. Therefore, treatment begins by addressing the origins of the problem. We begin by directly addressing the original mechanism that required a coping response in the first place.

We will use phobic behavior as a prototypical example. However, any of the above problems can be addressed similarly, with some specific variations. As we progress into a discussion of each of the manifest evolved symptoms, we will point out the differences in treatment methods. Note that phobic behavior is frequently a precursor to a full-blown panic disorder.

Session 1: Intake Evaluation

During the *first session,* a full evaluation takes place, and the target problem is identified. To initiate waking state reframing, explain the concepts of the conscious and the unconscious minds, how the unconscious learns, what hypnosis is and what to expect during hypnosis.

Session 2: Waking State Reframing

A typical reframing (in this example, involving fear of going to a supermarker) would be the following:

It is apparent that you are afraid of [going to the supermarket] because of the way thinking about going makes you feel. Fear of any kind is an exaggerated anxious feeling that is very uncomfortable and that you naturally want to avoid. As you described when you first felt panic in the supermarket, you said that you didn't know what happened that made you afraid.

We talked earlier about the conscious and unconscious minds. Something happened at one time that alerted your unconscious to feel afraid. It could have been a noise that you didn't hear consciously or a flash of light that you didn't register, or even a momentary noxious smell that only lasted a second. The unconscious mind related it to something similar that upset you a long time ago that you may have forgotten. It triggered a safety response that is called the fight or flight mechanism.

As we were evolving as humans, way back in time, living in caves and creating civilizations, we were constantly in danger. The danger could have been from wild animals, other tribes, the weather or the environment. In order to survive, we had to develop an internal alarm system to alert us to danger so we could fight and protect ourselves or run away and save ourselves. As we have continued to evolve and control our environment, most of the things that were a danger to us once, are no longer present. But the fight or flight mechanism has not changed. We don't need it now except if we are in a dangerous profession like a police officer, fire fighter, soldier or doing other dangerous work or if we step off a curb and quicker than we thought possible we jump back on again to avoid being hit by a car. That was the fight or flight mechanism causing a pumping of adrenaline into the blood stream, epinephrine into the lungs, increased heart beat, muscle tension, change of breathing and an instant response to perceived danger.

Because you have been taught to look for reasons for what happens, your conscious mind, unable to identify a reason, chose the setting as being frightening to you. So you left the supermarket and felt better, then avoided going back because of a fear that returning would make you afraid again. We naturally avoid what we are afraid of.

The fact is, it was not the supermarket that made you afraid. It was something that you heard or saw or smelled, that you were not consciously aware of, that triggered a long forgotten memory of the feeling of fear, and this made you anxious.

The physical and emotional opposite of anxiety is relaxation. When you are relaxed, you can't be anxious, afraid, angry, frustrated, tense or stressed. There is no pumping of adrenaline. You are not afraid.

I am going to help you learn to deeply relax yourself by regularly practicing self-hypnosis and later learning instant relaxation. While you are experiencing relaxation here in the office with me, with your permission, I can give information to your unconscious to better understand which signals are dangerous and which are not. This will make it easier for you to discriminate and to change the way you feel and how you behave.

You will be taught how to relax yourself to feel more comfortable and confident and resourceful and to build a memory of those positive feelings that will allow you to feel relaxed and unafraid for longer and longer periods of time. This feeling of relaxation becomes your feeling of choice and the anxiety feelings go away.

Later, you will learn how to bring about a feeling of instant relaxation, with your eyes open, without anyone knowing you are doing it. This will allow you to prevent panic before it even starts, when you may be in a stressful situation.

You will do your own self-relaxation twice a day. In the morning, before you start most of your activities, for about 10 minutes, and in the late afternoon, before you start to prepare or eat dinner. If you plan to exercise, do your relaxation before you exercise rather than after. By doing it before, you will have more energy and be less tired. Initially, your only goal will be to learn how to relax yourself, without the need for self-talk.

Typical Trance Induction and Suggestions

A typical trance induction in the second session (using this same example) would be the following:

Sit comfortably in the chair, with your head supported and your feet flat on the floor. Now, gently close your eyes and pay attention to your breathing. Your eyelid fluttering that you may notice is an indication that you are going into the relaxed state that we call hypnosis. After a while you will no longer notice your eyelids fluttering, but you will notice your breathing start to change all by itself. It becomes deeper and more regular, then a little more shallow and more regular, as you go deeper into relaxation.

Concentrate on your breathing and allow yourself to go even deeper into relaxation. If your mind wanders, the moment you notice that you are thinking of something other than your breathing, bring your attention back to concentrating on your breathing. When you do this, notice that your mind wanders less and you feel even more relaxed.

Soon you will reach a level of deep relaxation that brings about a balance of your mind and your body. When mind and body are in balance during this kind of deep relaxation, there is no wasted energy on stress or distress. This relaxed place is called the neutral place, or the healing place. Because there is no wasted energy on anxiety or fear, all of that energy is available to the mind–body system to be used for healing and change.

There is another important thing about this neutral place. It is difficult to go from negative feelings and behaviors directly to positive feelings and behaviors. It is too big a leap. But it is very easy to go from negative to neutral and then to positive. This experience in the neutral place is one of internal peace and quiet and relaxation. It is without pressure or tension or fear. It is when healing can occur, because there are no stressors or feelings of anxiety present.

This peaceful, safe, calm feeling is imprinted as a memory in the unconscious, so it is present and available in the future. Being able to carry this memory into the future means that you now have choices that you didn't have before. You can recognize that you will be able to feel this new way, calm and peaceful, instead of the old way, fearful, so you are no longer trapped. Remember, you are only trapped as long as you believe that you have no choices. Once you recognize that you have another choice, and you make that choice, you are no longer trapped.

Teaching Self-Hypnosis

During the second session, as a continuation of suggestions following the induction and deepening, self-hypnosis can be taught, as follows:

While you are feeling comfortable and safe, and the doorway to the unconscious is open, with your permission I am going to teach you how to enter this relaxed neutral place all by yourself. As you did here today, sit in a comfortable chair where you can be alone and undisturbed. When you are seated comfortably, gently close your eyes. Pay attention to your breathing without trying to change your breathing. You may notice your eyelids fluttering. You may notice your breathing becoming deeper and more regular, then more shallow and more regular. Your body will feel more and more relaxed as you continue to concentrate on your breathing. If your mind wanders, bring it back to concentrating on your breathing. As you do this, as you did here today, your body will relax more and more deeply. You will recognize when you have entered the neutral place, the healing place, by your feelings of greater inner peace and comfort. When that happens, as it will, allow yourself to drift in deep comfort and calm for a while, enjoying the freedom from fear and the building of the memory of safety and inner calm.

When you feel you are ready to awaken yourself, you can do so, as I will be doing with you very shortly, by counting slowly from 1 to 5. With each number you count, you will feel more and more alert. With the number 5, you will open your eyes and feel wide awake, yet still feel very relaxed, peaceful and calm for some time.

Remember to relax yourself twice a day on a regular basis, until I see you next. This will help you to continue feeling calm and comfortable between your regular sessions of self-hypnosis. Now, I am going to count slowly from 1 to 5. With each number that I count, you will slowly become more aware of your environment and more awake. With the number 5, you will open your eyes and be fully alert. The feeling of calm, peace, and comfort will last long into the day and evening. 1—2—3—4—5. Eyes open and wide awake.

The usual posttrance discussion of the experience takes place with a review of the patient's responsibilities regarding regular practice and encouragement to call the therapist if there are any questions. Repeating the instructions of self-hypnosis after trance is almost as effective as having the patient go back into trance without help, immediately upon awakening from the initial trance state. If time doesn't allow for an immediate patient-initiated self-induction, repeat the instructions posttrance.

Relaxation Rreplaces Fear

Note that, during the second session, which covers the use of hypnosis and the teaching of self-hypnosis, no specific suggestions are given that directly address the specific fear (in this example, going to the supermarket). That is, no direct suggestions are given regarding the object of the patient's fear. No systematic desensitization rehearsals are practiced. No suggestions to test the effectiveness of the relaxation are made. The first goal for the patient is to learn that the body and mind can experience relaxation without thinking of, or feeling, fear. You can then help the patient to reproduce this comfortable experience independently. The feeling of freedom from fear can then be extended in time by the patient and strengthened by repetition.

The patient, without prompting from you, usually will test this newfound feeling of peacefulness when ready, and in a relatively short time. It is more effective for the patient to bring a story of success than to be challenged to do so. Sometimes the patient may not actually test the use of trance as a coping skill by immediately confronting the feared object, but may do so in his or her imagination for a while before actually going on site.

The use of the hypnosis trance state and posttrance imprinting of the self-hypnosis coping skills takes advantage of a number of phenomena that are incompatible with anxiety. We've already mentioned the phenomenon of relaxation. When we are relaxed, we cannot be afraid, anxious, frustrated, tense or stressed.

Another trance phenomenon is the experience of time distortion. In trance, a person's experience of time is distorted. Time can seem to pass much more quickly, or much more slowly, than it really is. We can use this property of trance to shorten the time it takes to treat a particular problem. Thus, when we use hypnosis to imprint feelings that are incompatible with anxiety, we often do not have to take as many steps to help a patient overcome the anxiety as we would if we were not using hypnosis. The cognitive and emotional reprocessing that takes place draws mainly on the "right brain" experience.

The traditional behavioral protocol for systematic desensitization is very "left brain." It is carried out in a hierarchy of discrete steps and takes place over a number of sessions (Wolpe, 1982). It is ritualistic and complex, having to be followed in a fixed sequence of behavioral steps, and involves the construction of a hierarchy of feared situations that are addressed in a fixed sequence. Every aspect of these situations that are deemed significant has to be included in the hierarchy. Even though it attaches the experience of relaxation to each feared situation (first in the patient's imagination and then in reality), systematic desensitization does not take advantage of the uniquely special phenomena of the hypnosis trance experience other than for relaxation.

Session 3: Review and Expansion of Suggestions

The third session starts with an exploration of the patient's compliance with the regular practice of self-hypnosis and an examination, in retrospect, of any changes in the patient's feelings and thoughts about himself or herself and the environment. This is important because very often patients are not able to discern that changes have occurred except in retrospect, that is, by looking back to recognize differences in feelings and behavior.

If you are told that there has been little change, retrospective examination of the patient's current experience and comparison with what it was like before is necessary. Do not accept a patient's blanket statement that no change has occurred. Examine each of the presenting behaviors and ask the patient if they are still present, or are less intense or have changed in their frequency of occurrence. Discuss changes that the patient can directly relate to the daily practice of self-hypnosis and the experience of relaxation. If there have been any problems of any kind, they should be discussed and resolved now, or schedules for practice may be renegotiated, if agreed upon schedules have been difficult to comply with.

During the third session, invite the patient to enter the trance state by initiating self-hypnosis as it has been done at home and to signal by a head nod or verbalized "okay" when sufficiently relaxed, so you can then take over and continue the trance dialogue. Use suggestions to pick up on the patient's descriptions of change, and tailor them to relate this change to future action by the patient (in this example, going to the supermarket). After the patient signals that it is okay for you to help the patient "go deeper" into hypnosis or trance, proceed as follows:

> Thank you. As you are sitting in the chair and are already relaxed and listening to the sound of my voice, pay attention to your breathing and allow yourself to continue to go even deeper into relaxation, deeper with each breath that you take and deeper with each word that I say, regardless of the meaning of those words. As you continue to feel more and more comfortable and enter into this neutral healing place, the doorway to your unconscious opens. Once again, with your permission, I have the opportunity to give more information to your unconscious that it can use to help you to continue to change the way you feel and what you do.
>
> You told me that you were feeling much calmer and more comfortable within yourself as a result of our last visit together and your daily self-hypnosis sessions. You also told me that you had gone to the supermarket and parked in the parking lot, but had not gotten out of the car to go inside. During the time you were in the car, you were able to quiet the feeling of fear that was present, but you weren't yet

confident enough to go the next step. You did very well. What you succeeded in doing was proof of your progress in taking charge of how you feel and changing how you feel. Now that you know you have the ability to quiet the fear, you can continue to build your confidence. Today you are in very deep hypnosis relaxation. As you continue your own self-hypnosis, you will continue to experience deeper calm and comfort. This will carry over to your taking the next step and entering the supermarket without being afraid.

As deeply relaxed as you are now, take a few very slow, deep breaths and experience how more relaxed it is possible for you to feel. That's right. Very slowly. Nod your head for me to tell me that you do indeed feel even more relaxed. Thank you.

If a few slow, deep breaths can relax you even more when you are this deeply relaxed already, think of how powerful they can be as an interrupter of the start of discomfort.

Stay in relaxation for a while longer, and enjoy the experience of quiet comfort and confidence. Allow the things that I have said to you to be imprinted in your unconscious mind, so that they can help you be in charge. When you decide you want to awaken, you can do so.

Discuss the patient's experience during this session, and verbalize how well the patient is doing. The patient may say that he or she feels so great that right now he or she could confront the former object of fear without a thought of being afraid. If this is verbalized, suggest that this will certainly be the case when the patient decides to do just that. You can then schedule a fourth session in 1 or 2 weeks, suggesting that the patient call before the next visit if he or she has any questions. If the patient calls before the following visit expressing satisfaction about the changes experienced, and asks if it is okay to cancel the next appointment with the understanding that he or she can call if necessary, we agree. At that point, the patient usually thanks us for all of our help.

VARIATIONS AS APPLIED TO OTHER ANXIETY-BASED SYMPTOMS

Generalized anxiety, as you already recognize, may be treated with the same approach as described above, without specific reference to a chosen external object of fear, because the anxiety is pervasive, or "free floating." With generalized anxiety, however, there is a difference because there are a number of internalized feelings that become exaggerated. This is because the externalized objects of fear are vague and the feelings of fear are generally internal. They may vary from low level to more intense, depending on the patient's changing levels of awareness. There are usually more worrying thoughts than there are with the more focused phobic problem. These are patients who, like problem eaters, have some difficulty identifying the messages of their own bodies and thus tend to worry more.

An induction that allows the patient to gain a better understanding of his or her bodily messages while also focusing on externalizing the constant anxiety is desirable. Therefore, you will want to employ a kinesthetic and visual trance induction approach. Note that the previous induction for phobic behavior involved only attention to breathing. That is, the patient was asked to close his or her eyes and concentrate on his or her breathing. With generalized anxiety, add the eye fixation element for externalization and the attention to breathing for increasing awareness of body messages.

Case Study: Generalized Anxiety

A 46-year-old male accountant was referred to me (JIZ) by his physician because of high blood pressure that was not being adequately controlled by medication. There was no prior history of heart disease in the patient's family, and his blood pressure had been fairly normal until the previous year.

The intake evaluation revealed information that had not been discussed with his doctor. The patient was expanding his accounting practice and found that the increased financial demands were making him hesitant about having done the right thing. In addition, he found himself procrastinating and dreading going into the office. It was experienced as continuing anxiety and feelings of guilt because he was not doing what was needed to accomplish his stated goals. He had not shared these concerns with his wife or family, but had used the high blood pressure as his "medical problem" responsible for any difficulties he may have had at work. We decided that we needed to deal with his generalized anxiety, high blood pressure, procrastination, and guilt.

Note that this problem included, besides generalized anxiety, performance anxiety, procrastination, somatization (high blood pressure), worrying and guilt feelings. Rarely does a patient present with a problem that is not multifaceted.

Session 1

The usual waking state reframing started with a discussion of the various target behaviors that were to be addressed. The conscious and unconscious minds were explained. The concept of hypnosis and relaxation were discussed, with emphasis on relaxation being the opposite of anxiety and how self-hypnosis would put him back in charge. We discussed the patient's perfectionism and consequent guilt as a result of his not performing perfectly. I explained that these feelings were responsible for his procrastination and feeling trapped. He asked about his health problem, his high blood pressure, and was informed that he would feel much better quickly because the learning of relaxation would help his medication to work more efficiently and give him more control over how he felt. Because our time had run out, we made an appointment for him to come in again later in the week to experience hypnosis and learn self-hypnosis.

Session 2

When the patient returned for the second session, he was asked to describe to me what he thought about our earlier session together. He said that he felt encouraged and had tried to identify the various physical feelings that he had when he procrastinated and felt guilty. He described that he felt tightness in his chest and that his heart seemed to beat louder. This recognition was new because he had never really tried to be this specific before. I explained that he would be able to identify more of his feelings as we continued and that he would be able to recognize the contrast between anxiety and relaxation.

He was asked to sit back comfortably in the chair and look at an object not too far away. The eye fixation and attention to breathing induction was initiated, with the patient very quickly closing his eyes, with much eyelid fluttering. He quickly went deeper as he concentrated on his breathing. I encouraged him to control his wandering mind by bringing his concentration back to his breathing and going deeper into relaxation every time his mind wandered and he returned his attention to his breathing. I then delivered the following trance state suggestions:

> The purpose of this hypnosis–relaxation experience today is to introduce you to how it feels to be relaxed and not anxious and not trapped. You are trapped only as long as you believe that you have no choices. Once you are aware that there is another choice, and you make that choice, you are no longer trapped. Deep relaxation, as you are already recognizing, is such a choice. Notice also that it is easier to concentrate and your mind wanders less. As your mind wanders less, you relax even more. It is interesting that, with each mind wander, you relax more and with each control of that wandering, you relax more." [This is a double bind suggestion: Succeed if you don't and succeed if you do.]
>
> While experiencing this deep relaxation, the feelings of anxiety and guilt are no longer present. Look inside and feel the difference. Be aware that the tightness is gone and the breathing is more regular. Nod your head when you recognize this. Thank you. That's great. Build a memory of what it feels like to be deeply relaxed and free of anxiety and guilt. I am going to teach you, as we had discussed, how you can do this by yourself to continue to imprint the choice of relaxation over fear.

This may be viewed by the reader as substituting one feeling for another. Although we made a point of talking about not substituting symptoms, here we are replacing a negative experience and memory with a positive experience and memory. The fact that the patient is an accountant is important to this approach. He is concerned with making sure that things add up. This approach fits right into his way of thinking. Remember that it is essential to individualize the treatment to meet the way the patient processes information.

> You will be able to experience, this deep relaxation not only when we are working together here in my office but also at home or at your office twice a day. When you get to the office a little earlier, as we had agreed you would do, silence the

phone, close your door, and sit comfortably in a high-backed chair. Look at something not too far away as you did here today, and notice your eyes blinking faster and your breathing start to change. When your eyelids feel heavy, gently close your eyes without squeezing them tight. Then concentrate on your breathing and feel yourself going very deeply into relaxation, as your mind wanders less and your breathing deepens and your concentration improves. Stay that way for a while, allowing yourself to enjoy feeling so comfortable and quiet inside. This will help you build and strengthen the memory of feeling peaceful and relaxed that will last for a long time during the day.

You will be awakening yourself, the way I will be doing shortly, and feel really great. Then, late in the afternoon, before you leave for home or after you get home, do the same thing and extend this good feeling long into the evening.

You will notice that this feeling of calm and improved ability to concentrate will replace the tendency to procrastinate. In fact, you will find yourself eagerly doing whatever needs to be done, and you will feel more in charge and satisfied than you have in a long time. This newfound energy is a direct result of the replacement of the anxiety with the experience of feeling relaxed. There will be no wasted energy on stressful feelings, so that reserve of energy can be used to be more productive.

Now, I am going to awaken you from this deep relaxation and hypnosis by slowly counting from 1 to 5. This is what you will do, silently when awakening yourself. With each number, you will be more and more awake and aware. With the number 5, you will open your eyes and feel very peaceful and comfortable for a long time. 1—2—3—4—5. Eyes open and wide awake.

We discussed his experience, which was very positive and encouraging. It was suggested that he not check his blood pressure, because he would be seeing his doctor during the following week, when it would be checked. We made another appointment for a few days after the appointment with his doctor. He was advised to practice self-hypnosis twice a day, without self-talk, and to call me if he had any questions.

Session 3

The patient returned about 2 weeks later following his appointment with his doctor. His blood pressure was within normal range, and he was to monitor it once a week to report to his physician. He was feeling little or no anxiety and guilt. He was actively getting his work done and making plans to hire someone with bookkeeping experience to help him in the office. He had said that one of the reasons money was a worry was because he did not bill his clients quickly enough. This past week he had sent out all of his bills.

He reported that he had done self-hypnosis twice a day, except this past Saturday, when his family went out for a day of recreation. He enjoyed how it felt and was pleased at the changes. I congratulated him on his successes and encouraged him to continue to do self-hypnosis regularly, even after his problems were long gone. By doing this, not only would he be in charge and feel good, but he would eventually be able to reduce the dosage or eliminate the medication as his doctor saw his blood pressure stabilize. I also said that I believed that he would be more successful in his business because he would be able to apply himself in a more focused manner to a more productive work schedule.

I instructed him to sit comfortably in the chair and relax himself as he had been doing at his office and at home. When he felt he was as deep as he could go, he was to say "okay" to signal me to help him go deeper into hypnosis. When he did this, after about 5 minutes, I took him deeper by counting slowly from 20 to 1. Then I repeated all of the positive changes that he had been aware of and suggested that they were the foundation for his continuing success. I instructed him to add the 20-to-1 countdown to his self-hypnosis practice so he could deeply imprint his peacefulness and comfort and continue to improve his health. I then asked him to awaken himself. We discussed his experience and where we should go from here.

The patient stated that he wished to make another appointment in a month, to make sure everything was working. I agreed, and again reminded him that I was as close as the telephone. His doctor called me 3 weeks later and stated that the patient was doing very well. He thanked me for a job well done. The patient called a few days before his appointment and asked if I felt it would be okay if he canceled it. He was doing well and said he would call if he needed any help. He thanked me for teaching him how to take better care of himself.

The preceding cases were chosen for their quick response to treatment. Not all cases are resolved as quickly, however. Some require up to 10 visits to bring about the desired changes. Every clinician has patients who are not as willing to give up the strong support and dependency that often occurs through the transference process. Such cases may linger for some time, for support, encouragement and cathartic release. As new problems arise, these patients may come back for reinforcement of their learned coping skills to be directed toward resolving new discomforts.

OBSESSIVE THINKING

Obsessive thinking generally comes in two forms: repetitive "doom and gloom" thinking and ritualistic obsessive thinking. We will deal with "doom and gloom" thinking first.

Repetitive "Doom and Gloom" Thinking

Repeated "doom and gloom" thinking is depression related and one of the ways that people internalize anxiety. Expecting the worst and not being able to recognize the possibility of a better future are forms of feeling trapped. These individuals not only think negatively most of the time, but they also frequently verbalize their negative thoughts to others. This constant talking about how terrible everything is usually causes friends and family to avoid contact. This can further reinforce the feeling and belief that the person is not wanted or liked. It becomes a self-fulfilling prophecy.

These patients should be encouraged to externalize their negative beliefs by using half a session to express their anger at all the bad things they feel and expect. The other half of the session can be used for extensive waking state reframing. Reframing in this context involves discussion of the nature of depression. This could be done during the second session, with the first session being intake and evaluation.

> Depression is the internalization of anger. The more you send anger inside, the more thoughts become negative. Negative thoughts are a way to safely express the anger that is now experienced as depression. Depressed people cannot escape from believing that everything is bad, because they feel trapped. Feeling trapped means believing there are no choices available that could change the situation. That is your belief, but it is not true. It is distorted by your depression. Medication can help the depression, but medication doesn't change thinking that you are trapped.
>
> That way of thinking is a habit fed by repeated internalized anger. The feeling of anger can be changed. Feeling relaxed is the opposite of feeling angry. You don't have to give up your feeling of loss that may have sparked the anger and depression. But the feeling of loss can become a warm feeling of what was rather than an angry, self-punishing feeling of what isn't.
>
> Would you give us, together, the opportunity to demonstrate that what I have been saying to you is true? If you agree, you can first experience deep relaxation and how good it feels, then learn how to do this yourself to change the way you think and feel and become untrapped. Think about the possibilities this might allow. Is it okay to make another appointment to prove what I am saying?

The third session typically involves the explanation of the conscious and unconscious minds and about what to expect during hypnosis for relaxation. An induction using the marble (see chapter 5) can be used to allow the internalized anger to leave the mind and body and flow down the arm to the hand and into the marble, then dissipate into the air. In the same way that the marble absorbs warmth from the body and becomes warm itself, the marble can absorb negative thoughts and feelings and safely release them into the air. Using the marble for concentrating on something outside of oneself helps to externalize the angry feelings and quiet the repeated negative thoughts. Self-hypnosis and self-relaxation using the marble should be taught and the patient should be instructed to practice every day, twice a day, until the next session.

During the fourth session you will want to have the patient initiate the relaxed state, which you can then deepen. Validate and reinforce the patient's report of whatever changes have been experienced. Encourage the regular use of self-relaxation and the expectation of better and better feelings and thoughts of the present and the future. Suggest that, if the patient looks deeply inside, he or she will already be aware that the "loss" is less angry and more caring and warm. The memories are of good times with whatever or whomever was lost, and although these memories may produce tears, they are tears of past happiness, not tears of anguish. A fifth and sixth session may be needed to support and reinforce the new ways of thinking and feeling, and deal with the concern that "this just won't last."

This protocol is applicable in cases of unresolved and complicated grief.

Ritualistic Obsessive Thinking

There are two kinds of ritualistic obsessive thinking. As addressed earlier, one kind is obsessing about some specific problem, such as overeating. This is dealt with by addressing the behavior that is considered the problem, not the obsessive thoughts directly. The ritual is the repetitive behavior, such as overeating, with the thoughts (in this case, food) a secondary issue. A second type of ritualistic thinking is often exhibited as repetitive words or music that the patient cannot seem to get out of his or her head. This involves thought patterns that are an attempt, without conscious awareness, to deal with some unidentified auditory stimuli that were interpreted at some time by the unconscious as threatening.

In the extreme, this may be schizoid in nature and may require antipsychotic drug therapy. Interestingly, less intense specific ritualistic thinking is a common experience that many people have from time to time. On the normal end of the continuum, it can be transient and not bothersome. However, if it is persistent, there may some accompanying obsessive-compulsive behavior that develops. Such behavior does not necessarily evolve into an exaggerated form that becomes identified as a serious dysfunctional problem.

Ritualistic obsessive thinking is anxiety based and an attempt to feel more comfortable. Caught early, it can be treated as an auditory expression of unrecognized anxious feelings. The brief cognitive hypnosis approach involves the use of relaxation training and the suggestion for interruption of the thoughts by consciously changing them with concentration on each breath that brings more relaxation. Additionally, full concentration on breathing, or on an object held in the hand, such as a marble, can serve as a coping skill to interrupt the thoughts and "quiet the head."

Thought stopping (yelling as loud as you silently can the word *stop*) has been found to be helpful and effective. It can be introduced during waking state reframing, then repeatedly suggested during the trance state. It is often a convincing demonstration to the patient of his or her ability to stop bothersome thoughts (Cautela & Wisocki, 1977).

OBSESSIVE-COMPULSIVE BEHAVIOR

This is the most complicated form of the evolving outcome of an anxiety response to a perceived threat. Because of its complexity, extensive ritualistic treatments have been created to extinguish this dysfunctional behavior. As was indicated, there are essentially two forms this takes. *Repetitive behavior* and *ritual behavior* are the two ways that they may be manifest.

Repetitive Behavior

Behavior repetition such as frequent hand washing, or returning to make sure the lights are out and the door is locked are considered "incomplete rituals." That is, they do not fulfill the needs that rituals are designed to satisfy; namely, the ability to predict the future in order to feel secure. Because they are incomplete, and do not fill in the gestalt requirements of "closing the circle," or the loop, they are repeated until they do, even when the gestalt is only transient until the next time (e.g., as in "clean," germ-free, uncontaminated hands).

In the completed ritual circle or loop, closure occurs, whereas, with incomplete repetitive behavior, there are a series of only temporary closures, requiring repeated attempts at closure. In fact, that is the motivation, or "pay-off," for repeatedly repeating the behavior. However, because the ritual is not complete, and thus fixed in place, the resolution of the problem behavior may in fact be easier to accomplish.

Instead of developing extensive therapeutic rituals or tasks, such as thought stopping, to take the place of these incomplete compulsive dysfunctional behaviors, our approach is to go back to the "root of the problem," which is to treat the basic, initial anxiety.

Case Study: Compulsive Repetitive Behavior

A 39-year-old single male office manager was referred to me (JIZ) by his primary care physician because prescribed medication did not seem to be helpful in alleviating the the patient's compulsive repetitive behavior problem. The patient did not want to be referred to a psychiatrist for further medication "experimentation" because of his concern over possible medication side effects and the stigma of psychiatric treatment.

During the first visit, after the initial evaluation was completed, the waking state reframing process included an explanation of the conscious and unconscious minds and a description of hypnosis. Then the problem and treatment approach were explained to the patient, as follows:

> Sometime in the past something happened that alerted your unconscious to possible danger. You may or may not have been consciously aware of being frightened.

If you were aware of being afraid at the time, now that time and place and cause may be lost in memory. Do you remember anything that may have happened to you a long time ago that frightened you? It is okay that you don't remember, because by now whatever did happen is far in the past. We are going to help you change the result of that no longer present cause of your problem.

Your need to go back again and again to make sure everything is okay is your way of trying to assure yourself that nothing bad will happen. This behavior, which ties you up and causes you so much discomfort, is the present form, much exaggerated, of what you may have felt when that first fear message was picked up by your unconscious. It is like getting an infection that caused you only slight discomfort and wasn't treated, but which then became a major infection. The treatment for either form of the infection is still the same, it just takes a little longer to eliminate, because it wasn't treated earlier.

You will be taught a form of self-hypnosis, self-relaxation, that you will experience here in the office, then practice at home, just as you might take medication every day to control an infection.

This need to repeat behaviors is an attempt to control fear. Fear is an expression of anxiety that causes adrenaline to pump into your bloodstream, causing breathing changes, muscle tension, a problem swallowing, and tightness in your chest. You feel uptight. The opposite of anxiety, physically and emotionally, is relaxation. When your body and mind are relaxed, you do not feel anxious, afraid, tense, or uptight.

Because we will not have enough time left today to teach you to relax yourself deeply, what I will do is help you experience what it feels like to be relaxed and without fear, so you will have a better idea of what the future holds. We have been sitting here and talking together for a while, and you seem to be much more comfortable than you were when you first came into the office. Do you notice that? You are already beginning to let go of your fear because you are already beginning to feel more comfortable, just as a result of our talking together and my explaining some things to you. Isn't that so? Very good, so let us take it one step further.

Gently close your eyes and pay attention to your already more comfortable breathing. Notice that with your eyes closed and eyelids fluttering slightly, your feeling of being more relaxed is more apparent. Very good. You can now recognize that your body has let go of most of the tension you had felt earlier. By the way, if I ask you a question or make an observation that is true, and you want me to know that it is true, just nod your head for me. Thank you.

Enjoy this first experience of feeling relaxed and mostly free of fear. Let it build as a memory in your mind and in your body that you can freely borrow between now and the next time we get together. All you have to do, if you feel tense, is stop for a moment, pay attention to your breathing without closing your eyes, and notice that you feel less tense and less afraid. This is the beginning of your ability to take charge of how you feel and change the way you feel. During the next visit, you will learn to relax yourself even more deeply and feel even better. Now, just gently open your eyes and tell me what it was like to feel this much better.

The patient's experience was discussed and the positive outcome of the quick trance experience was reinforced. The patient was instructed to use attention to breathing as a temporary quick return to some level of comfort when needed. He was told that this might not stop the behavior repetition entirely, but that it would certainly reduce it and generally help the patient to feel more comfortable and less trapped. Another appointment was made for later that week to continue the patient's learning of controls and comfort.

Session 2

When the patient returned for his second session, he was asked to describe what the past few days had been like. Usually, the response is positive and includes a description of some reduced repetition and less feelings of anxiety, as it was in this case.

(If the patient had said that he felt no difference, I would have responded:

We only recognize change in retrospect, that is, thinking back to before your last visit and comparing how you felt and what you did then with your present experience. When you do that, are you aware of any difference in how you feel now and what you have been doing since your last visit?

This approach usually evokes some acknowledgment of positive change. In either case, the patient is told that what he experienced was positive and is the beginning of the change process.)

It was then explained that today he would be taught to go deeply into relaxation, for greater relief and how to practice this greater relaxation without help from me. The induction employed was an eye fixation and attention to breathing (see chapter 4), which emphasizes greater awareness of internal feelings and neutral thoughts. The patient was told:

Sit comfortably in the chair and pick something in front of you to look at. Choose something that will allow your eyes to fully see in its totality. You might choose to look at the creamy mineral ball on the windowsill or the small cactus plant there. Which seems to be better for you? The large creamy crystal ball; that is a good one. Fix your eyes on the crystal ball, and notice that your eyelids start to flutter, as your breathing begins to change. When your eyelids get heavy, gently close your eyes and concentrate on your changing breathing—deeper and more regular, then more shallow and more regular as you go deeper into relaxation.

Your breathing was one of the first things you noticed when you were feeling afraid. That part of your chest was the center of your discomfort. But, it is not like that now. Notice how comfortable your chest is now, how even your breathing is, and how this is very different from when you were experiencing anxiety. Remember that relaxation is the emotional and physical opposite of anxiety, fear and tension. Being relaxed and going deeper into relaxation with each breath that you take and each word that I say also means imprinting the feeling of relaxation in your unconscious mind. This more recent memory of relaxation instead of fear is the memory that will be available to you from now on.

You will be able to keep this memory and these comfortable feelings foremost in your mind, consciously and unconsciously, by practicing your own self-relaxation every day, twice a day.

Find a time before you leave the house for the day, about 10 minutes will be enough. Sit in a comfortable chair by yourself, in a quiet place and look at something not too far away. Fix your eyes on that object and notice that your eyes start to blink more frequently, as they did here today. Notice your breathing change and become deeper and more regular, then more shallow and more regular, as you feel the tension drain from your body. Your chest becomes more comfortable and you feel very relaxed. Stay in deep relaxation for a while, enjoying the experience. Build the memory of relaxation, the freedom from fear, and the release from the need to repeat yourself unnecessarily. That's right, it is no longer necessary to behave in the old way. The occasional thought of doing so is recognized as a memory remnant from the past that no longer has validity. Think about the meaning of what I just said to you. Your unconscious understands that you can be free from the need to keep checking to be sure that all is well. You can feel at peace as the feeling of peacefulness continues to be stronger and more present as you practice your own relaxation.

When you relax yourself at home, before you leave for the day, when you feel ready, you can awaken yourself, as we will do shortly, by counting slowly and silently from 1 to 5. With each number you count, you will be more and more alert, yet relaxed at the same time. When you reach the number 5, you will open your eyes and feel really great—getting up and going about your business, leaving the house feeling free and comfortable, doing what needs to be done once, and feeling relief as you let your breath out and leave your house safely behind you.

Your day will continue to feel relaxed and more productive throughout the day. Late in the afternoon, before you prepare to leave for home, find a quiet place to do your self-relaxation again. After you awaken yourself, notice how easy it is to leave your office behind and drive home in peace.

There may be occasional thoughts of repeating something. These remnant memories of the past, if they occur, will be fleeting. Paying attention to your breathing, should they occur, will continue to be helpful in sending them away quickly.

Now, I am going to count slowly from 1 to 5 to awaken you from this very deep relaxation experience here in the office. When you open your eyes, you will still be able to feel how comfortable you are, for the rest of the day. You will practice on your own before you leave your office today. 1—2—3—4—5. Eyes open, alert and awake, and still relaxed.

The patient shared his enjoyable deep relaxation experience and was then asked to go back into relaxation by himself. I sat back and observed while he took charge and experienced his own skill in doing this by himself. I told him that, when he felt very relaxed, he was to drift in deep relaxation for a while, then awaken himself with the slow, silent count from 1 to 5. The patient took about 8 minutes to complete this task, and upon opening his eyes expressed his pleasure at how easy it was. This success was reinforced as a posttrance suggestion with the comment that "this is what you will be able to do every time you do your own self-hypnosis to relax yourself at home, at the office, or anywhere."

A third appointment was scheduled for a week later. The patient was encouraged to practice regularly and to call if he had any questions.

Session 3

The patient returned 1 week later and did not call in the interim. He said that he had been almost completely repetition free and had done self-hypnosis every day, twice a day, with the exception of one day when he had to go to a meeting with a visiting client. He noticed that he still had not engaged in the unwanted repetitive behavior, but that he had thought about it more. The attention to his breathing, however, had been helpful in reducing and controlling these thoughts.

I complimented him on his success and asked him to describe what he did to relax himself and if there was any difference between his home relaxation and his office relaxation. His description was similar to the way he had been taught. He said that it took him longer to relax on his own at his office because of his concern that he might be interrupted. I explained that this was common and that today I would teach him how to go even deeper into relaxation and eliminate any concern about being interrupted.

I asked the patient to relax himself as he had been doing. When he felt relaxed enough, he was to say "okay." On his signal, I took him deeper into relaxation by counting slowly from 20 to 1. When I reached the number 1, I suggested that he could add this countdown to his own practice of self-hypnosis to go deeper into relaxation; by doing so, he would remove the remnants of past memories of anxiety. While he was in trance, I reviewed his success and complimented him on it. I gave him further suggestions regarding the value of the countdown for creating more extended feelings of peace and personal power. I said, "You are in charge." After awakening, we then arranged for another session in 2 weeks, and I instructed him to call in the interim if he had any questions.

Eight days later, after two weekends had passed, the patient called very upset because he had started the compulsive repetitive behavior again the day before. On the telephone, I suggested that he stop for a moment and pay attention to his breathing to calm down, then tell me what had happened. He stated that he was involved in a minor car accident over the weekend, and that he had received a ticket for going through a yellow light that had turned red while he was in the intersection. He was cited for causing the accident, and he became very upset. The repetitive compulsive behavior started again when he got home, slowly, then became as intense and frequent as it had been before.

I asked him if his attention to his breathing was helping him now and he said yes. He said my voice also seemed to help a lot. I suggested that we make an appointment for the next day, and that when he got off the phone, he should deeply relax himself and remain in deep relaxation a little longer than he had been doing. This would help quiet things down at the moment, and we would be able to correct any mistakes that were made when I saw him the next day.

Session 4

The patient came in the next day for his fourth session, and we discussed his first encounter with a stressful situation since we began working together. He stated that, after our phone conversation, things had improved. He wasn't repeating the behavior, but he was worrying that he would. I explained that he had not generalized his ability to relax and control his anxiety to things other than his stated problem. The stress from the accident and ticket had brought back the intense feeling of anger at himself, which he identified as anxiety and the problem returned. It was like having a flashback. I explained that this was not unusual early in treatment. When he became upset, he made a mistake and misinterpreted his feelings as being the same as before, so he became afraid and the behavior that he had control over returned.

The patient thought that he had failed. The label *failure* took him back to the mental state when he had a problem, so the problem seemed to return. I used the *"Labels Dictate Behavior"* reframe described earlier in chapter 2 and said:

The labels we place on the behavior we do dictate future behavior.

I explained that he had made a mistake because he misinterpreted the feeling of stress that he was experiencing from the accident as being the same as when he used repetitive behavior to reduce his discomfort. I told him that the feeling of upset that he had from the accident was *specific* to the accident. It was not related to what he had been experiencing. Mistakes can be corrected and we were going to correct his today.

He was asked to relax himself and to include the countdown from 20 to 1. When he felt sufficiently relaxed to have me talk to him, he was to say "okay" to signal me. About 5 minutes passed before he said "okay." i went on to say:

Now that you feel sufficiently relaxed, allow my voice to take you even deeper into relaxation and hypnosis. You will go deeper into relaxation with each breath that you take and each word that I say, regardless of the meaning of those words. You will recognize this deeper level of relaxation by being aware that whatever residual physical and emotional tension that you had is leaving you. It is draining out of your body, leaving you feeling loose and comfortable, very relaxed and peaceful inside.

Be aware of how quickly this peacefulness took place, how quickly you were able to recognize that you felt at peace, without anxiety and without fear. This is because the memory of freedom from fear is deeply imprinted and easily available to you. The label relaxation now means "freedom from fear." So, every time you do deep or instant relaxation, you reexperience freedom from fear. Even just paying attention to your breathing while recognizing that stressors are present will produce enough relaxation to bring freedom from fear.

Continue to enjoy this deep relaxation, and allow the things that I have said to you to be imprinted deeply in your unconscious mind. Every time you practice deep relaxation, or produce instant relaxation, or think the word relaxation, you will automatically reinforce what I have been saying to you while you and I have been talking together and while you and I have been working with hypnosis together. Because the change suggestions will be reinforced automatically, you do not have to talk to yourself during your own relaxation. You do not have to give yourself suggestions for change. All you have to do is enjoy the experience of relaxation and allow it to work for you to put you in charge.

Now I am going to back off and leave you in relaxation for a while. When you feel you have relaxed long enough, you can awaken yourself. After you open your eyes, you will feel great, fully awake, yet peaceful and comfortable inside.

When the patient opened his eyes, we again talked about his experience in trance and continued posttrance suggestions regarding his deep relaxation experience and how his continuing to do self-hypnosis would continue to fully imprint the process of change and his personal power to be in charge. Another appointment was made for 2 weeks later. The patient stated that he felt that he would not have any more problems.

Session 5

The patient came in for his fifth session 2 weeks later. He told me that he had contacted a lawyer, and the traffic accident had been handled with a paid fine, traffic school, and no points on his license. He had to appear in court and did so without anxiety. His insurance company took care of the costs less his deductible, but he suspected that the company would raise his insurance costs.

We discussed how he had been using deep relaxation and attention to his breathing for ongoing comfort. He said he was very impressed with his success in no longer having to repeat the compulsive behavior, but that he wanted to see me on a further extended basis, perhaps once a month, until he felt totally secure that the problem would not return. I agreed that this would be okay.

I asked the patient to relax himself again, and to let me know when it was all right for me to again talk to him. He said "okay" after a while, and I talked about the deep relaxation he was experiencing as the "healing place" that he could enter every time he did his own self-hypnosis.

In the healing place, there is no wasted energy on stress and distress, so all the energy is available to be used for healing, for growth, and for ongoing change.

I went on to suggest that the patient's practice of deep relaxation, attention to breathing, and thoughts of relaxation would continue to be fixed in place as a way of producing and accessing his inner peace, thus eliminating the need to repeat compulsive behavior as a way to be comfortable.

The patient came in for two more sessions a month apart, and we did the same thing regarding reinforcement, the healing place, and administering encouragement for building confidence in his own power. He did not experience problems during the 2 months, and we decided to set up another session for a month later, which he could cancel if he wanted. A week before his scheduled appointment, he called and canceled. He thanked me, and has sent me holiday greetings every year since.

RITUAL BEHAVIOR

Everyone who is able to stay well and successfully negotiate this complicated world does so by using ritual behavior. Rituals help us to maintain order, keep on schedule, take care of ourselves, do our work and reduce stress. Pocket planners, appointment books, and electronic gadgets help us stay on the right path to being responsible adults. As discussed in more detail in chapter 7, our society functions by employing various general and specific rituals.

Rituals become dysfunctional when they become overly obsessive-compulsive. The homemaker who cleans the house in an ordered way once a week is comfortable in her care for her home. The homemaker who scrubs from top to bottom every day is uncomfortable in the compulsivity of the need to be so obsessed with the exaggerated activity of cleaning. We may observe that all dysfunctional behavior is an extreme expression of normal behavior. This suggests that any treatment approach to dealing with dysfunctional ritual behavior and its obsessive components does not involve elimination of all such behavior. It involves the reduction of the intensity and frequency of such behavior. The ritual behavior needs to be tempered, moderated and made more normal.

As stated earlier, completed rituals are closed gestalts. That is, they are fully closed circles of behavior that allow a person to know the past and the future within the closed circle. Individuals who create these closed, complete circles of behavior are comfortable because they know what was and what will be. Breaking the circle or changing its contents produces discomfort and insecurity. The key label is *insecurity*. Let's return to the example of a homemaker who cleans incessantly.

Case Study: Obsessive Cleaning

A 32-year-old married woman was referred by her gynecologist because she had shared with her doctor a problem of obsessive housecleaning. Her doctor had discussed possible approaches to dealing with this problem, including antianxiety medication, a psychiatric consultation, a referral for long-term psychotherapy, or short-term cognitive behavior therapy with clinical hypnosis as an adjunctive treatment approach. The patient chose the latter and was given my card (JIZ) to call for an appointment.

Session 1

The woman called, and an appointment was made. The patient had been married for 3 years and had no children. Her husband was a high-powered executive for an insurance company and preferred that his wife not work because economically it was not necessary. They lived in a country club community with golf and other recreational and social activities available. The patient had been employed before marrying by a large department store as manager of the women's sportswear department. She had liked her work and her fellow employees, and that is how she had met her husband when she assisted him in a purchase for his girlfriend. The marriage, the move, and the resignation from her job meant a new home environment, a new social circle and new friends who were more acceptable to her husband.

This patient tried very hard to adapt to the changes and her new husband's wishes for about a year. However, she was not happy, nor could she become involved to a satisfactory degree in the social life of the community. She told her husband that she was not happy, and that she wanted to return to work and see her friends whom she had not seen in a while. Her husband convinced her to try to be more sociable and learn to golf. He offered his assurances that things would get better. However, the patient became depressed and spent more and more time redecorating the house. She also took up gardening instead of learning to play golf.

Eventually, the depression seemed to lift. She took a course in gardening and became engrossed in exercising her own skills as a gardener. Her husband was pleased that she found something that she enjoyed doing and complimented her on her beautiful garden. However, he complained to her that, because of the garden, she was neglecting the house and not keeping it orderly or clean enough. She explained that she felt crushed, and that was when she started neglecting the garden and cleaning and cleaning and cleaning the house.

We discussed her husband's behavior and their relationship. I asked about whether she had ever considered marital counseling. She said that she had decided against that course of action because she believed that the problem was hers, not her husband's. She believed that they both loved each other. She stated that her husband was good to her and very generous. Their sex life was reported to be very good. Her belief was that she had been suddenly transported into a new and affluent lifestyle, and that she needed to adjust to it and learn to enjoy it.

After the intake, which included the above information, I explained about the conscious and unconscious minds. I stated that the basis of her obsessive cleaning was her unconscious attempt to please her husband and make her life more comfortable. I told her that she had taken it to an extreme because she was very angry and turned that anger inward rather than on her husband because she felt responsible for the problem between her and her husband.

(Note: Obsessive cleaning is both repetitive behavior and ritual behavior. The process of cleaning involves a whole series of orderly step-by-step activities that need to be done in a specific order to complete the task. Although these two manifestations of obsessive-compulsive behavior are being addressed separately, they naturally overlap.)

Hypnosis and self-hypnosis was explained as a way to shorten the length of time it would take to resolve the target problem, namely, obsessive ritualistic housecleaning. It was also explained that the behavior she was uncomfortable with was unconsciously chosen to satisfy her husband's request for the home to be cleaner and more orderly. It was also her way of releasing her anger. I told the patient that she would be helped to feel more secure within herself and to be able to gradually move out into the environment to socialize more and feel comfortable doing so. I indicated that we would be discussing ways for her to communicate better with her husband.

The intake revealed that this patient was primarily kinesthetic in the way that she processed information. Her sense of smell was her secondary system and she was just beginning to use visual processing as a result of her work with colorful flowers. Her husband was visual and communicated in primarily visual language, whereas she talked about how she felt.

I explained that anger and anxiety were different expressions of the same underlying feeling, and that internalized anger was what we immediately had to deal with. I explained that when she was relaxed, she could not be angry or anxious because these feelings are physical and emotional opposites. I asked her if she understood my explanation and if she wanted to work together to help her with her problem. She indicated that she did, and I explained that I would ask for a verbal contract for five sessions, beyond this evaluation session. We probably would be able to complete the task in that length of time, but we would evaluate where we were as we progressed, and make decisions as needed. She agreed, so we made an appointment for a second session. She said that she was already feeling better because of our talk together and my explanation.

Session 2

The second session involved helping the patient into hypnosis using the marble induction (see chapter 5) so that she could use the marble to externalize and drain away her anger, as well as to do self-hypnosis. The marble would also provide her with an instant relaxation technique for interrupting feelings of anger, anxiety, and compulsivity.

During the trance experience, I talked about continuing the cleaning but with less intensity and less frequency. This would make her feel better and also would please her husband. I explained how to use the marble for her own self-hypnosis relaxation sessions first thing in the morning after her husband left for work and before she usually started to clean house. I also suggested that she take a break and spend at least an hour a day cleaning up and repairing her garden and enjoying the various and pleasant smells in her garden, to please herself. She might want to remember which of the flower odors gave her the most pleasure and remember that pleasurable smell when she was relaxed. She was instructed to do her relaxation again at least an hour before her husband usually came home from work. She could use the marble to drain her anger, as we had done in the office, and as something to hold onto to feel more comfortable during the day or at any other time.

I suggested that by doing the marble relaxation twice a day and by playing with the marble in between relaxation sessions, she would immediately recognize a change in how she felt and what she did. She would also notice that by bringing to mind that special odor from her garden she would feel even better.

I also suggested that being more relaxed and calmer would immediately improve her relationship with her husband, because her more relaxed body and her calmer way of talking would communicate subtly to her husband that she was feeling better and he would respond in kind without knowing why.

After she awakened, I asked her to reenter relaxation on her own, using the marble. I would be an observer and she could stay in relaxation as long as she wanted to, and awaken herself by opening her eyes and looking at the marble, the way we had a few moments ago. She did this and stayed in trance for about 7 minutes, then awakened herself. She enjoyed the experience of being relaxed and comfortable, and being able to do this by herself. She stated that she looked forward to continuing her relaxation practice during the coming week, and she said that she expected it to be very helpful. Another appointment was made for a third session a week later, with instructions to call if she had any questions.

Session 3

When the patient came in for her third sessions she was very happy because she had been able to reduce her cleaning to two times over the last week. She even divided the tasks to be done so that she could spend less time each of the 2 days and work on her garden. She expressed surprise that her garden still smelled so wonderful, even though it had been unattended. She was practicing her relaxation techniques and feeling much more relaxed. She also found herself rolling the marble between her fingers from time to time and enjoying the feeling of peacefulness.

I congratulated her on how well she was doing and asked her how things were with her husband. She said she wasn't sure, but that she felt less pressured by him, more relaxed. I asked her if the garden was back to its previous beauty.

She said it would take a while because she had to remove some plants and needed to replant. I then asked her if any of the women that she met at the club enjoyed gardening. (I "planted a seed" for improving her social contacts.) She replied that she didn't know, and asked why I had asked the question. I suggested that she might find it easier to make friends if they had similar interests, and that she might start a garden club to share skills and learn more. She stated that she thought that this was a great idea and that she would look into it.

The patient was then asked to relax herself using the marble, without my help, and signal me with a head nod when she felt relaxed enough for me to talk to her. When she nodded her head, I took over and helped her to go deeper into relaxation.

> You are already feeling very relaxed, but as you concentrate on the feeling of the marble in your hand, you will become aware of the marble getting warmer. The warmth from your hand is radiating into the marble and warming it. The marble is getting warmer and you are feeling even more relaxed and comfortable. The fact that the marble can absorb positive warmth from your body is important to be aware of because the marble was also able to absorb the negative feelings of anger from your body and dissipate them harmlessly into the air. That is one of the reasons that you felt so much better and more in charge this past week.
>
> After you have worked with the marble for a while for self-hypnosis and quick relaxation, you will begin to recognize and feel that just thinking about the marble will be helpful. So, if you don't happen to have it with you, you can imagine it in your hand and feel more comfortable.
>
> By now the marble is very warm and comforting and you are very deeply relaxed. During this kind of deep relaxation you are able to use all of the healing energy of your mind and body to heal and repair any physical or emotional problem that brought about your extreme behavior. Because there is no longer any wasted energy on stress or distress, all of that energy is available for healing and change.
>
> When you relax yourself using the marble for self-hypnosis twice a day, you will be able to reach this deeper level of healing relaxation as you feel the warmth radiating into the marble and the marble getting very warm.
>
> Now I am going to back off and leave you in deep relaxation for a while. When you feel that you have relaxed long enough, awaken yourself as you have been doing. When you open your eyes, you will feel wide awake and very calm and peaceful. You're in charge.

After she opened her eyes, we talked about her experience and made another appointment for 2 weeks later. I reminded her to call if she had any questions.

Session 4

When the patient returned for her fourth session 2 weeks later, the twice weekly partial housecleaning seemed most comfortable for her, and the step-by-step ritual requirements were no longer compulsive ingredients of her cleaning. She wanted to talk more about how she could continue to improve her relationship with her husband. She recognized that the relaxation had helped more than she thought it would, but there still seemed to be some problems in their communication. She didn't always understand his reasons for the decisions he made, and that caused her some discomfort. I dealt with this issue as follows

> Each of us processes information through our own sensory system. We see, we hear, we feel, we smell, and we taste. Often, one or more of those sensory systems are more dominant than the others. Most often, most people process learning through the visual or kinesthetic system. The choice of system involves using language that relates to how they think. For example, when we talked about you and your husband and your relationship, I determined that he processes visually and thus uses mostly visual language. He probably says things like 'Can't you see what I mean?' and 'I can see that.' You, however, are primarily processing information with the kinesthetic system, and you say the same thing in a different way. You say 'Can't you feel what I'm trying to say?' and 'It doesn't feel that way to me.'
>
> So each of you hears the words, but you can't always understand them very well because you process information differently and use different words to describe things. This can be very frustrating because it is almost as if you are each speaking a different language. Because of this, the meaning and intent of what you say to each other may evoke a question such as 'What did you mean?' How often has that happened to you, and how often have you been upset because he didn't seem to understand what you were telling him? And vice versa? He can enjoy the visual beauty of the colors of the flowers in your garden, but you enjoy more the handling of the plants and the smell of the flowers. The odors give you pleasure because you also use your sense of smell to process information. You are more aware of something that goes bad or is dirty by the smell that disturbs you. That is one of the things that led to your doing so much cleaning. The odors of dirt and dust were unpleasant to your nose.
>
> Listen to the language your husband uses when he explains things to you, or when you are talking to each other. Recognize the visual predicates he uses, and try to translate their meaning into your own feeling words. When you respond to him or explain something to him, take your time, and choose seeing words instead of feeling words.

We did some word exchange exercises to get her used to the idea of being aware and changing her words to meet her husband's way of thinking. She said that she really had no idea that their language use could cause so much misunderstanding and that she would pay more attention to how they communicated.

During her self-hypnosis work in the office during this session, her trance experience was deepened, as was done in earlier sessions, and suggestions were given to further fix in place her success at controlling her compulsive ritual cleaning behavior. The waking state reframing information on sensory language differences was paraphrased in a simpler format, and it was suggested that she would find it very easy to translate her husband's language into her feeling language as she paid greater attention to the language exchanges between the two of them.

The patient returned for two more sessions, 2 weeks apart, to fine-tune her behavior and anxiety control and her language skills. She has called a few times since then to tell me about her progress. Her new "normal" cleaning rituals have become comfortable for her. She started a garden club and has made a number of friends with similar interests. She and her husband continue to communicate better and have fewer major misunderstandings. She took up golf and is playing with her new women friends. She even reported that she may eventually play with her husband when she feels that she is skilled enough.

IMPULSE CONTROL PROBLEMS EXPRESSED AS FREQUENT LOSS OF TEMPER

The discussion of obsessive-compulsive behavior leads naturally to some consideration of more specific issues of impulse control. Obsessive-compulsive behavior is naturally a problem of the inability to control one's impulses. Almost all dysfunctional behavior, from habits to compulsions, really are impulse control issues. Here, however, we will deal with another form of extreme behavior, anger externally expressed in words or deeds. Anger is often externalized in the form of a temper tantrum, as with children, or as an emotional, sometimes violent, loss of temper with adolescents and adults.

Case Study: Anger Management

A 36-year-old, recently married white male called my (JIZ) office from my yellow pages advertisement to inquire about help with his violent temper. A short discussion on the telephone indicated that he was shopping for help because his wife of 6 months was very upset with his frequent loss of temper and threatened to leave him if he didn't get help. I asked if he was calling only because of her threats, or if he recognized he had a problem and really wanted help. He responded that he recognized that he had a problem and loved his wife and wanted help. An appointment was made for an evaluation a few days later.

Session 1

The patient indicated that he was employed as a manager of an auto parts supply store and that his wife worked at a women's clothing store. They had met at a party of a mutual friend and had dated for about 8 months before getting married. He reported that, although he had had a bad temper for many years, he had been able to control it during the premarital courting period. Once they were married, however, his temper became apparent while they were setting up their household.

He was asked about his family upbringing and his medical history. His father had a bad temper, and although he never hit his mother, he was verbally abusive to her and to his children. The patient had a younger sister and brother.

The patient indicated that he was generally healthy and that his doctor was not aware of his bad temper. He said that, by the time he got home from work, he was very tired and usually in a bad mood. He was easily set off by demands made on him to help with the housework or to go out shopping or socializing in the evening. He only wanted to have some junk food, then supper, then watch television. Their sexual relationship was good and seemed to be a way for him to ask forgiveness for his angry outbursts.

I asked questions about his family medical history regarding diabetes and other blood sugar problems. He was asked about his eating patterns and his intake of alcohol, coffee, sugar and heavy foods. His mother was diabetic, but the diabetes was under control with medication. His father had suffered from a heart attack but had recovered. The patient drank beer two or three times a week but not to excess. He drank at least five cups of coffee a day with 2 teaspoons of sugar. He did not eat breakfast, had a quick fast-food lunch at the counter, and was famished by 5:00 P.M., when he usually left for home. Upon arriving home, he would immediately have a sweet snack, or potato chips or candy. Dinner was at 7:00 P.M. and was usually large and heavy, including dessert. He did not snack after dinner. He was not overweight and seemed to have a lot of nervous energy despite his reports of feeling tired and grumpy after work.

The patient was asked if he had ever had a 5-hour glucose tolerance test for hypoglycemia. He wasn't aware of ever being tested and asked me to explain what hypoglycemia was. I explained that a person could be overly sensitive to sugar. This caused the body to manufacture insulin to absorb excess sugar. When that happened, there was often a marked drop in the blood sugar level that caused a person to feel grumpy and out of sorts and sometimes easily angered. For most people, blood sugar levels usually drop between 4:00 and 5:00 P.M. For this patient, the lower blood sugar level left the patient feeling lousy and he would eat sugary food to make himself feel better. When there is too much sugar in the blood, insulin dissipates it. Then the person has more sugar. A sort of biochemical and emotional seesaw is set up. I also said that watching his father blow up and get angry so often probably established a model of behavior that may have contributed to the patient's bad temper.

I explained that two major changes needed to happen. First, the patient needed to change his eating behavior. He needed to have a small breakfast, a better choice of lunch, and a smaller dinner. As part of this, he needed to reduce his sugar intake. That included reducing his coffee intake and using a nonsugar sweetener for a while. Second, he needed to learn to control his temper by learning deep relaxation and instant relaxation techniques.

I explained that, when he was relaxed, he could not be angry because relaxation and anger are physical and emotional opposites. I explained about the conscious and unconscious minds, about hypnosis and self-hypnosis, and that we would probably have to work together for at least five sessions. The patient responded that he would have to discuss this with his wife because of the amount of money involved. I indicated that if he decided to continue, his wife could come in for part of the next session so that everything could be explained to her. He paid for the session and said that he would get back to me.

A few days later, his wife called to talk to me. She told me what her husband had reported to her about our session together and asked if I felt I could "really" help her husband control his anger. I explained that this was a fairly common problem that I treated quite often with a good deal of success. I explained that I could not guarantee her success, and that her husband would need to actively participate in the treatment because he wanted to change and not because she wanted him to change. I told her that she was welcome to come in with him for part of the next session, but that she could not sit in for all of the session or for future sessions. They would only be responsible for one session at a time. Payment would be expected at the end of each session. They could expect changes to start to be apparent within two or three visits. She thanked me for the information and said her husband would call if they decided to proceed.

A few days later, he called to make an appointment. He said that they both wanted him to be able to control his temper. He said they talked to his doctor, who agreed with my assessment and suggested that this approach might be helpful. Their doctor also said that there were medications that could be used to control his temper if he wanted to go that route instead. He said that the medication approach might be less expensive at first, but could be required for a long time and so might be more expensive in the longer term. An appointment was made for the following week.

Session 2

At the start of the second session, I asked if his wife had wanted to come in, and he said that she did not feel that she had to because she was comfortable with what I had told her on the telephone and with what their doctor had said. He was asked if he had any other questions, and he told me not at this moment.

Because the patient processed information kinesthetically and needed to direct his anger out harmlessly, I chose the marble induction (see chapter 5). I asked him to pick a marble from the large jar on the table near him. During the induction, I directed him to be aware of the marble getting warm, and to feel the warmth coming from his hand and into the marble. It was suggested that in the same way the marble could absorb positive warmth from his body, it could also absorb negative anger from his body and dissipate it harmlessly into the air.

He was taught how to do self-hypnosis before going to work and immediately after he arrived home in the afternoon. Suggestions were given for him to consciously choose to have a small but good breakfast, to bring lunch to work, such as a tuna or chicken sandwich on whole wheat bread with an apple or other fruit, and to have a less heavy and smaller dinner. It was suggested that he could have fewer cups of coffee and use a small amount of sugar substitute to sweeten the coffee. It was also suggested that the afternoon self-relaxation session he did when he arrived home would interrupt and control the need for any junk food snacking. Before the start of this relaxation, he was to have a small glass of orange or grapefruit juice to satisfy any sugar hunger his body might have. I then suggested that he carry the marble in his pocket. If he felt the beginning of the feeling of anger, he was to immediately reach into his pocket and take the marble in his hand, close his hand around it without closing his eyes, and feel it getting warmer in his hand. I suggested that, with the warmth, the start of the feelings of anger would dissipate. I told him how to awaken himself and that he would feel a continuing sense of relaxation and peace for a long time into the day.

After he opened his eyes, he expressed pleasure at how he felt. This was reinforced by my commenting that the pleasure would get even better as he did self-hypnosis. I stated:

> In fact, why not do it on your own right now? Look at the marble, play with it, and relax yourself the way we did a little while ago. I will just observe. After you have relaxed for a while, awaken yourself and feel how you have relaxed even more than you are now.

The patient was in self-trance for about 6 minutes. When he opened his eyes, he had a big smile on his face and said, "Wow." I complimented him on how well he had done and reminded him that he had two things to do before our next session together. He was to relax himself twice a day and he was to consciously change his eating behavior and his sugar intake. A third appointment was scheduled for the following week with the usual *invitation to call if he had any questions."*

Session 3

During our review of his past week, the patient said that he had been practicing his self-hypnosis twice a day and that he had had only a few mild losses of temper. Holding the marble at work had made a big difference in his relationship with his employees. He hadn't realized how much their constant questions were making him angry. He had been controlling his anger with them but had taken it home with him. He was drinking less coffee and consuming less sugar but was having a problem with having breakfast every morning. He tended not to give himself enough time between getting up and getting to work. I told him not to worry about this and to have breakfast as regularly as he could.

His wife had been very nice to him over the past week because things had been much calmer between them.

Next, I asked him to sit comfortably and to take out his marble and start self-hypnosis, as he had been doing at home. When he felt he was as relaxed as he could be, he was to nod his head for me or say "okay," so that I could help him experience an even deeper level of relaxation. He was also to pay close attention to concentrating on the marble to control his thoughts. If his mind wandered, he was to bring his mind back to the marble.

After about 6 minutes, he said "okay," and I asked him to lightly squeeze the marble in his hand five times as I counted out loud from 5 to 1. I suggested that with each light squeeze, and each number that I counted, he would feel himself going much deeper into relaxation and hypnosis. After the number 1 was verbalized, I said:

> Now that we have reached the number 1 you feel so much more relaxed than you did when you told me okay. It didn't take very long to reach this much deeper level of relaxation, and you can do this for yourself every time you do your own self-hypnosis. When you feel you are as relaxed as you can be, count slowly and silently to yourself from 5 down to 1. With each number that you count, lightly squeeze the marble. Let the squeeze linger for a moment, and with each squeeze you will feel more and more relaxed and comfortable.
>
> This much deeper level of relaxation is called the neutral healing place. It is difficult to go directly from negative to positive. It is too big a leap. But it is easy to go from negative to neutral, as you are now, then feel more positive about what you will be experiencing. This is also a time for healing. All of your energy resources are in balance and available to be used for healing and change. There is no wasted energy on thinking and feeling angry, so that energy is free to be used to change how you feel now and in the future.
>
> That means dissipating the anger before it can hurt you or others, eating differently to reduce your sugar intake, and realizing that for the first time in many years you are in charge. You do not have to behave the way your father did. You are your own person. You are a better person and you feel good about that. In fact, you are treating yourself with more care, with more dignity, and with more self-respect. Because you are treating yourself this way, you will also be treating your wife and others this way, with more care, with more dignity, and with more respect. When you awaken yourself, you will be very aware of how comfortable and peaceful you have been. You will feel that the future will also feel very peaceful and comfortable, with you in charge of you. Awaken yourself when you are ready to do so.

We discussed his experience, and another appointment was made for 2 weeks later. He was reminded to consciously pay attention to his eating behavior and to regularly practice his relaxation and use the marble to keep things comfortable. He was also told to call if he had any questions.

Session 4

When he returned for his fourth session, the patient told me that he had a blowup at work when one of the people who worked for him "screwed up an invoice." However, he quickly cooled down and apologized to his employee and suggested ways to avoid the mistake in the future. He said he had never done that before, and everyone at worked seemed happier as a result of his change in behavior. There were no loss of temper episodes with his wife, and he was drinking less coffee and eating better. He was feeling better in the late afternoon, the evenings were much calmer and more enjoyable. In fact, he and his wife had gone out to a movie after dinner one night and were planning on doing something at least one evening a week or during the day on the weekend.

The patient returned for two more sessions 3 weeks apart, to further build his confidence and to reinforce his self-control skills. At the time of his last visit, his wife came with him, and I talked with them together about what he had been doing and how to enjoy the changes that had been accomplished. I suggested that they become more involved with other young couples through their work associates, or others, to add to their social contacts. Until now, she had been reluctant to widen their circle of friends because of his explosive behavior and the tension that existed between them. They both thanked me and said that they would keep in touch.

PERFORMANCE ANXIETY

The brief suggestive hypnotic approach can be effective in treating various performance anxiety issues, such as test or examination anxiety (Stanton, 1993). Performance anxiety issues are handled in a similar way. The problems of test anxiety, concentration difficulties, such as these experienced by professional musicians, "freezing," and public speaking anxiety are usually treated with this approach. However, the treatment plan is always individualized to meet the needs of the patient and the particulars of the presenting problem. We will address each of these categories of problems.

Case Study: Test Anxiety and Concentration Difficulties

A 42-year-old divorced real estate associate had a pending real estate licensing examination coming up in a month and a half; however, she was having trouble concentrating and learning the material. She had taken the exam twice before and had not passed some sections of the exam. She failed different sections each time. She needed to pass this time or change her profession. A former patient who had a similar problem with an examination for a different profession referred her to me (JIZ). She was seen for three sessions. The goals were improved concentration for studying and retention, reduced anticipatory anxiety regarding the pending exam, which had tended to freeze her in the past, and more confidence in her own ability to succeed at this and future challenges. She was bright and outgoing and felt that she should be able to do this, so positive motivation and reason were present.

The first session included an evaluation, waking state reframing, and an eye fixation attention to breathing induction (see chapter 4) that included the teaching of self-hypnosis. This was accomplished in the first session because the evaluation was shorter than usual and the establishing of goals was very specific. The suggestions during the trance experience were directed at taking a few slow, deep breaths at the start of each study session. Each half hour, the patient was to get up, stretch, and walk around the room, then sit down and take two or three slow, deep breaths again, with eyes open, before tackling the study material.

The patient was to practice self-hypnosis each afternoon, after work and before she did her regular exercise sessions of fast walking. On weekends, when she was planning to study longer, she was to do self-hypnosis in the morning, before she started studying, and in the afternoon when she took her break, before her exercise walk. It was suggested that the daily practice of relaxation would control her anxiety and fear because relaxation was the opposite of these feelings. It also would improve her concentration and retention because she would find herself better able to focus on what she was studying rather than worrying about flunking again. The deep breaths before each study session were to be used to bring back the feeling of relaxation she experienced from self-hypnosis and focus her attention on the material to be learned.

The patient returned for a second session a week later, reporting a great improvement in her mental state, having less anxiety about the upcoming examination and studying better. She said that she found that her exercise activities were less tiring when she did self-hypnosis first and that she enjoyed her fast walking more. She was proceeding with her study material at a faster pace and believed that she was retaining it better. At the start of each study period, she was giving herself a short test to check her retention and was scoring well.

I directed her to put herself into relaxation and let me know when she was ready for me to talk to her. I reinforced her previous week's successes and directed her to pay attention to her breathing if her mind wandered.

She came back for one more session 2 weeks later. She reported that she had finished her study material and was now reviewing the two sections that she had previously failed. The patient was feeling comfortable and confident that she had everything in place and would do well on the examination. After she relaxed herself, I reinforced the idea that she felt good about everything and emphasized her increased confidence in herself and her ability to succeed in whatever task she chose. The session concluded with my expression of confidence that she would pass the exam with comfort and confidence. She called the day after the test to thank me and to report that she had "aced" it. The examinations were electronically scored at the test site, so she knew her results right away.

Case Study: A Professional Musician's Performance Anxiety

The second violinist of the local concert orchestra called me (JIZ) because she was worried about her recent "freezing" during rehearsals and the fear that she would "really mess up" during a full performance of the orchestra. A physician friend had suggested that she call me. An appointment was made.

The patient was a 48-year-old accomplished concert violinist with much talent, proficiency and experience. Orchestras are made up of many talented musicians who are constantly vying for recognition and promotion, so the competition and the backbiting were integral parts of the scene. Lately, however, she had been having lapses in attention and fingering while reading music that she knew by heart. The conductor had recognized some of her slipups and had singled her out for correction. This made her more nervous and caused her more concern and anxiety. She could not remember ever having this problem before. She was becoming fearful that she would be unable to perform well because it would get worse.

The intake during this first visit included questions about her health and other stressors that might be in her life. Neither seemed to be a problem, so we decided to concentrate on the issues of concentration, anxiety and confidence.

We were able to include the initial evaluation, waking state reframing and induction and self-hypnosis instruction in the first session. The induction was simple eye fixation with attention to breathing (see chapter 4). When she was very relaxed, I asked her to concentrate on her breathing and to listen in her head to her best violin performance of her favorite short musical piece.

I told her that, as she did this, she would be able to talk to me and respond to my questions and suggestions without affecting her recall of the music and her satisfaction with her remembered performance. I suggested that this musical remembering would be enjoyable and without effort. Her recall and hearing of the music would be very powerful and real, although a part of her mind would also be able to be aware of her breathing and my words.

> As you listen to yourself playing, you will feel very comfortable and pleased with the easy flow of your music and the flawless fingering of strings and the smoothness of your bow. Gradually, you will change the music to the current concert program while continuing to hear and even see yourself playing it smoothly and effortlessly. During hypnosis, time is interpreted very flexibly, so that, although you may experience a long time passing while playing the full musical score, only a few minutes will have actually passed. As you are playing the same piece that you have been rehearsing, flawlessly, describe to me what you are doing and how you are feeling.

She described the technical aspects of her playing, and that everything was going so smoothly that she was really enjoying playing the music. She felt calm and comfortable and part of the music. I encouraged her to finish the piece and to tell me when she was done. When she said she was done, I asked her to come back to paying attention to her breathing and how relaxed she felt. I suggested that she was to do this same relaxation herself at home that afternoon and before she left her home to attend rehearsal that evening. She would find it easy to pay attention to her breathing and to feel relaxed, without anxiety, and hear herself playing the various compositions that were to be included in the program being rehearsed.

Her rendering of the compositions in her head and in her ears would be flawless and effortless. When she sat at rehearsal and during the performance of these works, she would automatically recall and perform the same program with skill and perfection. Her concentration would be exceptional and her coordination smooth. She was awakened with a simple eyes open directive and looked at me. When her eyes opened, she said with surprise in her voice that she had just performed better than she ever had and that "it was great!"

We discussed this experience. It was suggested that she also practice relaxing and performing during relaxation a few times a day over the next week, then return for a second session.

She returned a week later and told me that everything went smoothly. The fear and embarrassment were gone and the rehearsals were without flaws. Her concentration and confidence were back and she enjoyed her mental rehearsals. I complimented her on her success, then asked her to relax herself here in the office the same way she had been doing at home, but to not rehearse the music. She was to keep her concentration on her breathing.

When her breathing was relaxed and regular, I suggested that she regularly practice this kind of relaxation at least once a day without hearing or concentrating on her music.

> Every day, when it is most comfortable to fit it into your schedule as a regular part of your daily routine, relax yourself by closing your eyes and paying attention to your breathing. You may hear some of your music softly in the background, but you will pay little attention to it as you continue to go deeper and deeper into relaxation. This quiet, peaceful time is your daily self-healing. It is the time that you treat yourself with more care, with more dignity and with more self-love. It is the time when you allow any feelings of stress or worry or discomfort to melt away as you experience relaxation and comfort, physically and mentally. It is a time for renewal and rejuvenation. It is your special daily retreat into self-care and self caring. Enjoy it, and use it to take better care of yourself and to feel good about yourself.

I asked her to awaken herself when she was ready and to open her eyes to a great sense of well-being. She did so, and with a smile and a deep breath, she told me just how delightful this experience had been. She did not need to return, but became a friend who has often sent tickets to symphony performances over the years.

Case Study: Public Speaking Anxiety

A 45-year-old married man was referred to me (JIZ) by a former patient. He worked as a regional sales manager for a large furniture company and had been asked to prepare a presentation for a sales meeting to take place in 2 months. He had written out and prepared a Microsoft Windows Power Point program that he felt was "very powerful," but he was anxious that he would be unable to speak to the large group without making a lot of mistakes.

The patient was scheduled for three sessions. During the first session, the usual evaluation was done and waking state reframing information was given, with emphasis on a discussion of the fight or flight response and relaxation as the opposite of anxiety and fear. I used an eye fixation with attention breathing induction and taught him self-hypnosis. I instructed the patient to slow his breathing while looking at an object across the room, then to gently close his eyes and feel his breathing become more regular. He was to do this himself once a day and to pay attention to how the anxious feeling left with each normal, comfortable breath that he took.

The patient intended to practice his presentation before a few friends. I instructed him to take a few slow, deep breaths before he started, then to lightly squeeze the remote control he was using to control a computer and projector. The light squeezing of the remote was used as a posthypnotic cue that would give him control and allow him to follow his verbal script more smoothly and comfortably. I suggested that, as he proceeded, he would be aware only of what was on the screen and what he was saying, in perfect cadence with his material. He would feel very relaxed and peaceful, and would be confident in his ability to present the information. I also suggested that, after the visual presentation, he would easily field questions because he felt so good about his command of the material.

I told him not to try to verbalize what I said to him when he practiced self-relaxation. The very experience of being able to do self-relaxation would automatically reinforce what I said to him when we were working together.

During the second session, a week later, he said he felt more relaxed from the daily self-relaxation practice and was more comfortable with his presentation practice sessions. He used the deep breathing and the light squeezing of the remote. It worked.

I asked him to relax himself and say "okay" when he felt as relaxed as he did at home. I then took him deeper into relaxation with a 20-to-1 countdown, and instructed him to use the countdown as part of self-hypnosis. I asked him to come back in 3 weeks for a follow-up and to call if he had any questions.

The patient returned after 3 weeks for a third session and reported that he felt very sure that he could do his presentation without difficulty. He relaxed himself again including a silent countdown, and said "okay" when he was ready for me to talk. I reinforced his confidence and feelings of relaxation, asked him to take a few slow, deep breaths and to recognize how powerful the deep breaths were to relax him even more. He said that he felt "great" after awakening. He thanked me and said that he would call after the presentation to tell me how it went. He did call and the presentation went off without any problems. He said that, because of his success, he was asked to make the presentation again to a different group.

SUMMARY

This brief approach to anxiety control can be applied to other problems that are anxiety based. Although we do not specialize in sports psychology, for example, there have been occasions when golfers, bowlers, and other athletes have consulted with us for help in controlling their anxiety, which had impaired their performance. This has been true for amateurs and professionals alike.

Because anxiety is a central feature of most psychological disorders and psychiatric illnesses (Kaplan & Sadock, 1981), the experienced clinician most likely can think of many more problems for which this approach can be helpful. As stated earlier, anxiety is a signal that something is disturbing the internal psychological equilibrium. It is a symptom of internal conflict, an indication that something unacceptable is pressing for conscious representation and expression. As a signal of an internal or external threat, it originally called for some coping behavior to ward off the perceived threat. The chosen coping behavior may or may not have been adaptive and functional at the time. Yet it may continue, even though the original circumstances are no longer present and the original coping behavior is no longer necessary. The ongoing dysfunctional coping behavior may have been imprinted emotionally at the time of its origin, and through repetition became a dysfunctional habit.

The form that anxiety takes and the individual's pattern of symptoms are determined by the nature of the original unconscious and conscious inner and outer threats (i.e., objects of fear), and the complexity of the interactions and conflicts between the original sources of fear and the individual's evolving attempts over time to cope with them. Therefore, there are two key questions that are helpful to ask in order to develop a useful understanding of the dynamics of a patient's specific anxiety symptoms: (1) What are the specific inner drives, impulses, thoughts, feelings, and experiences that the patient fears or feels threatened by? and (2) What consequences does the patient fear will occur if those dreaded experiences are expressed, acted out, or continue to occur?

11

Medical Problems Including Pain, Preparing for Medical Procedures, Self-Healing, and Coping with Treatment Side Effects

Brief cognitive hypnosis is used primarily to change dysfunctional behavior. It cannot be used to treat medical problems. Cognitive approaches combined with the tool of clinical hypnosis however, can address the double-sided issues of medical problems being exacerbated by emotional overlay created by the patient's reaction to health problems, as well as medical problems that result from extreme or chronic emotional distress.

By reducing the emotional overlay, anxiety, fear, anger, and depression, that accompany serious and chronic medical problems, medical symptoms can be lessened. This can promote the body's ability to heal and help the patient to benefit more from medical and pharmacological interventions. With chronic, continual, or persistent pain, the main emotional overlay is depression and anger. In either case, the emotional meaning of the pain experience is significant and needs to be addressed. Emotional overlay exaggerates and intensifies the experience of pain and other chronic medical problems. It also creates the expectation that these problems will never improve.

Hypnosis is a valuable tool in changing the emotional meaning of pain and chronic illness, but it is not the primary change agent. Reframing and relabeling, changing belief systems, recognizing choices, and acknowledging possibilities are the change agents. The patient's learning experience of acquiring the ability to personally participate in changing feelings, thoughts, and behaviors is a valuable agent of change. The patient initiates some action that improves feelings, which leads to change in the belief that the patient is helpless. This allows the patient to feel more in charge.

Living daily with chronic illness can create a huge emotional and physical toll on any individual. In addition, patients facing chronic medical problems often endure negative and iatrogenic experiences in their contacts with the medical system. Many treatment situations inadvertently encourage patient passivity, and others can be very unpleasant. Most produce unwanted negative side effects. One of the most pathogenic results is the development of learned helplessness (Peterson, Maier, & Seligman, 1995; Seligman, 1975).

The brief cognitive hypnosis approach addresses and reframes patient beliefs that contribute to learned helplessness. Coping tools are used to reduce or interrupt chronic, continuous and persistent beliefs about being trapped and reduce the side effects and iatrogenic nature of the medical treatment process.

PAIN ISSUES

Acute or acute posttraumatic pain serves as a signal to the brain that the body needs help in an injured area so that it can start the process of healing and repair. With chronic pain, the signal continues long after the need for an emergency response is over. Often, chronic pain continues because physical healing has been inadequate or compromised by physical factors such as scar tissue, which can create pressure on nerve endings or blood vessels.

The continuing noxious stimulation (termed *nociception* or *nociceptive input*) associated with persistent chronic pain conditions is a powerful force that shapes the afflicted individual's response patterns over time. The individual's behavioral responses in turn affect responses by other people and conditions in the individual's environment. Those other responses shape the hurting individual's response habits, which are then imprinted through repetition in the individual's unconscious mind. In addition, the emotional overlay associated with the pain imprints certain pain beliefs and behaviors. Thus, chronic or continuing pain has a very powerful learned component. This learned component needs to be addressed and changed if we are to help the pain sufferer obtain some relief from the pain and improve functionality.

It is important to make certain that full and appropriate medical evaluations of the patient's pain have been conducted before any treatment for pain amelioration with hypnosis is attempted (Hunter, 1987). To proceed with hypnosis for relieving pain that has not been adequately medically evaluated is inappropriate and unwise.

Pain can be intensified or exacerbated by the patient's emotional state, cognitive expectations, beliefs, learning and coping skills (DeGood & Shutty, 1992; Hanson & Gerber, 1990). The patient's discomfort is intimately related to the patient's ways of thinking about himself or herself and problems. We invariably encounter and direct our efforts at counteracting issues of anxiety, depression, desperation and anger, unhelpful beliefs in absolutes, unintentional iatrogenic statements by physicians and previous unsuccessful treatment experiences.

Thus, the treatment of chronic pain differs markedly from the treatment of acute pain (Eimer & Freeman, 1998; Hanson & Gerber, 1990). The factors that exacerbate the pain need to be incorporated into the reframing process. Given that many of these factors can be changed or controlled, it should be suggested to the patient that the current pain does not have to be experienced at such a high level of intensity and does not have to be debilitating. However, the brief cognitive hypnosis approach requires that all suggestions given to the patient be individualized based on the patient's needs, personality and sensory and cognitive processing style.

Part of doing this requires that the clinician listen carefully to the language the patient uses to describe the pain and the experience of pain (Bassman & Wester, 1984; Eimer & Freeman, 1998; Melzack & Torgerson, 1971; Turk & Melzack, 1992). This language usually provides significant leads for choosing the appropriate change language, induction procedure and suggestions for helping the patient gain control of his or her pain and symptoms. Our goal is helping the patient to get back in charge. Chronic pain patients typically feel hopeless and depressed because they have lost their sense of self-efficacy (Bandura et al., 1987; Blanchard et al., 1993; Eimer & Freeman, 1998; Turk, Okifuji, & Scharff, 1995). Hypnosis can help these patients regain some of their lost sense of control and self-mastery by teaching them ways to gain control over their symptoms (Bassman & Wester, 1984).

Brief cognitive hypnosis can make all of the treatment strategies we use work better. It can alter the patient's pain experience and imprint more functional pain-coping skills. However, the degree to which the patient with chronic pain can be helped to experience the pain differently depends on a number of significant interacting factors. These include the patient's personality and coping style, the level of hypnotic responsivity, motivations, particular problems in living, the treatment context and living situation and economic and social influences (Eimer, 2000a, 2000b; Eimer & Freeman, 1998; Eimer & Hornyak, 2001).

Depending on the patient's level of hypnotic responsivity, which itself is affected by many of the other factors listed above, brief cognitive hypnosis can:

1. heighten the patient's ability to distract himself or herself from the pain by diverting the patient's attention to some other aspects of his or her ongoing or past or future experience
2. imprint alternative sensory impressions that reshape the patient's perceptions of the pain and distort the nociceptive input in the direction of less negative and less disturbing experiences
3. amplify the patient's ability to disconnect and separate the pain from his or her ongoing experience (thus, moderately to highly hypnotically responsive patients can be helped to dissociate from the pain; when it is deemed appropriate, they can be helped through hypnotic techniques to experience the pain as something that is separate and distant, or removed, from their ongoing perceptible sensory input)

4. imprint positive cuing systems to produce alternate, adaptive ways of thinking, feeling, and behaving and help the patient to think, feel and behave in different ways

The patient's ways of processing information via the sensory system is important to all of the above and to facilitating successful change results. Therefore, we pay close attention to this issue when evaluating a pain patient and formulating a brief cognitive hypnosis pain treatment plan. Remember, as nonmedical clinicians, we cannot treat the pain directly, but we use the term *pain treatment plan* for lack of a better way of saying it.

In our discussion of pain in this chapter, we will not be presenting extended case histories and treatment plans as we have done in other chapters. Rather, we will offer an overview and a description of a number of brief cognitive hypnosis procedures in enough detail so that they can be adapted for use by the experienced clinician.

A detailed presentation on the uses of hypnosis for the control of pain can be found in *Pain Management Psychotherapy: A Practical Guide* (Eimer & Freeman, 1998). Interested readers are also directed to detailed texts by Barber (1996), Bassman and Wester (1984), Brown and Fromm (1987), Hilgard and Hilgard (1994), Spiegel and Spiegel (1987), and Turk, Meichenbaum, and Genest (1983), and may wish to consult informative articles by Alden and Heap (1998), Crawford et al. (1998), Weisenberg (1998), Eimer (1988, 1989, 2000a, 2000b), and Eimer and Hornyak (2001). The text by Bassman and Wester (1984) is especially useful in light of the helpful annotated session-by-session trance scripts provided.

Additional Information Gathered during Intake

After obtaining the standard intake information described in chapter 1, we obtain additional information pertinent to understanding the patient's chronic pain by asking the following types of questions.

1. Please tell me about your discomfort.
2. How "high" or "strong" or "intense" is your typical or usual level of discomfort, on a 0 to 10 scale, with 0 being *the most comfortable,* and 10 being *the least comfortable*? What is the least comfortable you have felt? How often do you feel this way? What is the most comfortable you have felt? How often do you feel this way? What is your level of comfort right now?
3. How would you describe the discomfort? Do the sensations of discomfort that you get usually feel sharp or dull? Throbbing or steady? Stationary or moving? Jumping or shooting? Drilling or stabbing? Pinching, pressing, gnawing, biting, cramping, crushing? Spreading or radiating? Penetrating

or piercing? Tingling itchy, stinging or numb? Hot or cold? Light, heavy, or pressing? Aching or sore, or both? Tender and sensitive or numb? Tiring or exhausting? Sickening? Frightening? Punishing or cruel, vicious or killing, or neutral? Annoying, troublesome, miserable, intense, or unbearable? Mild, discomforting, distressing, horrible, or excruciating? Brief, intermittent, or constant?

4. How long does the discomfort usually last?
5. Are there any physical remedies or other ways that give you relief? What helps you feel more comfortable? What helps you feel better? What causes you to feel greater discomfort?
6. How long have you had this discomfort? How did it start?
7. What have you done in terms of treatment (medical and/or alternative)? How about medical work-ups? How have you been coping with this? What helps you cope?
8. What do you and your doctors think is happening?
9. What medications are you taking now? What do you take for the pain? How much and how often? What have you taken? How much relief do your medications give you?
10. What do you think hypnosis is?

HYPNOTIZABILITY AND BRIEF COGNITIVE HYPNOSIS FOR PAIN

As we stated in chapter 4, we do not routinely test for hypnotizability, with the exception of some pain cases. A clinician employing the brief cognitive hypnosis approach will already have prepared the patient to experience hypnosis by the time the clinician is ready to formally induce trance. Hypnotizability (in terms of the questions "Can the patient be hypnotized?" and "How hypnotizable is the patient?") is not really an issue, because the patient's readiness to enter hypnosis and hypnotic responsivity will already have been primed and conditioned. Therefore, in our practices we generally do not use formal measures of hypnotizability, but instead prefer to naturalistically assess hypnotic responsivity during the intake evaluation process, during and following the waking state reframing process, and during the administration of the initial trance induction, the teaching of self-hypnosis and the deepening of the trance state.

However, with pain patients, BNE, who specializes in pain management psychotherapy (Eimer, 2000a, 2000b; Eimer & Freeman, 1998), does prefer to administer a brief standardized measure of hypnotic responsivity after conducting the initial intake. The reason for this exception, is that, with chronic pain patients, formal hypnotizability assessment often helps to predict the degree of hypnotic analgesia likely to be realized. It also can inform about the types of hypnotic strategies that are likely to be most effective in inducing hypnotic analgesia, and for helping the patient cope with, and gain control over, the pain symptoms (Eimer, 2000a, 2000b; Eimer & Freeman, 1998; Eimer & Hornyak, 2001). The patient's pattern of responses on a formal test of hypnotizibility yields an individual hypnotic response profile. This can help guide the clinician's choice of specific suggestions, cognitive reframes, hypnotic metaphors and pain relief imagery.

A brief assessment of the patient's hypnotic responsiveness is not conducted until after waking state reframing is done with the pain patient regarding how hypnosis can help in controlling pain, and how when the patient is relaxed he or she cannot be uncomfortable, tense or stressed.

For measuring hypnotic responsivity, BNE usually uses the Spiegel Hypnotic Induction Profile (HIP; Spiegel & Spiegel, 1987). The HIP takes just 5 to 7 minutes to administer and score. It is important to note that the patient always does well.

The HIP can be used as a diagnostic tool (Eimer, 2000a, 2000b). The patient's responses show (1) how quickly the patient can relax, (2) how easily the patient can let go of the need to control the interaction and allow things to happen, (3) how trusting the patient is, (4) how suggestible the patient is, and (5) how motivated and compliant the patient will be.

As part of the initial waking state reframing, I (BNE) usually state the following:

> Hypnosis is a relaxed state of attention that allows your critical mind to rest so that you can be receptive to positive comfortable thoughts. In this relaxed state, you use your imagination to change your experience in a positive way. You gain more control. Hypnosis is not sleep. When you are in hypnosis, you are awake and alert, but you feel deeply and pleasantly relaxed. When you are deeply relaxed, you cannot feel uncomfortable.
>
> Pain perception has two parts. First, there is the sensation of something happening to a specific part of the body. Second, there is your reaction to this information. This is the "hurting" part, the part that signals discomfort. Acute or new pain serves an important function. It warns a person that damage is being done to the body. But when pain continues long after it has done its job of giving warning and long after the physical problem has been medically treated, it is no longer needed as a warning. The discomfort may be needed as a reminder not to overdo things or strain, but it is no longer needed at the same degree of intensity or strength. It can still remain as a reminder and be less intense and less uncomfortable.
>
> Hypnosis for pain control works in two ways. First, when you are deeply relaxed in hypnosis, you cannot be uncomfortable. That is because relaxation is the opposite of discomfort. So, when you are deeply relaxed, you can filter out uncomfortable sensations and tune in more comfortable sensations. Second, when you are deeply relaxed, you cannot be angry, anxious, scared or depressed. So, hypnosis can reduce the emotional impact of chronic pain.

Hypnosis works best for appropriately medically diagnosed physical pain. We do not want to use hypnosis to mask medical conditions that need to be addressed. We want to use hypnosis to diminish unnecessary pain and discomfort.

The first thing that we want to do is to find out about your ability to relax—how quickly you can enter deep relaxation and how easily you respond to therapeutic suggestions. Then, after you come out of hypnosis, I can help you back into deep relaxation and hypnosis, and teach you an exercise in self-hypnosis and self-relaxation that is specially designed to meet your individual needs. After we accomplish this, we can explore what methods of coping with discomfort can be most helpful for you.

What do you think about what I've told you? Do you have any questions?"

After the patient's questions are answered, the Spiegel HIP is then administered. Then the patient is told, "You did very very well." No patient is disqualified for the use of hypnosis on the basis of their performance on the HIP. No matter how the patient scores clinically on the HIP, hypnosis is used. However, the clinician may want to adjust his or her hypnotic pain management strategy based on the patient's HIP profile (Eimer, 2000a, 2000b; Eimer & Freeman, 1998; Eimer & Hornyak, 2001).

After administering the HIP, the patient's responses and experience can be used to do further waking state reframing of several issues that are pertinent to relieving pain and discomfort. For example, the results of the HIP assessment (Spiegel & Spiegel, 1987) can be interpreted to the patient as follows:

This is what it's like to experience hypnosis. It is a state of relaxed, easy concentration. Your imagination is working, and it is focused and more powerful. Your unconscious mind is responsive to acceptable suggestions. You do not have to try to respond. It just happens all on its own. You can just permit yourself to let go, and let interesting and comfortable things happen.

You imagined along with my suggestions, and you discovered a difference in how you felt. Isn't that so?

Isn't that interesting? A response occurred in your sense of perception, yet you had no idea that the response was due to my giving your unconscious mind a prearranged signal. This is what happens to you when you react to things without being aware that you are reacting.

Some of these reactions cause discomfort. Many of the things that increase the discomfort occur outside your awareness, unconsciously. Therefore, when you learn to use self-hypnosis to go into deep relaxation, you harness the power of your unconscious mind to lessen the discomfort and replace it with comfort.

Interested readers are referred to the original text by Herbert Spiegel and David Spiegel, *Trance and Treatment: Clinical Uses of Hypnosis* (1987) for a full description of the Hypnotic Induction Profile, its rationale, development, and validation, and the verbatim administration instructions and verbal scripts. Thorough study of the information in that book or taking a workshop on the

HIP (Frischholz & Spiegel, 2000) is essential to learning and mastering this highly portable and clinically useful method for assessing hypnotic responsivity in a standardized manner.

If the patient was not responsive to the items on the HIP, the clinician should still assure the patient that he or she did well and go on from there. For example::

> You did fine. Now, let's explore another method for helping you to become deeply relaxed. With this method that we are going to explore now, there is less for you to do. Everyone can discover the best way to relax for them. Once we discover the best method for you to deeply relax, it will feel so pleasant to use your method, because when you are deeply relaxed, you no longer feel uncomfortable.

At this point, the clinician will have learned a good deal about how to proceed and about what "level" of hypnotic pain control strategy to explore further with the patient. "Low hypnotizables" usually respond best to distraction-based strategies. "Medium hypnotizables" usually respond best to distortion-based strategies (i.e., sensory distortion or "transformation" of the pain sensations). "High hypnotizables" usually respond well to dissociation-based strategies, as well as to direct suggestion (Eimer, 2000a, 2000b; Eimer & Freeman, 1998; Spiegel & Spiegel, 1987). In any case, the clinician may say:

> In hypnosis, the doorway to your unconscious mind opens, so that, with your permission, I can give your unconscious mind the information that it needs to have to help you to become more comfortable and to learn how to do this on your own. This is what makes hypnosis such an excellent tool for pain management, for relieving discomfort.

For "low" and "medium hypnotizables":

> When you are deeply relaxed in hypnosis, you can diminish your awareness of the discomfort by focusing on something else. You can follow along with pleasant, easy suggestions that help you focus your attention elsewhere, away from the discomfort. It is this openness to positive suggestions, this willingness to pay attention and think and imagine along with my suggestions, that can bring you comfort and relief from discomfort.

For "medium" and "high hypnotizables":

> When you are deeply relaxed in hypnosis, you can change and transform discomfort to something more comfortable, or make the discomfort feel less uncomfortable. You can do this by following along with some pleasant, easy suggestions that help you to discover a difference in sensation. You build on that difference in sensation, and increase that difference in sensation by concentrating on the changing sensations and imagining things that relieve the discomfort.

For "high hypnotizables":

> When you are deeply relaxed in hypnosis, you mentally can be in more than one place at the same time easily and without effort. You can be aware of the discom-

fort on one level, yet on another level be totally elsewhere. You can follow along with pleasant, easy suggestions that help you focus your attention elsewhere, away from the discomfort. It is this openness to positive suggestions, this flexibility in your attention, that can bring you relief from discomfort.

With your permission, let's come up with an individualized exercise that you can practice to gain more control over your discomfort.

DIRECT BRIEF COGNITIVE HYPNOSIS TECHNIQUES FOR PAIN SYMPTOM TRANSFORMATION

After we have conducted an intake evaluation, assessed hypnotic responsivity, done waking state reframing, induced trance and taught the patient self-hypnosis, if appropriate, we begin to work with the symptoms of discomfort directly. The goal is to help the patient to diminish the intensity of the discomfort and/ or experience it in a different way. Initially, we emphasize direct hypnotic techniques for pain alleviation and pain symptom transformation. These techniques do not involve uncovering, age regression, or hypnoanalysis. Below are scripts of some of these directive procedures.

Changing Patient Perception of Discomfort Intensity

One procedure that we use incorporates the subjective measure of levels of comfort or discomfort before and during the trance state. This is usually done during the first trance induction experience. It can be used with almost any of the inductions described, or any other that the clinician prefers.

Before the induction begins, the patient is asked to judge his or her current level of comfort or discomfort on a 1 to 10 scale. Again, 1 represents *most comfortable*, 10 *least comfortable*. The patient's number choice establishes the level that needs to be reduced during the trance experience.

The example that follows was taken from a transcript of a patient of mine (JIZ) who was helped into trance and taught self-hypnosis using the marble induction. After I was satisfied that the patient was comfortably relaxed and in the neutral or healing place, I went on to state:

> Now that you are in the neutral or healing place, where change can begin to occur, check your level of comfort once again, the way you did earlier. It will be okay for you to talk to me during this deep relaxation without disturbing the experience of hypnosis. Which number would you choose from 1 to 10, 1 being *most comfortable* and 10 being least comfortable? [In the waking state, the patient had chosen the number 7 level of lesser comfort.]
>
> You just told me that you are at the number 5 level. There has already been an improvement in how you feel, because before you started to relax, you chose the number 7. You have brought the comfort level down to 5. Any number 5 and lower is now called the "comfort level" rather than the 'less comfort level."

Concentrate on the marble in your hand and take yourself deeper into relaxation. As you do, you will relax even more and feel more comfortable. When you reach number 4, tell me. I'll just sit here quietly and let you do this all by yourself. Thank you, that's just great. Now take yourself down to the number 3 level of comfort, while concentrating on the marble and relaxing deeper. Take as much time as you need. Time is very flexible during hypnosis, so what seems like a long time to you may actually be a very short time. When you reach comfort level number 3, please tell me. Thank you. That was very good; it only took a few minutes. Now that you know how to do it, take yourself down to number 2. Let me know when you are there, then linger there for a while and enjoy it. Thank you. That was even faster. Enjoy the number 2 level of comfort for a while longer. When you are ready, you can move down to 1 or not, as you choose. Whatever you do, tell me about it, so I can know where you are.

The patient stated that she did not want to go down to number 1. I asked her to explain this, and she said that she was afraid that if she reached the number 1 level and was completely comfortable, the feeling would not last. I responded:

That was a very important recognition on your part. You are probably correct. It would not last, but not because you reached number 1. Any increased comfort that you feel today is not the final outcome of what we are doing. Today you have learned that you can, in fact, feel more comfortable. When we first talked, you told me that you always hurt. Now you realize that you can hurt less. You also realize that you can change the way you feel. This improvement in how you feel, that is, feeling better and more comfortable, is a new experience and is building a new memory of a new level of comfort that you will be able to reach again and again and eventually maintain.

Now I am going to teach you how to use the marble to do your own self-hypnosis and while relaxed continue to take yourself from less comfort to more comfort, at home or almost anywhere.

I explained the use of the marble for self-hypnosis and self-relaxation while the patient was still in trance, as has been described in previous chapters. I then instructed the patient to do self-hypnosis twice a day, in the morning and late afternoon. I instructed her to examine her level of comfort using the 1-to-10 scale, before initiating self-hypnosis, then when very relaxed, to determine again where she was on the scale. I told her that she would experience an improvement as a result of her self-hypnosis and could take herself down to number 2, as she had done in the office. She was to remain at the number 2 level of comfort for a while before she awakened herself. I also suggested that each time she did this, she would continue to feel more comfortable for longer periods of time after awakening from self-hypnosis.

I then instructed her to awaken herself, here in the office, when ready, by opening her eyes and looking at the marble. We discussed her experience of changed perception of comfort. I asked her to put herself back into self-hypnosis using the marble, without my help, and to stay relaxed for a while, monitoring her level of comfort, then awakening herself. We talked about her own ability to relax herself and I encouraged her to do this daily, then return for another session in 1 week.

Over a period of three more sessions, the patient came in for encouragement and reinforcement of her own ability to feel better for longer and longer periods of time. She learned how to use the marble to improve her level of comfort while in the waking state, by holding the marble and rolling it around in her hand, if she felt she needed it to interrupt or control any specific moment when she felt her comfort level decreasing.

By the last visit (a total of five, including the evaluation visit), the patient said that she was comfortable enough to continue on her own. She decided not to go down to number 1 because her level of comfort at number 2 was enough to allow her to do things she had not been able to do for a long time. I told her that this was a wise decision and that, as time went by, she would move in and out of number 1 from time to time and only realize this in retrospect. When she thought about how she used to feel, she would be aware of how good she was feeling in the present.

Comfort Transfer Techniques

In the practice of brief cognitive hypnosis, we make use of the association between gentle and soothing tactile stimulation and the transformation of pain sensations and pain relief. We call our method of hand-on application of gentle tactile stimulation a *comfort transfer*. When it is deemed clinically indicated, we teach patients to do this as part of their self-hypnosis. Whatever the actual physiological mechanisms are, these comfort transfers do in fact transfer novel sensations that can counter the noxious pain sensations.

There are two kinds of comfort transfers that we use often in our brief cognitive hypnosis model. The first involves "warming" or "numbing" a hand, then placing the hand on the area of pain, if it is accessible, and transferring the feeling to the area where the major discomfort resides. This is done in the waking state prior to trance and again in the trance state with eyes either open or closed. The hand transfer is effective with topical and internal pain problems. A variation of this involves transferring warm or burning feelings from the area of pain into the hand and producing a feeling of cool numbness in the affected area.

The second type of comfort transfer involves having the patient place one hand palm down on the arm of a chair or a flat surface, then having the patient concentrate and become aware of a strong pulse in one or more fingertips of that hand. This is initiated in the waking state. The patient is instructed to place the strongly pulsing fingertips, or the whole hand, on the affected area and transfer the healing power of the strong pulse to the area of discomfort. This is repeated in the trance state.

If the patient has difficulty experiencing the strong pulse, the patient is asked if the therapist can touch his or her hand. The patient is asked to turn the hand palm up. The therapist first concentrates on developing a strong pulse in his or her own hand, then places the strongly pulsing fingertips on the fingertips of the patient. The patient is asked if the strong pulse from the therapist's hand can be felt by the patient. Usually the response is positive. If it is not, the therapist should back off and do something else. Then it is suggested to the patient that the pulse is now felt in the patient's fingertips, and the therapist's hand is removed. After the patient is aware of the strong pulse, he or she is asked to place the fingertips or hand on the affected area and transfer the healing power of the strong pulse to the area of discomfort.

The patient will be able to do this again in the trance state without needing the therapist's touch.

A simpler variation of these techniques is to have the patient, during trance, place the palm of one hand on an area of the body closest to some internal health problem and to apply light pressure to the skin surface. It is suggested that the light pressure will penetrate deeply into the body into the area of illness or disease and direct the immune system to concentrate healing energy to the needy place. This has been effective in reducing pain and discomfort that is internal and related to some physical trauma or disease. While in hypnosis, the patient is instructed that this improved feeling will also be effective when the patient does this during the waking state. Regular practice during self-hypnosis will make it even more powerful when used as needed.

An Exercise in Controlled Dissociation from Pain

With patients who are highly hypnotically responsive, controlled dissociative techniques can be used to reduce their experience of pain. After asking the patient to start the relaxation process, the clinician deepens the relaxation and begins talking about dissociation as a form of detachment from feelings in the body. It is then suggested that, as the patient feels more and more relaxed, he or she will also feel more and more dissociated from his or her body, "like a shadow."

The shadow metaphor is invoked because a shadow is attached to the body, yet it is not an actual part of the body. The following is suggested:

> You see, a shadow is attached to your body, to your arms, your feet, or wherever it is. It is a part of you, yet it is not inside of you.

Having the patient imagine himself or herself connected to a shadow allows the patient to feel dissociated from the physical body. While the patient is already in an altered state (trance), this imagining changes the patient's body experience and deepens the altered state of trance. It allows the patient to sense himself or herself floating slightly out of his or her body. It is explained that this way of dissociating (or detaching) from the body and the discomfort is a way to help the patient feel better; to feel more comfortable.

It is also suggested that the patient can experience further dissociation, or detachment from the discomfort, and greater comfort, by putting the discomfort into his or her shadow, that is, out of his or her real body and into the shadow body. The patient can be told,

> You can further detach that shadow from your total being even though it is still a part of you.

Patients who are responsive usually enjoy this hypnotic experience. Practicing it as part of their self-hypnosis adds to their sense of self-efficacy.

During the trance work session, the patient is also instructed to raise an index finger as an indicator of the degree of dissociative experience. It is suggested that the higher the finger is raised, the more dissociated the patient will be. The patient is also given the option of acknowledging and describing his or her dissociation verbally to the therapist while in trance.

It is then suggested that the level of comfort attained will continue for some time after the trance experience (posthypnotic suggestion). It is also suggested that practicing this technique as part of his or her own self-hypnosis will improve the patient's skill in detaching (or dissociating) from the discomfort.

An Example of Mind–Body Healing: Hypnotic Removal of Warts

As described by Ewin (1992b), "the 'charming' of warts was enshrined in American folklore by Mark Twain in his Tom Sawyer stories (1936 edition), and he described three different methods as successful" (p. 1). Ewin goes on to point out that "[curative] hypnotic techniques vary, from suggestions to 'stop the blood supply to each wart on your body'—make it cold (Clawson & Swade, 1975)—to 'increasing the blood supply to bring in more antibodies and healing substances'—make it warm" (p. 1).

The key factor in all of these strategies is the conviction by the patient of the efficacy of the treatment (DuBreuil & Spanos, 1993). The case reports on the use of hypnosis in the treatment of warts reveal that the word *cure* is appropriate, as there are no reports of their recurrence after they disappeared. Warts often recur after standard medical-dermatological treatments (Ewin, 1992b).

The literature on the treatment of warts mostly consists of direct suggestive hypnosis approaches. For example, in a study by Surman, Gottlieb, and Hackett (1972), as stated by Ewin (1992b, p. 2), "*all* nine patients who improved had in common the ability to image the sensation of tingling in their warts. Hypnotiz-ability was not a significant variable." Ewin, in contrast, describes an effective brief hypnoanalytic uncovering treatment strategy for wart eradication without teaching the patient self-hypnosis. His approach combines ideomotor question-ing, age regression to wart onset, cognitive and expectational restructuring and reframing in trance, followed by direct healing suggestions. He emphasizes that it is important for the patient to not pay conscious attention to eradicating the wart or warts.

Our brief approach to the hypnotic treatment of warts involves direct skills shaping that also includes sensory imagery, redirection of attention, fraction-ation, reframing, direct healing suggestions and elements of surprise. Like Ewin (1992b), we suggest that the patient need not pay conscious attention to the wart-affected limb. Here is the step-by-step procedure:

1. To begin, direct the patient to learn how to reduce the blood flow to and cool the limb opposite the one affected. For example, say:

   > It is not necessary to pay attention to the hand with the wart. Instead, pay attention to your other hand [surprise and redirection of attention). Now tell me what level of warmth that hand feels using the scale 1 to 10, with 10 being most warm and 1 being least warm.

2. Next, ask the patient to concentrate on decreasing the blood flow through-out the nonaffected limb (e.g., from the shoulder down to the left hand). For example,

   > Just look at your hand. You don't even have to close your eyes. Tell me when your hand is feeling a level of warmth at 5. It's at 6? Well, that's okay. Now tell me when it's at 5. Just look at it and feel it getting cooler, and tell me when it's down to 5. Think of the blood not flowing down there [Imagery], and that the arm and the hand are getting cooler, and tell me when it's down to 4. [fractionation; repeat using levels 3 and 2]

3. Proceed until the patient answers affirmatively when you ask,

   > Is it feeling pretty cold right now?

   Ask the patient if you may feel it. After you feel the patient's limb, say,

   > It is in fact feeling pretty cold right now

   [if it indeed is]. You may add for reinforcement

   > By the way, my hand is pretty cold now, too, as I'm feeling yours.

4. Next, say

   > Okay, continue to concentrate on the hand [or foot] that doesn't have the wart. Now concentrate on the hand [or foot] with the wart and tell me what the level

of warmth is in your hand [or foot) with the wart [surprise and redirection of attention].

5. If the patient reports that the hand or foot feels cooler, ask the patient how that happened. Then say,

> Well, I guess it must be that both hands [or feet] are connected somehow, aren't they [reframing]? You have a right hand and a left hand. Your right hand is the one with the wart, but you weren't paying any attention to it, were you? It got cool all by itself, didn't it? Well, it's going to continue to get cool all by itself, without your having to pay attention to it [direct suggestion]. As it continues to get cool all by itself, there will be a reduction of blood flow to that hand, just like there was today. Gradually, the wart will no longer be fed from the flood flow, and it will shrivel up and fall off. But you didn't do any hypnosis. Would you like me to do some hypnosis with you?

What you have suggested at this point is that the patient no longer needs to pay any attention to the wart. You've also demonstrated that by not paying conscious attention to it, but rather by paying conscious attention to the unaffected limb, a transformation in physical sensation occurred in the affected limb.

6. This next step involves doing a hypnotic induction. After the patient is in trance, repeat the same process, except suggest that the hand or foot with the wart is going to continue to remain cool, and continue to reduce the blood flow to the wart. Then say the following:

> You're not going to pay any attention to it. The wart is going to shrivel up and fall off [building a desired expectancy]. It may happen today or tomorrow or next week or 10 days from now, but it's going to happen, because automatically, without your having to pay any attention to it, you are going to divert the blood flow away from the area. The wart is going to stop being fed. And because the wart is not going to be fed, it's not going to be able to exist without being fed [reframing]. The wart is going to shrivel up and fall off [direct suggestion]. Is that okay with you? Yes? Thank you.

In summary, the procedure involves using the unaffected limb to demonstrate that the patient can exercise control over the blood flow and the temperature of that limb. Then, you demonstrate that the two limbs are connected in terms of the effects of the process. In other words, when the patient checks the other limb (the one with the wart), he or she is likely to notice that that limb is cool also. Then, you give a very simple suggestion to the effect that

> Now that you haven't paid any attention to that limb, it has become cool, because the blood flow has been cut off. It will continue to cool without your having to pay any attention to it [suggestion for continued healing].

BRIEF COGNITIVE HYPNOSIS TECHNIQUES FOR "UNCOVERING" WITH PAIN PATIENTS

Many clinicians who work with patients dealing with chronic pain emphasize age regression and verbalization during trance that is cathartic and that uncovers and releases strong emotions that occurred at the time of the original trauma (Cheek, 1994; Ewin, 1986, 1992a; Watkins & Watkins, 1997). Others uncover and "peel away" the protective emotional overlays that metaphorically resemble one Band-Aid on another, completely insulating the emotional wound so that it cannot be exposed and allowed to heal (Hunter, 1996). These are often very powerful and effective approaches in dealing with pain of long duration.

In brief cognitive hypnosis, we attempt to emphasize the word "Brief." So, we have developed some procedures that utilize those important concepts, and allow for some limited "uncovering" to occur, but these procedures take significantly fewer hourly sessions. They also do not necessarily require specific regression to the time of the original trauma. We have scripted some of these procedures.

The Scrolling Blackboard Technique

This procedure usually is used after the patient has been working with self-relaxation for a few weeks to lessen the anxiety and emotional overlay that accompany chronic and continuous pain.

Now that you have relaxed yourself and are experiencing a very deep level of relaxation and hypnosis, you have entered the neutral place, the healing place. This is the place where there are no pressures or tensions or discomforts. This is where we can begin to erase the problems of the past and leave them behind, where they can do no harm.

Do you remember when you were in school and each classroom had a blackboard? You could write on it with chalk and erase what you wrote whenever you wanted to? Can you imagine such a place with a blackboard that you will be able to write on today, in your imagination? When you have that blackboard fixed in your mind, say "okay," so I can continue. Thank you. Now, imagine that this is a modern blackboard that has a scrolling feature that will allow you to write a lot, and it will scroll to produce more space as you need it. Do you have the scrolling feature on the blackboard? Say "okay" when you do. Thank you.

Now, take that chalk on the blackboard ledge and go back as far as you can in your mind and begin to write everything that you can remember that happened to you that was hurtful, harmful, fearful, uncomfortable or severely emotional. Include your physical hurts as well as your emotional hurts. Be as detailed as you can be. Include people and places and things.

Don't be concerned about how long it will take for this task to be accomplished. During hypnosis, time is flexible. What seems like a long time to you could be a short time during hypnosis, and what seems like a short time could really cover a long time in your life. Be as complete as you can, and take as much time as you seem to need. Notice that, as you finished a section of the blackboard, it automatically scrolls up, and a clean panel is available for your writing. Is the blackboard working okay? Thank you.

When you have written everything that you possibly can, right up to the present time, tell me "okay." Thank you. Now, look at the blackboard and note that it is scrolling back to the beginning. Check over everything that you have written and make sure that you haven't left anything out. If you need to add anything, extra space will appear for you to fill in what you want. When you have completed this, let me know. Thank you.

Take the eraser on the shelf and, starting with the bottom, most recent thing that you have written, begin to erase it. Notice that the blackboard scroll is working in reverse. Erase every bit of chalk writing that you see. Wipe the slate clean. Remove all of the things that you wrote that happened to you that caused hurt, whether it was physical or emotional. Wipe it out. Remove it. Leave no trace. Take whatever time you need and erase every bit of it. Don't leave anything. When you have wiped the slate clean, go back and remove any remnants that may be left. Please tell me when you have finished. Thank you.

Now, just sit there for a while, relaxed and feeling very clean and comfortable. When you are ready, you can awaken yourself and tell me about this interesting experience.

Discuss the patient's description of the blackboard experience and the way the patient feels after awakening compared to before the trance and blackboard experience. Instruct the patient to add the scrolling blackboard to one of the two self-hypnosis sessions that are already part of the patient's daily ritual. Explain that this will not add much time to the self-relaxation session because the purpose is to deal with any "left-over remnants" that are brought to mind. Usually the patient's pain level is significantly reduced because the buildup of "trauma" (stated as "hurt") causing emotional overlay has been mostly dissipated.

The patient should do this for a week, then return for another session. At this time, use further waking state exploration to help the patient become aware of his or her present experience of level of comfort. Whatever instant relaxation procedure has been taught should be reinforced in the waking state by having the patient practice the procedure in the office to consciously control the level of comfort. A scale of 1 to 10 can be used, with 10 being *least comfortable* and 1 being *most comfortable*. It is rarely necessary to continue the scrolling blackboard procedure again in the office. If treatment continues, return to training the patient in self-hypnosis skills and personal control.

The Silent Abreaction Method

This age regression procedure is used only after the patient has been working with self-relaxation for a few weeks to lessen the anxiety and emotional overlay that accompany chronic and continuous pain. It can help an individual to scan past hurts (or traumas) and to have a silent abreaction in relationship to these past hurts. This allows the patient to work through some of the past experiences and things that may have contributed to the continuation of his or her pain experience.

This technique can be helpful with a patient with whom you've been working for some time. It is not a technique to be used after one or two sessions, but rather after you've established a relationship with a patient, taught the patient self-hypnosis and had the patient practice self-hypnosis and self-relaxation. Silent abreaction should not be confused with silent abreaction technique developed by Helen Watkins (1980) for helping a victimized or abused patient safely express, defuse and release his or her anger against a perpetrator.

When introducing the technique, indicate to the patient the following:

> After you've entered deep relaxation and self-hypnosis, with your permission, we're going to be doing some exploration of the past. I'm not going to ask you to verbalize what you discover. I'm not going to ask you to detail in any way to me what you discover, although you can describe what you discover to me if you wish. This method will help take you back into the past by using a very strong hypnotic deepening procedure. You will begin to explore in your own mind, visually, kinesthetically and emotionally, those things that have occurred, that you need to put closure on, that you need to work through, that you need to feel comfortable about, and that you need to allow to be left in the past in order to be able to change your experience of the present, in terms of the discomfort, and your experience in the future, in terms of your having more and more comfort.

Have the patient put himself or herself into self-hypnosis using whatever method has been used so far, so that the patient can start the process. Then instruct the patient to signal when he or she wants you to take over.

> Allow yourself to go very deeply into relaxation, which you can do. You've already had the opportunity to learn and practice relaxation procedures, which have helped quite a bit in terms of reducing the experience of discomfort. You can feel more in charge of yourself. As you continue to go deeper into relaxation, allow yourself to feel more and more comfortable. Now I'm going to back off and leave you to do that. When you feel that you have reached the level of comfort that you can today, just lift a hand to indicate that you've reached that level of comfort and I will take over once again.

Deepening and Age Regression

Sit quietly as the patient continues the process of self-relaxation. When the patient signals that he or she is ready, say the following:

> I'm going to count from 30 to 1. With each number that I count you will go deeper and deeper into relaxation and hypnosis. You'll find yourself not only going deep-

er into relaxation and hypnosis but also moving rather quickly into the past, to the earliest time that you can remember when you felt hurt, when you felt extreme emotional and physical pain, when you felt great fear or a great deal of guilt. When you are there, you will encounter those experiences, and with the knowledge that you have today, the safety of my presence here in my office, silently work them through, and change their meaning so that they no longer have any validity or influence on your present and future feelings. If that feels okay to you, lift your hand to let me know. Good. Thank you.

Just listen to the numbers, and let yourself go. Find yourself going back in time, back into the past, as you go deeper and deeper into relaxation and hypnosis. 30—29—28—27 . . . [continue the countdown until you've reached the number 1. It should be a slow, gradual, deepening process.]

Silent Exploration and Abreaction

Once the patient is in deeper relaxation, you can say:

Now that we've reached the number 1, you can start the process of exploring those past experiences and begin to work through to resolve and to change the meaning of those past experiences. Remember, time has no meaning when you're in hypnosis. It may feel as if you're taking an hour or two to do that, but it may in fact be a very short period of time. When you've reached the present once again, when you work through all of those experiences and reach the present, just lift a hand to signal that you've completed the process.

As the patient explores these things, silently observe the patient's posture, movements and changing features. As the patient explores the past, he or she will give nonverbal feedback. You may observe smiles, grimaces, raised eyebrows, head nods, and so on, in response to the things that the patient is encountering. You may even watch as the patient carries on conversations, sometimes aloud, sometimes silently, with the individuals or circumstances in the past. This whole process may take anywhere from 10 to 30 minutes to accomplish, depending on how many traumatic experiences (hurts) the patient encounters and how intense those experiences are.

Reframing the Experience

When the patient has completed the task of exploration from the earliest time remembered to the present, he or she will lift a hand to inform you that the process is finished. At that point, say the following:

You've explored all of the things from the earliest past you can remember to the present that have had some effect and influence on the continuing chronic discomfort that you've been experiencing. As a result of this exploration, you can now leave behind you, as only a memory, those things that contributed to the problem that you brought to me when you came to see me here in the office. Because of that, you can begin to experience a greater sense of comfort, a greater sense of resolution, a greater sense of optimism and a greater sense of closure on those things that may have contributed to your discomfort problem.

Post-Hypnotic Imprinting

Next, use suggestion to imprint the feeling of comfort.

You are going to be able to realize that you have freed yourself from most of that emotional overlay that has contributed to the ongoing intensity of your discomfort and pain. From now on, every time you do your own self-hypnosis and relaxation, without having to go back into the past, you are going to be able to recognize and experience a greater sense of freedom, a greater sense of comfort and a greater sense of well-being.

Awakening

Let yourself be relaxed. When you're ready, you can awaken yourself. Very good. Now, please tell me how you are feeling.

Allow the patient to talk about how he or she is feeling, but do not encourage conscious detailed verbalization or description of the patient's hypnotic age regression experience. It is best left unstated, unless the patient feels the need to talk about it. Follow the patient's lead on this.

PREPARING FOR MEDICAL PROCEDURES, SELF-HEALING, AND COPING WITH TREATMENT SIDE EFFECTS

In the practice of brief cognitive hypnosis, we have often been called upon to assist individuals in coping with the unpleasant, uncomfortable and stressful aspects of various medical treatment procedures, such as surgery. There is substantial agreement in the literature that psychological preparation for surgery is beneficial for patients and improves their psychological and physical postoperative function (Blankfield, 1991; Johnston & Vogele, 1993; Kessler & Whalen, 1999).

Hypnosis can be an effective tool for producing analgesia for acute procedural pain. It is an ideal tool for preparing patients psychologically for surgery. Research reviews by Blankfield (1991) and Kessler and Whalen (1999) show that successful hypnotic preparation for surgery shortens hospital stays, reduces postoperative pain, results in less need for narcotics, reduces both pre- and postoperative anxiety, results in less blood loss and facilitates earlier return of normal gastrointestinal, bowel, and urinary tract functions.

Psychological preparation provides the patient with needed support and reassurance, as well as understandable information about the upcoming procedure and what to expect during each stage of the experience. The appropriate use of the hypnosis tool empowers the patient by increasing the patient's sense of control of his or her own experience, thus facilitating the patient's coping abilities. It can make the experience of undergoing a medical procedure more tolerable. Appropriately taught, clinically applied and supervised, the hypnosis tool can help ease the patient through surgery by reducing postoperative side effects and by speeding the patient's recovery (Kathy Platoni, personal communication, January 2001).

It has been shown that the tremendous apprehension, fear, and anxiety normally experienced by most patients before surgery or other invasive medical procedures negatively influence the body's physiological functions by inducing the fight or flight reaction (Fredericks, 2001; Kessler & Whalen, 1999). This increases the output of stress hormones, such as adrenaline and cortisol, and results in increased need for anxiolytic sedation, chemical anesthesia and narcotic analgesics, as well as untoward complications (Fredericks, 2001).

In the hands of the experienced clinician, the hypnosis tool can counter these undesirable reactions by preparing the patient for the medical procedure in several ways. The following steps are suggested:

1. Through the use of direct suggestion, imprint cue words or images that re-create comfortable, pleasant sensations previously experienced and that are associated with analgesia.
2. Use deep relaxation to calm the patient's fight or flight reaction and to counter the anxiety response. This results in a lower output of stress hormones, such as adrenaline.
3. Use hypnosis to put the patient back in charge and to build self-efficacy. By learning self-hypnosis before the medical procedure, the patient can practice inducing relaxation, turning off the fight or flight response and controlling and reducing anxiety. The patient also learns to selectively deploy his or her attention. This is an important skill for the patient to use both before and during the procedure. During surgery, for example, the patient needs to be able to focus his or her attention on selected aspects of the experience and to ignore sounds and conversations in the operating room that are not meant for the patient's awareness.
4. Instruct the patient to use self-hypnosis to rehearse the experience of going through the impending surgery, feeling in charge and in control. This repeated practice imprints a positive experience in the patient's unconscious, which then allows the patient to have that experience in the actual situation.
5. Provide the patient with a positive anchor to rely on before, during and after the experience. Go through several rehearsals in the office before the procedure is to take place.

Steps 1 through 5 teach the patient that the surgical procedure and its aftermath can be dealt with comfortably. Steps 6 through 8 below involve taking the clinician's presence one step further into the operating room.

The presence of the clinician in the operating room is necessary only for extensive, invasive, or lengthy procedures, or if the patient doesn't feel comfortable going through the procedure on his or her own and the surgeon is agreeable.

6. If you and the patient determine that your presence in the operating room is important to the patient, seek permission from the surgeon. If the request is denied, help the patient to imagine your presence and use the deep trance experience to satisfy the need for additional help.
7. If the request is granted, have a brief conference with the surgeon before the procedure is performed. During this conversation, discuss with the surgeon what he will be doing and ask for the surgeon's collaboration in terms what he or she can say that will help and what he or she ought not to say that could undermine the hypnotic suggestions and images.
8. Your reassuring and supportive presence can then be taken into the operating room, to be relied on during the procedure, to make sure that the patient remains comfortable, calm, and safe and to deliver the necessary hypnotic suggestions to the patient. You will be present at the patient's side during the entire procedure to coach the patient through it. You should be prepared to assure the patient that everything that happens, expected or not, is okay and can be handled. At times, when anxiety-provoking stimuli occur during the procedure, you can creatively reframe those stimuli to the patient in trance, so that they are perceived as something neutral or positive.

Case Study: Pain Control during a Colonoscopy

A 70-year-old patient who was using self-hypnosis for pain control needed to have a colonoscopy and wrote me (JIZ) of her experience:

"I was scheduled for a colonoscopy as part of a yearly physical. My mother had colon cancer when she was 72 years old. She was treated with surgery and died a peaceful death at age 86 from heart failure. My doctor told me that I would be sedated, so I would have no pain and no recollection of the procedure. I thought about that overnight and decided that sedation was unnecessary, that I would prefer going through the procedure using self-hypnosis. It took several days for me to reach him to ask if he would allow me to do that. He agreed with no reservations except that the IV needle would be inserted just in case. I was very pleased and surprised that he would agree so readily.

"During the precolonoscopy visit to his office, he asked me many questions, including my skills with self-hypnosis."

"On the day before the scheduled procedure, my therapist (who uses clinical hypnosis) and I went through a 'dry run' in his office. We looked up colonoscopy in a family health book and found an excellent illustration and explanation of the whole procedure, so I knew exactly what to expect. My therapist suggested that we use a numbing process of the whole colorectal area. During the dry run, I placed myself into self-hypnosis using my 'magic marble,' and I accomplished full numbing of the area while my therapist described the whole procedure.

"I arrived at the hospital at 9:00 A.M. the next day. I was quite calm and relaxed. Blood pressure 130/72. This really surprised my very nice nurse. She remarked that 'most people come in for this procedure off the wall.' The procedure was scheduled for 10:00 A.M., but since they did not have to wait for the sedation to take place, we were ready to begin by 9:30 A.M."

I felt a bit rushed in taking myself into trance, but we were off and running very quickly, so I had to go quickly. Through the whole procedure, I was very comfortable and watched it on the television screen as it was progressing. At the sharp turn into the bowel, I started to feel the beginning of a cramp, but when the doctor said to pay attention to my breathing, that feeling immediately went away. I forgot to mention that my therapist had told me to ask my doctor to say that if he detected a problem. When he said that, I heard my therapist's voice, the discomfort was gone, and they kept right on going."

"The doctor told me that on the way out, he was going to do some 'housecleaning.' He found five polyps at the proximal end of the bowel, nearest to the rectum, and he said he was going to remove two by cauterization and three with the loop on the instrument. My answer to him was 'Be my guest, I am feeling nothing.' So it was done. It was a veritable piece of cake."

"The nurse practitioner told me afterwards that invariably, even with sedation, the bowel tightens up at that last turn and makes it difficult for all concerned, but not this time. They were able to get through quickly. I felt like a 'star.' The doctor and the nurses, in fact the whole outpatient surgical staff, were very helpful and supportive and amazed at the ease of the procedure. They had never seen a patient use self-hypnosis before."

"I was back in my room at 10:00 A.M. and hungry. The doctor walked in with a tray with half a toasted bagel, a slice of cheese, butter, jelly, and a big cup of coffee, very happy about how things had gone. It all tasted delicious."

"I was home by 12:30 P.M., had a small can of light fruit, and had no side effects at all. No cramps, no pain, and no soreness, just very tired. I slept most of the rest of the day, played mah-jongg in the evening, and lost 20 cents. A fine ending to a fascinating experience."

"The method I used to induce self-hypnosis was my beautiful magic blue marble. I use it on a daily basis to deal with a chronic pain problem that I have. That too improves day to day. I place the marble in my hand, either one, and pay attention to the texture and warmth I feel, slow my breathing, and am in as deep a trance as I need to be for whatever I have to deal with at that moment. A truly 'magic marble.'"

SUMMARY

All of the techniques detailed in this and earlier chapters help the patient in feel relaxed, more comfortable and more in charge of how he or she feels. It is not a long leap to consider how these techniques can be used to help patients deal more comfortably with medical procedures and the numerous described side effects of medications.

The first thing that needs to be addressed is the patient's acceptance of the many descriptions from physicians and other medical professionals of what uncomfortable things to expect from any given medical treatment or medication. These always negative descriptions produce iatrogenic negatively charged suggestions that often represent to the patient prophecies of what the patient needs to suffer in order to suffer less. The statement that "most people experience" these side effects is powerful enough to make sure that they do in fact occur. This intensifies anxiety in anticipation of the procedure, or the use of the medication. It also intensifies any real or imagined uncomfortable side effects.

Health care professionals must describe the possible side effects to cover themselves against any possible ethical or legal ramifications of not obtaining the patient's informed consent for treatment. However, clinicians who use hypnosis already know that they can reduce and often control these predicted results of treatment. This seems self-evident, but it needs to be emphasized. The keys to accomplishing this include:

1. reframing the beliefs that the patient has regarding the warnings he or she received from other health care professionals (this means changing the negative absolutes to "maybe," "sometimes," "less noticeable," and "you can control how you feel and learn to change how you feel."
2. using waking state reframing, trance, self-hypnosis training and instant relaxation to reduce the anticipatory anxiety, to remove the emotional overlay and to teach the patient controlled relaxation to minimize the side effects to establish patient controlled comfort.

Having come this far in our book, readers are much more cognizant of the wide range of hypnotic procedures that can be applied to various medical problems. We will complete this chapter with a personal anecdote that illustrates the use of self-hypnosis in dealing with cancer treatment.

A PERSONAL ANECDOTE: CANCER TREATMENT, SELF-HEALING, AND THE USE OF SELF-HYPNOSIS AND RITUAL

Several years ago, I (JIZ) was diagnosed with prostate cancer. In consultation with my oncologist, I reviewed various treatment options. I established certain criteria that the treatment method had to meet so that my life could continue as normally as possible. At the time, I was in full-time private practice, teaching nationally at least four times a year and physically active. The least disruptive treatment chosen was 26 weeks of radiation therapy, 5 days a week, that could be done for about a half hour at the hospital on my way to my office each morning. My office was in a medical building near the hospital. This would also allow me to take a break from treatment to go to San Diego to teach at the International Society of Hypnosis (ISH) meeting.

Although a support group and other cancer information programs were offered, I decided to keep my life as normal and as regular as possible by not participating in these programs. I had been doing short sessions of self-hypnosis twice a day for many years to help me deal with the normal stressors of a busy clinical practice and active family life, I decided that self-hypnosis was an important procedure to use to assist in my recovery process.

In reviewing the literature on approaches to "tweak" the immune system to help the recovery process (Hall, 1983; Ruzyla-Smith et al., 1995; Simonton, Matthews-Simonton, & Creighton, 1978), I decided that the approaches I reviewed were too obsessive in nature for me. I felt that all of them concentrated on putting too much energy into thinking about the cancer and destroying it. My belief was and still is that the more one dwells on a problem, the less success one has in solving it. Instead, I decided to develop an approach that could become automatic and unconscious, without my thinking about it, in the same way that my autonomic nervous system keeps me alive without my having to pay conscious attention to it. I devised the following procedure.

I wrote down everything that I did from the moment I woke up in the morning to the moment I went to sleep at night, in as exact detail as possible. I then inserted into my daily ritual list the Monday through Friday early morning trips to the radiation department at the local community hospital. When I finished, my daily rituals looked something like this.

A.M.

Get out of bed. Put on a robe. Go to the bathroom. Turn on the coffeemaker. Read the morning paper with coffee and a small breakfast. Kiss my wife good morning. Clean up my breakfast mess. Shower and shave if I didn't shower before going to bed. Shave, if I did. Apply deodorant, gargle, use aftershave lotion, comb hair and get dressed.

(Usually I would do self-hypnosis when I arrived at the office, before I saw my first patient. Because I was adding the trip to the hospital, I decided to do the morning self-hypnosis at home before I left for the hospital treatment. So, after getting dressed, I added self-hypnosis to the ritual. Then I would drive to the hospital.)

After arriving at the hospital, I sign in. Wait to be called for radiation therapy. Walk into the dressing room. Change to a hospital gown. Lay on the radiation table. Close my eyes and listen carefully to the sounds of the technicians and the placement of the projector and the hum of the machine, while relaxing deeply. When the treatment finished, I get up, get dressed, confer with the radiation oncologist, thank everyone and leave the hospital.

Drive to my office. Pick up my phone messages and return calls. Prepare for my day's patient schedule by selecting records, starting new pages and opening filing records in order. See my morning patients and make notes after each patient. Answer phone messages, if any.

P.M.

Have lunch or take a long walk. Return to the office and check for phone messages and return calls if necessary. See afternoon patients and make notes. Check messages again and return calls.

Do afternoon self-hypnosis and leave stress behind before leaving the office and driving home. Drive home. Park my car. Go into my home. Greet my wife with a kiss and inquiry about her day. Set the table, or discuss dinner out.

Evening

Have a drink before dinner and watch the news on TV. Enjoy a good meal at home. Wash the dishes. Talk about our day for a while. Read, or watch some TV, or do some studying or work. Prepare for bed, brush my teeth, maybe shower, watch late TV news, read fiction in bed. Put out the light. Kiss my wife goodnight, etc. Sleep.

Naturally, the ritual changed from day to day and on weekends, but this was the general daily ritual.

I wrote down a number of possible suggestions to give to myself before the induction and trance experience. When I do self-hypnosis, I never try to self-suggest during trance. I always repeat my self-suggestions silently four or five times before starting the self-induction.

I decided on the following self-suggestions to be mentally verbalized before the induction and trance. This particular choice was made because it was short, simple, and direct.

1. Everything that I do every day to take better care of myself, from the time I get up in the morning to the time I go to sleep at night, including my sleep time, will positively augment and overlay my cancer treatment program.
2. All of my healing energy will reduce and control any radiation side effects and will direct the radiation to where it is needed most."

This was repeated four or five times before each of my two daily self-hypnosis sessions. I continued the suggestions for 4 weeks, then stopped mentally verbalizing them. For the balance of the treatment, I did self-relaxation without self-talk.

I live and socialize in a condominium community. No one there knew that I had cancer. I didn't look like a cancer patient, nor act like a cancer patient, nor feel like a cancer patient. I had no side effects from the radiation therapy except some increased tiredness during the first few weeks of the treatment. When the treatment was interrupted for 2 weeks for my trip to San Diego to teach at the ISH meeting, none of my colleagues knew I had cancer. During the 2 weeks, I felt more energized.

When I returned, the radiation was continued to completion. My doctors knew of my use of self-hypnosis as part of my treatment process and were surprised at the lack of the usual side effects and the positive results of the outcome. Many referrals have been made since to help others with similar diagnoses. I have been free of any indications of cancer for over seven years as of this writing.

Smoking Cessation and Keys to Change

12

A Single-Session Smoking Cessation Program

More than 25 years ago, I (JIZ) was asked by a family practice residency program medical staff in Syracuse, New York, where I was teaching family practice second-year residents the use of clinical hypnosis as an elective, to develop a smoking cessation program. Over a 4-year period, patients were referred from the two hospitals that sponsored the residency program for help in stopping smoking. By the end of the first year, a smoking cessation protocol was established that appeared to be effective.

Telephone follow-ups were conducted at 3-month intervals for 3 years with patients who were seen by me for one session to stop smoking. The patients were asked what their nonsmoking status was at the time of these calls. During the second and third year, patients who had started smoking again were invited back for an additional single session. Review of the follow-up data revealed that, by the end of the third year, approximately 70% of those patients who were seen for one visit were able to stop smoking for a period of 1 year or more. The percentage of success was even greater with those patients who had started smoking again, but who had not yet resumed smoking the original number of cigarettes they had originally smoked and who returned for a second visit.

Since that time, the smoking cessation program has been further refined with the addition of new scientific information and extensive feedback from former patients. Although no further formal follow-ups have been done, the anecdotal responses by the patients who have called back or returned have been even better than the previous reports.

Numerous workshops have been conducted over the years, with excellent reports from clinicians who have adopted or included key elements of this protocol in their own clinical treatment of smokers. The detailed protocol follows.

ESSENTIAL INGREDIENTS OF THE SINGLE-SESSION SMOKING CESSATION PROGRAM

The following constitutes an outline of the single-session approach. We will go into each section in detail and provide scripts later on in this chapter.

1. Intake Evaluation

A thorough intake evaluation is conducted to obtain the following information so that the single-session approach can be geared to the individual patient's needs: the patient's medical history; family and social environment; family medical history; others residing with or frequently with the patient; smoking and other substance use; frequency of use of tobacco and other stimulants, coffee, and medication (prescription and over-the-counter); recreational drug use, if any; motivation for the decision to make the appointment; patient's desire to stop smoking and reasons; any previous attempts to stop smoking (number of times and methods); if previous attempts to stop were made, length and probable reasons for success or failure. (See the discussion of intake evaluation in chapter 1.)

2. Initial Waking State Reframing

First, patient's belief system regarding the built-in dangers contained in cigarettes and other tobacco products is reframed. We accomplish this by going over the following information with the patient right after the intake evaluation is completed:

1. the four different U.S. Surgeon General's warnings printed on every pack of American-produced cigarettes (if available, a reading of the major warning on British-produced cigarettes is also discussed) (i.e., "Smoking Kills.").
2. newspaper articles regarding the health problems, poisonous contents, research studies, and U.S. Surgeon General's published report on the effects of cigarette smoking
3. information and printed confirmation regarding the healing results of no longer smoking

3. Additional Waking State Reframing

We then go on to address and reframe the following concepts:

1. The concept or belief that "the problem is an *addiction* to cigarettes and nicotine" is reframed as "the problem is that smoking is a h*abit.*" Addictions are hard to change. Habits can be changed.
2. The concept that "the ex-smoker will have to fight the *urge* to smoke" is reframed "the ex-smoker will from time to time have *memories* of having

smoked in the past." The point is that *urge* is a word that implies the need to take action, whereas the word *memory* does not imply any need to act (i.e., to start smoking again). A memory is just another thought.

3. The concept that "once the smoker stops smoking, he or she will experience *nicotine withdrawal*" is reframed as "the symptoms that people who have stopped smoking often label as 'Withdrawal' are really a "stress reaction."

4. Explanations and Corrections of Misconceptions about Hypnosis

At this point, we elicit the patient's expectations about the hypnosis experience and we clarify any misconceptions and update the patient's understanding of hypnosis. Next, we explain what the patient can expect after experiencing hypnosis and after changing "smoking behavior" to "nonsmoking behavior."

5. Choice of Trance Induction

We are then ready to choose an induction method and use it to help the patient into hypnotic trance. In our single-session protocols, we do not teach the patient self-hypnosis. Instead, we choose an induction that is not designed for the patient's self-application. In most cases, the chosen induction is rapid and emphasizes the "kinesthetic" sensory system. However, we always gear the approach to the individual patient. There are cases when we might feel that it is necessary to choose an induction that emphasizes additional sensory representational systems (e.g., visual in addition to kinesthetic). (See chapter 5 for a discussion of induction methods.)

6. Trance Dialogue and Change Language

Once the patient is in trance, we verbalize carefully chosen trance dialogue and change language. There is a general script (given below) that we always follow. However, once again, we gear the contents of our trance state suggestions, informational presentation, change language and reframes, as well as the order of their presentation, to the individual patient. This is based on the information gathered during the intake evaluation, which includes the patient's level of intelligence, verbal sophistication, how the patient processes information, and the patient's unique history, medical factors, motivational factors and psychological and life issues.

7. New Coping Skills Taught during the Trance Experience

During the patient's trance experience, we teach the patient alternative coping skills for coping with stress instantly and effectively as an interrupter of stressful feelings.

8. Posttrance Reframing and Imprinting of Change

During the trance experience, we administer verbal suggestions for the patient's conscious use of the newly taught coping skills and concepts after he or she awakens from trance, leaves the office and in the future. After awakening the patient from trance, we focus the patient's attention back onto the pleasant relaxing aspects of the trance experience and reinforce them. We reinforce the patient's expectations of success and also inform the patient of the availability of our support from that point on.

SMOKING CESSATION REFRAMING

The patient comes to the treatment setting with an agenda and belief system that are often unrealistic and distorted. This can prevent or delay a successful outcome of treatment. The patient may have beliefs about hypnosis, cigarettes and smoking behavior that are not valid or realistic. The patient's expectations and motivation may be unrealistic or insufficient. Previous attempts to control smoking behavior may have established a mindset that may negatively or positively affect the outcome. How the patient came to treatment may be important in this regard. The referring source could have established positive expectations or iatrogenic fears.

Hypnosis and the trance experience are only tools to facilitate change. The trance state is only part of the change process. The gathering of information (intake evaluation), waking state reframing, and the trance experience, with accompanying change language, are the three equal partners in our single-session smoking cessation program. Most of the waking state reframes that are presented below are contained in the script that follows. Note that some are used only if the patient asks about or expresses concern about those specific issues.

THE U.S. SURGEON GENERAL'S WARNINGS

The four U.S. Surgeon General's warnings discussed below are printed one to a pack. Every brand of cigarette must have all four, one to a pack. If cigarettes are purchased by the carton, all the packs in the carton have the same warning. The process of initial waking state reframing confronts the patient with key facts about these warnings that many smokers either do not know, are unaware of, or have chosen to ignore.

"Cigarette Smoke Contains Carbon Monoxide."

Fact: Carbon Monoxide is a Poison

It can cause brain damage, lung damage, severe respiratory problems and can reduce oxygen into the bloodstream, thus reducing immune function, and can even kill.

Fact:

Smokers take in 300 times more carbon monoxide from a single cigarette than from the exhaust of a running automobile or truck over the same length of time it takes to smoke a cigarette.

Fact:

All of these warnings are compromise statements negotiated between the tobacco companies, which wanted no warning, and the federal government, which wanted an extreme warning. This means that each warning is less than all of the facts.

"Smoking Causes Lung Cancer, Heart Disease, and Emphysema, and May Complicate Pregnancy."

Fact:

This warning contains a simple declarative sentence that says in no uncertain terms that cigarette smoking *causes* these diseases. It doesn't say maybe, or occasionally, or sometimes. It says *smoking causes* these diseases. This is a compromise statement. Therefore, we can assume that smoking causes more diseases than are listed here.

"Smoking by Pregnant Women May Result in Fetal Injury, Premature Birth, and Low Birth Weight."

Fact:

Once again, this is a compromise message. Smoking by pregnant women may cause other serious complications, such as miscarriage, high-risk pregnancy, and risk to the life of the pregnant woman.

Fact:

The seriousness of carbon monoxide and its effect on the fetus cannot be emphasized enough. Carbon monoxide intake from cigarette smoking significantly reduces the amount of oxygen transmitted to the fetus through the bloodstream of the mother. This reduction of oxygen can cause brain damage, serious physical deformity, and premature birth.

"Quitting Smoking Now Greatly Reduces Serious Risks to Your Health."

Fact:

This is a compromise warning that reduces the significance of the research proving that when a person stops smoking, that person's body immediately begins the process of healing and repair of much of the damage caused by smoking. Remove the carbon monoxide intake, and the increased oxygen invigorates the immune system by increasing the manufacture of antibodies.

Fact:

Research studies that examined groups of 100 people who never smoked and 100 people of similar background and ages who stopped smoking for 5 years showed both groups to be equally healthy.

"Smoking Kills!"

This message is found in large, bold type on the back of packs of cigarettes manufactured and sold in Great Britain. A visitor from London was brought to my (JIZ) office by a former patient. The patient brought a pack of cigarettes with that message. In my workshops, I give a photocopy of that package and message to participants with the handouts. It cannot be reproduced here because of copyright and trademark restrictions.

BENZENE AND OTHER POISONS IN CIGARETTES

After reframing the U.S. Surgeon General's warnings, reference is made to several newspaper articles and research studies regarding the poisonous contents of smoking tobacco, the health problems caused by smoking and the healing results of no longer smoking. Reference is also made to the U.S. Surgeon General's published report on the effects of cigarette smoking.

Fact:

In 1990, Perrier bottled water, a French import, was removed from stores, restaurants, and bars all over the world because bottles tested for purity contained benzene, a known cancer-causing chemical. Benzene is an industrial solvent often used by bottlers to dissolve leftover residues in recycled bottles before sterilizing and filling.

Fact:

In 1986, a U.S. Surgeon General's report indicated that tobacco products contained as much as 2,000 times more benzene than was found in the bottles of Perrier water that led to their recall.

Fact:

The same report listed 42 other known carcinogens also found in cigarettes and 200 known poisons contained in the smoke inhaled, such as benzene, DDT, arsenic, formaldehyde and carbon monoxide.

ADDITIONAL SMOKING REFRAMES

The reframes that follow are not part of the regular script that is used during the smoking cessation waking state reframing process. These are add-ons to be used if the patient makes statements or asks questions regarding these issues. They address common erroneous beliefs about smoking and its consequences.

Erroneous Belief 1: "It Won't Happen to Me"

Many smokers believe that because they have been smoking for a long time, and smoking a lot, without developing serious health problems, they are not at risk to develop such problems if they continue to smoke. The thinking goes something along the lines of "It hasn't happened yet, so I guess I'm safe."

Fact:

Many smokers ignore almost invisible warnings of health problems by identifying them as a normal part of aging, too much sun, not enough exercise, something that was eaten, and so on.

For example, cigarette smoking causes premature aging of the skin. It causes crow's-feet around the eyes, furrows around the mouth, and pronounced lines and wrinkles caused by drying of the skin. Plastic surgeons, in most cases, will not perform facial surgery on smokers. They tell the patient that nicotine is a vasoconstrictor that narrows the arteries and blood vessels, thus reducing circulation throughout the body and especially the face. Plastic surgery usually requires the lifting of the skin. For this skin to remain alive, it requires normal blood circulation. When skin is covered, tucked, or stretched, the skin often dies, leading to infection and other complications.

Erroneous Belief 2: "I'm Too Old to Stop, and It Won't Help If I Do"

Many smokers believe that, because they have been smoking so long and are over a certain age, stopping now will make no difference to their health and will not improve their existing medical problems.

Fact:

Women and men who do stop smoking, whether age 35 or 70, whether they smoke five cigarettes a day or five packs a day, whether they smoke filters or nonfilters, lights or regulars, can significantly cut the risk of a heart attack or early death.

Fact:

A 6-year study (U.S. Surgeon General, 1990) was conducted that kept track of all deaths and nonfatal heart attacks among 1,693 people age 55 and over, all long-time smokers. Of the group, 807 of them quit smoking at the start of the study, and 1,086 kept smoking. Six years later, 42% of the smokers had died or had a nonfatal heart attack, compared with less than 35% of the former smokers. When the researchers translated these figures into relative risks, they found that those who had stopped smoking had reduced their chances of heart attack or early death by between one-third and one-half.

Erroneous Belief 3: "Smoking Relaxes Me"

People believe and almost always explain that cigarette smoking relaxes them.

Fact:

Cigarettes contain nicotine. Nicotine is a stimulant. Stimulants send adrenaline into the bloodstream, increasing all of the physical changes associated with anxiety and stress. The sense of relaxation starts to occur as a result of the interruption of some activity, as well as the time and ritual leading to and lighting the cigarette. With the first puff, it takes only 6 seconds for 25% of the nicotine to reach the brain. That is enough stimulant to give a lift in feeling that exaggerates the experience of relaxation. Each puff enhances that feeling for a while. However, by the time the smoker has finished the cigarette, all of the nicotine has reached the brain and the person begins to experience nervousness. The nicotine then leaves the brain, and the smoker feels let down. The system slows, the smoker feels tired, then wants another cigarette to bring himself or herself back up. This sets up the cycle of chain smoking. Chain smoking creates the feeling of need that leads to more smoking.

Fact:

Nicotine causes the heart to beat faster, blood vessels to constrict, blood pressure to rise, and pulse rate to increase. Free fatty acids pour into the blood. These effects, combined with the stress caused by carbon monoxide, cause 120,000 excess heart attack deaths a year among U.S. smokers.

Nicotine's Contradictory Effects

Nicotine has various contradictory effects. At first, it sharpens thinking, but soon the smoker feels tired and let down. The heart rate slows, the blood pressure drops and the mind loses its keen edge. Hitting the brain first, nicotine galvanizes nerve connections, then blocks them. It invokes the discharge of adrenaline and similar catecholamines, then shuts them down. It stimulates nerves in muscles, but this quickly gives way to a kind of paralysis. In small doses, nicotine causes tremors; in large doses, convulsions. Small doses stimulate breathing; large ones have the opposite effect. Nicotine excites the vomiting reflex in the brain and in the stomach nerves. It has an antidiuretic effect, but in the intestines it is initially stimulating. This explains why many smokers depend on the first smoke of the day for bowel regularity.

Erroneous Belief 4: "Cigarettes Are Addictive"

Most smokers believe that cigarette smoking is addictive, and that when they try to stop smoking, the various discomforts they experience are "withdrawal symptoms." Without arguing the label *addiction*, it is important to reframe the concept of withdrawal as stress reaction. This reframe will be noted in the smoking cessation script to follow.

It is our position that the label *addiction* has been too often generalized to include almost all behavior that individuals have difficulty changing. The early research on cigarette smoking used the label *habituating*, and dictionary definitions of addiction use the label *habit* when applied to compulsive behaviors that are object or behaviorally directed.

Erroneous Belief 5: "If I Stop Smoking, I Will Eat More and Gain Weight"

Many smokers believe that if they stop smoking, they will eat more and then gain weight. This belief is related to the that eating food will become a substitute form of oral gratification. As long as an individual holds these beliefs, that individual is likely to bring his or her behavior into conformity with them. Therefore, the beliefs need to be reframed if they are brought up by the patient.

EXPLANATIONS AND CORRECTIONS OF MISCONCEPTIONS ABOUT HYPNOSIS AND THE HYPNOSIS EXPERIENCE

As has been stated, the patient often comes to the hypnosis experience with many misconceptions. They often expect to be "zapped," "put out," or "put under" so that they are unconscious and not aware of what is taking place. They may expect to hear the suggestions given by the therapist but not remember what has occurred afterwards. Posttrance, they may question the reality of the trance experience by saying: "How come I heard everything you said, and only felt relaxed?"

As contained in the script that follows, during the waking state reframing, emphasis is placed on the cooperation between the two parts of the mind—the conscious and the unconscious. The patient is also told that he or she may indeed hear everything that is said, but if the mind wanders, the unconscious will still hear everything. If the patient asks this question after "awakening," the clinician should remind the patient about this earlier explanation.

After the intake evaluation, the smoking cessation waking state reframing process starts. It is scripted below.

THE SMOKING CESSATION WAKING STATE REFRAMING SCRIPT

The session starts with the following question:

> Why do you want to stop smoking? What have you done to stop smoking in the past? Tell me about those times. What did you do? When was that? How long did it last? Why did you start smoking again? Why did you now choose hypnosis and your current visit to see me?
>
> Do you have any cigarettes with you? If you have, please put the pack or packs on the table. Thank you.

Look at the U.S. Surgeon General's warning on the patient's pack of cigarettes, then reach into the table drawer to remove additional packs to complete the four warnings. Place them on the table with the carbon monoxide warning first, then the lung cancer warning, followed by the pregnancy warning and the quitting smoking statement. A copy of the British "smoking kills" warning can be put on the table for later use. You then continue:

> When was the last time you read the Surgeon General's warning on a pack of cigarettes? Do you remember the message?

Very often the patient will reply, "Cigarette smoking may be dangerous to your health." If so, your reply is:

> That message hasn't been on a pack of cigarettes for many years.

Continue:

> There are four different messages, one message to a pack, on every brand of American-made cigarettes. Every brand must have four different messages, one message to a pack. If you buy them by the carton, every pack has the same message, because that is how they are packaged. If you buy four or five packs off the rack, they usually have the same message because they come out of the same carton. This is important to what we are doing, so please bear with me.

Hand the patient the pack with the carbon monoxide warning and say:

Please read the Surgeon General's warning out loud" [Surgeon General's warning: "Cigarette smoke contains carbon monoxide"].

Thank you. Is carbon monoxide a poison? Of course it is. It is what comes out of the exhausts of automobiles and trucks. In sufficient amounts it can kill you. That's how people die in a closed garage with the motor running. In lesser amounts, it can cause brain damage and breathing problems, by reducing oxygen in the brain and lungs.

What is important about this message and all of the others that I will be sharing with you is that they are all compromise messages—compromise between the federal government, which wants an extreme message, and the cigarette companies, which want no message. They got together, they negotiated, and they reached a compromise.

So, if the cigarette manufacturers admit that cigarettes contain carbon monoxide, and carbon monoxide is a poison, that's the least dangerous poison they have to admit to. There is no current law requiring the listing of contents or ingredients, so they don't have to tell you what is in their cigarettes. Let's talk about carbon monoxide for a moment.

If you were to stand outside inhaling the fumes from a running car for 5 minutes, or stand outside and smoke a cigarette for 5 minutes, you would take in 300 times more carbon monoxide from the cigarette than you would from the car. That is a fact. What you smell from the exhaust of the car is not carbon monoxide. Carbon monoxide is odorless. What you smell is the burning gas and oil. By the time carbon monoxide reaches you, it is mixed with a lot of air. But the moment you light up the cigarette, that combustion immediately releases carbon monoxide directly into the smoke that you inhale.

That carbon monoxide reduces oxygen to your brain and to your lungs, but more importantly, it reduces oxygen into your bloodstream. The blood needs oxygen to manufacture white blood cells, which in turn manufacture antibodies that are moved throughout your bloodstream to heal and repair your body. So, with every single cigarette, you reduce your immune system's ability to heal and repair your body. You are more tired than you may need to be. You have more aches and pains than you need to have. You get sick easier and stay sick longer.

Take the cigarette pack from the patient and set it down flat on the table so that the Surgeon General's warning is facing the patient. Then get ready to refer to a newspaper article that was originally published in the *Palm Beach Post* entitled "Cigarettes Have More Benzene Than Perrier" (Spires, 1990, p. 1E). In a moment, you will pick up the article (A copy of this archived article can be obtained by logging on to the Palm Beach Post website address, www.palmbeachpost.com. Search Final Edition online Archive for author name, "Spires," headline, "Benzene.") and read portions that are excerpted below. First, say:

Do you remember when they took bottled Perrier water off the shelves because it contained benzene? I collect newspaper articles on cigarettes and smoking, and here is one that says "Cigarettes Contain More Benzene Than Perrier."

Show the headline to the patient and say,

Let me read a few paragraphs to you.

Begin to read the following excerpts from the article:

"When traces of benzene, a known carcinogen, were found in some samples of Perrier bottled water, the Environmental Protection Agency and the Food and Drug Administration reacted quickly and immediately removed the product from retailer shelves. There was no such action in 1986, however, when a Surgeon General's report measured almost 2,000 times more benzene in tobacco products as was found in the imported bottled water." (Spires, 1990, p. 4A)

Do you know what benzene is? Benzene is an industrial solvent that causes cancer. When bottlers recycle glass bottles, dried up in the bottom of the bottle is residue from the previous contents. As the bottles are going around the rack in preparation for filling, benzene mixed with pure water is injected into the bottle. The bottle is mechanically shaken to dissolve the residue, and then it is washed and dried in preparation for filling.

Apparently, in the bottling process in France, there was some problem with the machinery. When samples were taken to test for purity, trace amounts of benzene were found. Because benzene causes cancer, the company had to remove millions of bottles from shelves all over the world, costing it millions of dollars.

The tobacco leaf is shiny. It has a waxlike coating that protects it from weather conditions, insects, and disease. The coating doesn't burn very well. In the curing process, the tobacco leaf is sprayed with benzene to dissolve the coating. Tobacco is porous. It absorbs benzene. You can't wash it out. Then that tobacco is used for cigarettes, cigars, pipe tobacco, chewing tobacco and snuff.

Let me read two other parts of this article:

"The same Surgeon General's report listed 42 other known carcinogens also found in cigarettes. Tobacco smoke contains 4,000 chemicals, including 200 known poisons such as DDT, arsenic, formaldehyde and carbon monoxide." (Spires, 1990, p. 4A)

Every single cigarette, regardless of the brand or style, has almost 2,000 times more benzene, a cancer-causing chemical, than each of the bottles of water removed from the shelf. It also contains 42 other cancer-causing chemicals and 200 known poisons. When I said that this was a compromise message, that was an understatement, wasn't it?

After this, hand the patient the next pack with the lung cancer warning, then ask the patient to read it out loud. (Surgeon General's warning: "Smoking causes lung cancer, heart disease, and emphysema, and may complicate pregnancy")

That says cigarette smoking causes those diseases. It doesn't say maybe, or occasionally, or sometimes. It says, in no uncertain terms, that cigarettes cause those diseases. This is a compromise message. It causes many more diseases than are listed on that pack of cigarettes.

Take the second pack from the patient and stack it on top of the first pack so that the Surgeon General's warning is facing the patient. Then hand the patient the third pack with the pregnancy warning and ask the patient to read the message out loud. (Surgeon General's warning: "Smoking by pregnant women may result in fetal injury, premature birth and low birth weight")

> This message may not apply to you personally [stated if the patient is male or an older woman]. But it is important for you to be aware of it. That warning clearly says that cigarette smoking causes problems of pregnancy. That is also a compromise message. The carbon monoxide reduces oxygen into the bloodstream of the mother, thus reducing oxygen into the bloodstream of the fetus. Without sufficient oxygen, the baby can be born with brain damage or physical deformity, and is usually prematurely born. It has to be placed in an incubator for oxygen to start its own immune system working. Plus, all of those cancer-causing chemicals and poisons go directly into the bloodstream of the fetus, causing additional health problems at birth. These are usually considered high-risk pregnancies.

Take that pack from the patient and stack it on top of the other two packs with the warning facing the patient. Next hand the patient the fourth pack and ask the patient to read the message out loud. (Surgeon General's warning: "Quitting smoking now greatly reduces serious risks to your health")

> This is the most important message printed on a pack of cigarettes. Stopping smoking now greatly reduces serious risk to your health. Isn't that a rather extraordinary message to be on a pack of cigarettes? Remember that I said that this is a compromise message? What it ought to say is, When you stop smoking, your body immediately begins the process of healing and repair. That's what the research says beyond any question. But that would be too dramatic a statement to appear on a pack of cigarettes, so the compromise message is "Quitting smoking now greatly reduces serious risks to your health."

If you have a pack of British cigarettes with the message "Smoking kills," bring it out now and say the following:

> I had a patient recently who lived in England. He brought me this pack of cigarettes. [Hands the pack to the patient.] Please read this message out loud. ["Smoking kills."] Isn't that an incredible message? You can't get any more specific than that, can you?" [If that pack is not available, the clinician goes on without it]

Now take all of the packs, with the exception of the one brought in by the patient and place them back in the drawer or out of sight. Pick up the patient's pack and say:

> Let me explain why I did this. The mind is made up of two parts. One part we call the conscious mind. You have control of the conscious mind. When you buy this pack of cigarettes and pay money for it, that is a conscious behavior. You can't do it without knowing that you are doing it. Behavior can't change without the cooperation of the conscious mind. I can't make you do something that you do not want to do. So it is important for the conscious mind to be fully aware of all of the

issues relating to smoking behavior. You know that smoking is not good for you, or you wouldn't be here. But you were not aware of all the information that I just shared with you. Isn't that so?

We tend to not want to read about what we don't want to know about, so we ignore the messages on the packs and the newspaper articles. We don't want to be told or reminded that we are doing something wrong or bad or unhealthy.

Well, now your conscious mind has this information. It cannot ignore it any longer. Now your conscious mind has a greater motivation to want to help you stop smoking.

The other part of the mind we call the unconscious or the subconscious mind. Both names mean the same thing. The unconscious mind controls all of your automatic functions. It controls your breathing, heartbeat, pulse rate, blood flow, all of the things that keep you alive that you pay little or no attention to. They are automatic.

Plus, the unconscious controls all of the other things that you do that you have little or no control over; like your habits, your automatic behaviors, your smoking, even such behaviors as which side of the bed you sleep on and which shoe you put on first when you get dressed in the morning.

One of the problems is that we assume if we know something consciously, we also know it unconsciously. The fact is, we may not. And the reason we may not is that the unconscious is not easily communicated with, so it may not always have enough information to make some judgments for us. One of the ways to communicate with the unconscious is repetition. We do something over and over and over again, and the unconscious gets the idea we want to do it. It takes charge of it and makes a habit of it. Once it is a habit, we have little or no control over it.

Another way to communicate with the unconscious is through a shock, a traumatic experience, a serious illness, or a death in the family. This causes an imprint into the unconscious that can cause fear or anxiety or depression or whatever is appropriate to the particular shock experience.

Still another way to communicate with the unconscious is the way that we will be using here in the office today. When a person is in a deep state of relaxation, and for the moment I use the words relaxation and hypnosis interchangeably, the doorway to the unconscious opens. With your permission, I can then talk to your unconscious and give it information it needs to have in a language and form that it will accept, to help you change the behavior that you want to change. That is why I asked questions, so I can determine the language and form to use specifically for you.

Once the unconscious has accepted this information, it can't ignore it and has to act on it to change the behavior that you want to change, namely, to be a nonsmoker. But it is not quite that simple. The reason it is not that simple is because there are two parts of the mind, the conscious and the unconscious.

Make two fists and face them toward each other. Hold up your left fist and say:

The conscious mind wants to change.

Then hold up your right fist and say:

The unconscious doesn't yet know it needs to change.

Push both fists together two or three times and say:

This causes a conflict between the conscious and the unconscious. This conflict causes stress. This stress is what makes it so difficult to stop smoking. From my point of view, there are no withdrawal symptoms when a person stops smoking. If there were, I wouldn't be able to help so many people stop in one visit.

So, I'm convinced that what people call "withdrawal symptoms" are their own individual unique stress reactions. You hear people say, "When I tried to stop smoking, I became irritable and short-tempered and hard to get along with." When they are asked "What happens when you are under stress?" they usually say, "When I'm under stress, I am irritable and short-tempered and hard to get along with." Someone else may say, "When I try to stop smoking, I gain weight." When they are asked "What happens when you are under stress?" they usually say "When I'm under stress, I eat a lot." These are stress reactions unique to the individual, not withdrawal symptoms.

Place your hands vertically, palms facing each other, then slowly bring your hands toward each other, fold them together, and says:

You consciously want to stop smoking, and I gave more information to your conscious mind. I also give the right information to your unconscious mind, and it accepts that information. Now the two parts of the mind join together, in cooperation with each other, like my two hands folding together, without pressure or tension or stress. So the behavior changes easily and comfortably, without pressure or tension or stress and without withdrawal symptoms.

The reason we talk about hypnosis and relaxation in the same breath is because we are not talking about loss of awareness and being powerless. We are talking about helping you into the kind of relaxation that you experience just before you fall asleep at night and just as you are waking up in the morning. You know the feeling, loose and limp and relaxed. You know you can move if you want to, but you just don't feel like doing it.

That presleep, postsleep relaxed feeling is called the hypnogogic state. The reason it is called that is because it is similar in brain wave function to when someone is in hypnosis. Your mind is active, but your body is relaxed. You are aware of everything that is going on. Sounds are off in the background. If your mind wanders, it doesn't make any difference because your unconscious will still hear everything that I am saying to you. That is when the doorway to the unconscious opens, and with your permission, I can talk directly to your unconscious and give it the kind of information it needs to have to help you be a nonsmoker.

When we are through, you will have no wish or desire or need for a cigarette. You may think about smoking from time to time because we can't get rid of the memory of something you did so often, for so long, that quickly. You will recognize those thoughts as only a memory. They won't bother you. You will let them alone, they will go away very quickly and you will feel perfectly fine.

Even now, you may think about smoking but not smoke. You may be in a place where there is no smoking allowed, or with friends who don't smoke, or you are busy doing something. You may think about smoking during these times, but you don't get up every time you think about it and go outside to light up a cigarette, do you? You may do that sometimes, but most of the time you don't. Isn't that true?

What you just told me is very important. You just told me that you can think about smoking but not smoke. You have a behavioral system in place that says, "I can think about smoking and not smoke." It is operational. It is functional. It works. It just doesn't work all of the time. But because it works, we technically don't have to change your behavior. We can take an existing behavior that already works and stretch it into those times that you used to smoke. That makes it easier to do.

Imagine for a moment that behavior is a straight line.

While you are saying this, touch the thumb and forefinger of each hand together, then stretch your hands apart as if drawing a straight line. In the middle of that imaginary line, place your extended thumbs together, with the first and second fingers extended, then move both sets of fingers like two pairs of scissors and say:

This little part here is smoking behavior. We snip it here and we snip it here and we take it away. Then we take the two ends and tie a knot. [The clinician ties an imaginary knot.] This knot is the memory of your having smoked, but the behavior is gone. You don't have to change anything that you did while you smoked. You just won't smoke.

There is something else I want to mention. While we were talking, you said or implied that you smoked more when you were under stress. Well, you won't need to smoke anymore. I am going to teach you a way of dealing with momentary stressors, in seconds, without closing your eyes or having anyone knowing that you are doing it. That will come in handy, won't it? Do you have any questions?

SMOKING CESSATION INDUCTION AND TRANCE SCRIPT

At this point, you can choose a brief induction that you usually use or choose one of the inductions described in this book. However, it is important that it be short. We do not usually teach self-hypnosis for single-session behavior change. For smoking cessation, the induction that we use most often is rising and falling arms (see chapter Four).

Smoking Cessation Trance Dialogue

When the patient's arms are both on the arms of the chair or in the patient's lap, continue with the following:

As you are sitting in the chair, already relaxed and breathing normally, and listening to the sound of my voice, you will find yourself going even deeper into relaxation and hypnosis—deeper with each breath that you take, and deeper with each word that I say, regardless of the meaning of those words. As you go deeper with each breath, and deeper with each word, the doorway to your unconscious opens. With your permission, I have the opportunity to talk directly to your unconscious and give it information it needs to help you change the behavior that you want to change, namely, to be a nonsmoker.

When you light up that cigarette and inhale, that smoke contains poisons. Those poisons condense on the large tissues and organs of your body. As they do, they slowly begin to eat away at body tissue, causing that tissue to break down. A wide range of health-related problems can begin to occur.

The poisons from cigarettes affect other parts of your body in different ways. The narrow passages of your body—your sinuses, your breathing tubes, your digestive tract, your blood vessels, your intestines—all of the narrow passageways are blocked by the poisons. This can cause sinus problems, breathing problems, high blood pressure, heart valve problems, even a heart attack. If these poisons block the connecting link between the heart and the brain, they can cause headaches and sleeping problems, even problems of concentration and memory.

The human body is designed to heal itself. If you cut yourself, that wound heals. If you catch a cold, you may take some medication to help you feel better. But that medication doesn't cure your cold. Your own body does that by manufacturing antibodies that are moved through your bloodstream to the various places where there may be an infection and damage. They kill off the infection and repair the damage. They do that very well. That scab on a wound contains antibodies building new tissue to repair the wound.

But as long as you continue to smoke and take in all that carbon monoxide and all those poisons, your body can't do the job it is designed to do. It tries, but it can't. It is like taking one step forward and two steps backward. It tries, but it can't.

Once you stop smoking today, as you will, your immune system kicks in and your body immediately begins to heal and repair itself. There was a research study done a number of years ago. It compared 100 people who had never smoked, with 100 people of similar ages and backgrounds who had stopped smoking for 5 years. Both groups were given the same health and physical examinations. The results were rather surprising. The people who had stopped smoking were just as healthy as the people who had never smoked. Researchers believed that it took less than 5 years for the healing to occur, so they did some more research. They have since discovered that the healing starts immediately after the cessation of the smoking behavior.

When you stop smoking today, as you will, your body will immediately begin the process of healing and repair.

Let me tell you something else about smoking. Cigarettes are designed so that they affect your sense of taste and smell, so that you will not be aware of the poisons contained in them. Hypnosis has the ability to heighten your sensory awareness. It can return your sense of smell and taste. If someone is smoking around you, in most normal circumstances their smoking won't bother you. But you will become more aware and more sensitive to the smell of burning tobacco and the sight of the smoke from that burning tobacco. Even though that won't bother you, the sight of the smoke and the smell of the burning tobacco will act as an ongoing reminder to you, consciously and unconsciously, that this is not something you ever want to do again with a cigarette or any other tobacco product.

You came in today because you decided it was time to stop smoking. Now your unconscious knows it is time to help you stop smoking. So both parts of your mind, the conscious and the unconscious, can join together in cooperation with each other, the way my two hands joined together, easily and comfortably, without pressure or tension or stress.

You need not smoke again. You won't miss it, or want it, or care for it at all.

If you occasionally think about smoking, you will recognize that thought as only a memory. It will go away very quickly and won't bother you. In fact, the word poison may pop into your head and you will immediately think of something else.

Sometimes you may have smoked to deal with some stressful situations. Well, you don't need to smoke anymore, so I am going to teach you how to deal with those momentary stressors, in seconds, without closing your eyes and without anyone knowing that you are doing it.

You are sitting in that chair, already relaxed, feeling very comfortable and building a memory of what it feels like to be relaxed. When you are relaxed, you can't be upset or angry or stressed or frustrated because relaxation and those feelings are emotional and physical opposites of each other. When a person begins to feel pressured or tense or stressed, he or she usually feels it someplace in the upper part of the body—the chest, the shoulders, the neck.

The moment that happens to you, and you may be more aware of it more quickly, look at something not too far away, to focus your attention, and take two or three very slow, deep breaths. Breathe in relaxation through your nose, and slowly let out the tension through your mouth. That will bring back a part of the memory of this very deep relaxation and quickly melt away, dissolve away, any feelings of pressure or tension or stress.

Now, you are already sitting here very relaxed. Take a few very slow, deep breaths right now and feel how much more relaxed you become. That's great. Slow down the next one even more. Very good. That one was almost invisible. You took those slow, deep breaths and they relaxed you even more. If they did, just nod your head for me. Thank you.

I am going to awaken you from this deep relaxation. I use the word awaken because I don't have a better one. You are not asleep, just very relaxed and very comfortable. I am going to count from 1 to 5 slowly. With each number that I count, you will be more and more aware of your surroundings. With the number 5, you will open your eyes and be wide awake, yet still feel very relaxed and you need not smoke again.

1—2—3—4—5. Eyes open, wide awake. How did that feel? You did feel even more relaxed from the deep breaths, didn't you? You did really great. Do you have any questions?

The following can be used to wrap up the session. You would alter the script to reflect your own professional circumstances.

Here is my card with the number that you called. It is a 24-hour answering number [if that is the case]. If you have any problems over the next 2 weeks, there is no charge to come back within that two-week period. If you have any problems after that and call me the same day, I can usually help you deal with it over the phone. I don't charge for phone calls, so remember that I am a resource and use it. Here is a brochure that tells you more about me and what I do, for your information.

The patient may have questions or comments.

TELEPHONE APPEALS FOR HELP AFTER THE SESSION

If the patient calls you after the session and says that he or she has started smoking again, ask the following questions:

When did you start to smoke again? What was going on? Where did you get the cigarette? How much are you smoking now?

Typical scenarios are that the patient was out drinking in a bar, or eating in a restaurant, or socializing at a party where everyone was smoking, and the patient had a few, or more than a few, drinks. In any event, the patient may have been offered a cigarette, accepted it, and smoked. Or the patient may have asked someone for a cigarette and smoked it. Then the patient may have smoked a few more cigarettes while in that setting. The patient may have taken a few cigarettes home to smoke later, or bought a pack and smoked a few more cigarettes, or smoked the whole pack. Or the patient may have been in a low mood, or experienced a stressful event or series of events, and gone out and bought a pack of cigarettes and started smoking.

The key issue to determine on the telephone is whether the patient has smoked only a few cigarettes, has gone back to smoking as much as he or she was smoking before seeing you, or is smoking an amount that is somewhere in between.

If the patient has gone back to smoking almost as much, or as much, as he or she was before seeing you, it probably will be necessary to schedule an in-office follow-up session. Remember that our protocol stipulates that there is no charge for the patient to come back for a follow-up, if necessary, within the 2-week period following the patient's first session. We will explain the procedure to follow below. First, we explain the procedure to follow if the patient has smoked only a few cigarettes, or the number of cigarettes smoked is significantly less than it was before. This usually can be handled by telephone.

Telephone Procedure and Reframes

Let me explain a few things to you. First of all, you did not fail; you made a mistake. Had you failed, you would be smoking as much as you did when you came in to see me. You had the cigarette, and in your head you called it a failure, so you continued to smoke. But you just made a mistake. What happens when we make a mistake? Mistakes can be corrected. We can back off and start all over again. Had you called it a mistake, you probably wouldn't have smoked any more. The labels we place on the behaviors we do dictate future behaviors. So, what we call something leads to what we do about it. Calling it a failure continues the behavior. Calling it a mistake leads to correcting that mistake.

[If the patient started smoking again in a bar:] Second, you were drinking in a bar where a lot of people smoke. Alcohol is a central nervous system depressant, and nicotine is a stimulant. The alcohol brings us down, and the cigarettes bring us up, like on a seesaw, trying to find a balance. So, the more we drink, the more we smoke. That's why bars are all smoking areas. Smokers drink more.

You made a mistake, so let us now correct the mistake. Did you use the deep breaths that I taught you? They only worked for a while, but not when you were drinking. Okay, we can fix that. You realize that stopping smoking means controlling your drinking for a while—at least in crowded smokey bars. Okay? If you really want to stop, back off, and give it a chance to work for you.

Are you sitting down? Good. Take three very slow, deep breaths, then close your eyes lightly. Tell me when you close your eyes, by saying "okay." Good. Now, pay attention to your breathing without trying to change it, and feel yourself going much deeper into relaxation. Keep concentrating on your breathing. That is very good. Really relaxing. The doorway to your unconscious is open once again, and we can correct the mistake.

We know you made a mistake because you had only a few cigarettes [If this is the case]. We know you want to correct the mistake, because you called. You are already a nonsmoker. You stopped, then made the mistake because of the downer effects of the alcohol. As we correct the mistake so you no longer need to smoke, you will also no longer need to drink as much, or be in bars. That way the mistake will stay corrected. Remember to take those very slow, deep breaths if you start to feel stressed. They will relax you. Now, open your eyes. How did that feel? Terrific, call me if you need me.

The following procedure and reframes are employed if the patient calls and reports that he or she had a fight with a family member who smokes, "bummed" a cigarette in anger, and went outside to smoke to quiet the anger. It is also employed if the patient used to do this before, has not smoked since, but is concerned at this point.

I guess you were really taking the anger out on yourself, rather than on [person's name]. You came in to stop smoking and you did. That one cigarette was like saying, "You'll be sorry when I'm gone, you bastard you." But you were really only hurting yourself, not [person's name]. You calmed down and haven't smoked since. Did you use the deep breaths that I taught you? You did, and they helped a lot. Okay. Are you sitting down? Good. Take those same slow, deep breaths now that relaxed you before, then close your eyes and say "okay" so I will know you are relaxed. Thank you.

Pay attention to your breathing without trying to change it, and allow yourself to go deeper into relaxation, deeper with each breath and with each word that I say. That's very good. You are a nonsmoker. That single cigarette was an expression of anger that you internalized and only hurt you, not [person's name]. You stopped smoking because you want to take better care of yourself. It is time to treat yourself with more care, with more dignity and with more self-respect. Smoking is poisoning you. You no longer want to poison yourself, so you no longer want to smoke.

Your body has already started the healing process. Enjoy the feelings of more energy, better breathing, and easier physical activity. Be well. Now, open your eyes and be wide awake. How was that? Very relaxing. Good. You will be fine. Call me if you need me.

There are other reasons for a call, from "I didn't stop" to "I stopped, but I'm back to smoking as much as I did before" to "I really have an urge but haven't smoked" to "I really have the urge to smoke and can't resist it" to "I have been eating a lot more." A no-charge return visit within 2 weeks is part of the contract. Therefore, you need to ask the patient whether he or she would like to have the problem resolved over the telephone, still having the option to return in 2 weeks, or whether he or she would prefer to make an appointment for a quick return. That is a judgment call based on the patient's expressed needs and your availability.

If a return visit is scheduled, a typical session protocol is detailed below.

Case Study: Protocol for Return Visit within 2 Weeks

The Telephone Call

A patient called after a week and said that she had started smoking again. She was not smoking as much as she had been but she wanted to stop completely. An appointment was made for a half-hour time slot. Usually a half-hour time frame is sufficient.

The Session

The patient explained that she had been "fine" for about 4 days after her visit. She and her husband used to go out on the patio after dinner and have a cigarette together, then sit and talk. For the first few days, she didn't go out with him. She did the dishes instead. However, on the fourth day of not smoking, she went out with him and sat in her chair while he lit up. He knew that she had stopped smoking, yet he offered her a cigarette. She said, "No thank you," but her husband persisted. She felt he was testing her. She got upset and took a cigarette. Her husband then said, "See? I knew you couldn't stop."

She smoked and seethed. She felt like a "failure." Over the next few days, she had three or four cigarettes during the day but none after dinner. Then she increased it to more each day, but not to the full pack she had been smoking before her first visit. Finally, she called for help. She said that the deep breathing helped her early on, but once she started smoking again, she stopped using the deep breathing. I (JIZ) said the following to her in session:

Sometimes, smokers don't like to see people with whom they smoked stop smoking. They feel guilty that they don't stop. Without doing it consciously, they may try to get the other person to smoke so that they will feel less guilty. That's probably what your husband was doing. It is important for you to tell your husband that smoking is a personal choice. If he decides to smoke, even though you are concerned about his health, there is nothing you can do about it because you don't want to fight with him. But he should honor your decision to not smoke. After saying that to your husband, back off.

You did stop smoking. You were being encouraged to smoke and you did, so you felt that you had failed. You were also angry and may have repeated the smoking because you were angry. The repeated smoking reinforced the belief that you had failed, so you continued to smoke. But I can prove to you that you didn't fail. If you had failed, you would now be smoking as much as you did when you first came in to see me, a pack a day [if that is the case]. You are not smoking that much, so something must have happened that controlled your smoking. The unconscious must have gotten the message. But the unconscious needs your conscious cooperation to help you remain a nonsmoker. That is why you came in today—because, consciously, you really do want to be a nonsmoker. You didn't fail. You just made a mistake, and mistakes can be corrected. You are here today to correct that mistake. Okay?

Good. Now, sit more comfortably in the chair, and gently close your eyes. Take those three very slow, deep breaths that helped before, and allow yourself to relax with each deep breath that you take. Slowly inhale, and slowly exhale. That's right. Very good. Notice the fluttering of your eyelids. That indicates that you are already in hypnosis. Concentrate on your breathing to go deeper into relaxation. Don't try to change your breathing. Let your breathing change all by itself. Very good. Deeper and deeper. If your mind wanders, bring it back to your breathing. The doorway to your unconscious is open and I have the opportunity to again talk to your unconscious and give it more information to help you remain a nonsmoker.

You stopped smoking. Then you made a mistake. Mistakes can be corrected by backing off and starting all over again. You came in today to correct that mistake because you don't want to continue poisoning yourself. You liked the days you were not smoking because you felt so much better. You really do want to take better care of yourself. Now is the time to treat yourself better, with more respect, and with more self-love, to allow your body to heal any damage caused by the smoking behavior.

Because we have corrected the mistake, you need not smoke again. Any thought of smoking will be recognized as only a memory. It will quickly go away, and you will go about your business. If someone is smoking around you, that smoking will not bother you. Because you will be more aware of the smell of the burning tobacco and the sight of the smoke from that burning tobacco, you will be reminded that this is not for you. Relax and allow these words to be imprinted deeply in your unconscious mind. Remember to use the slow, deep breathing, as needed, to quiet down any stressful moments, as a way of taking charge. When you feel you have relaxed long enough, just open your eyes and be wide awake and feel really great.

That was very good. You really looked very relaxed. Here is another card. Call me if you need me. Remember, if you do have a future problem, but I don't think you will, and call the same day, we can immediately correct the mistake over the telephone. I don't charge for telephone calls.

Other reasons for a return visit can usually be dealt with using these approaches with individual variations and creativity.

Insert portions of this protocol into your own approach, or use the whole protocol. Whichever you choose, your success rate will improve. The choice is yours.

13

Review: Keys to Change

In this chapter, we will review the basic principles of brief cognitive hypnosis, and the essential reframes that are part of our behavior change protocols. We list and summarize them below following a brief review. It is our belief that these basic principles and reframes constitute the keys to change and are the essential ingredients for doing effective brief therapy. This chapter is intended as a concise review of the essential material covered in this book.

REVIEW

According to our model, most dysfunctional behaviors are anxiety based. These dysfunctional behaviors are coping behaviors that were originally invoked to reduce anxiety. They were imprinted in the unconscious initially by some form of marked hurt or trauma, then further imprinted by repetition. They became labeled as dysfunctional and negative when they become consciously recognized as a problem. Although the original initiating hurt or trauma may no longer be present and no longer identifiable, the continuation of the negative coping behavior, now labeled dysfunctional, has become a habit by repetition.

Because the initiating cause is no longer present, the negative coping behavior may no longer be needed, and may be labeled *empty habit* or *simple negative behavior*. Empty habits can be removed without the need for substitution. This is called *symptom removal*. It was used sparingly in the past because of the concern for possible symptom substitution. However, we have found that empty habits or simple negative behaviors can be removed in a single therapeutic session without symptom substitution. Their treatment usually does not require the teaching of self-hypnosis.

When dysfunctional behaviors continue because the original stressors, or new stressors, are present, the current dysfunctional behavior may be an exaggeration of the original coping behavior. According to our conceptual model, the original behavior arose as an attempt to cope with anxiety. The continued presence of stressors requiring strong coping behaviors caused the original coping behavior to be repeated and eventually to evolve into a more complex behavior pattern. We recognize that anxiety produces avoidance behavior. Avoidance behavior often becomes generalized, and as it does, it evolves in complexity if it is not treated.

We identify these dysfunctional behaviors as complex habits or complex negative behaviors. They require more than a single session to treat and usually necessitate teaching the patient self-hypnosis. These evolved more complex anxiety-based behaviors may include dysfunctional behaviors such as overeating, agoraphobia, obsessive-compulsive rituals, alcohol and drug abuse, depression, anger problems, exacerbation of pain syndromes and other medical problems.

THE BASIC PRINCIPLES OF BRIEF COGNITIVE HYPNOSIS

The Intake Evaluation

A brief but thorough intake evaluation forms the basis for doing brief cognitive hypnosis. It is required to understand the patient and the patient's presenting problem. It gathers pertinent information about the patient and the patient's current and past family and social constellations. Our intake evaluation places emphasis on the patient's belief systems, patterns of behavior, personal labels, habits, rituals, sensory processing systems, language use, goals, motivation, choice of coping behaviors and functionality. This list includes the patient's previous attempts to deal with the presenting problem as well as with other related or implied problems. Often, during an intake evaluation, the patient, in addition to talking about the presenting problem, verbalizes or demonstrates other problems.

The Conscious and Unconscious Parts of the Mind

We start with the concept that the mind is made up of two functional parts, the conscious and the unconscious. We conceptualize the conscious mind as essentially under the active control of the individual. We conceptualize the unconscious mind as that part of the mind that controls all automatic behaviors over which the individual has little or no active control.

Hypnosis as an Altered State

We view hypnosis as an alteration in internal perception, which is initiated at the start of a unique process of communication that can be verbal or nonverbal.

Natural everyday altered states we label *hypnoidal states* and therapeutic altered states we view as hypnosis states or trance states.

In the clinical setting, an informal hypnosis state is differentiated from a formal trance state which is induced by performing a trance induction procedure. The former may occur without a formal trance, during the intake evaluation process. It is a waking state, but it has trancelike qualities that arise from the early experience of relaxation, which naturally develops during the patient's comfortable interaction with the clinician. This comfort, the patient's growing sense of trust in the clinician, and the patient's expectation of eventually entering a formal trance, all help create the experience of relaxation, which leads into the informal hypnosis state.

Waking State Reframing

The communication process that takes place during this waking state is designed to start the process of change that is later fixed in place during the trance state. The term *reframing* used in this context refers to the purposeful verbal intervention by the clinician to assist the patient in changing the meaning of beliefs and labels that propagate dysfunctional behavior.

During waking state reframing, the patient begins to change beliefs, labels and misconceptions. The belief of being trapped is changed to the possibility of changing. The expression of absolutes becomes "sometimes" rather than "always," and erroneous and iatrogenic beliefs are corrected and changed. This is when most of the change work actually takes place, in preparation for the trance experience, which acts as a sort of fixative.

The waking state reframing procedure consists of redefining problems, clarifying real versus imagined causes and challenging and changing the patient's beliefs through the careful use of reframing, the provision of new corrective information and the changing of negative labels. This is accomplished while communicating with the patient's conscious and unconscious simultaneously during the waking state. This is when most of the change work occurs in preparation for the use of the trance state as a fixative.

The waking state reframing experience is an altered state during which the patient is more receptive to suggestions. It may also be described as an anticipatory trance state or expectant trance state in that it sets up the desired expectancies. It starts with a simple explanation of the conscious and unconscious minds. It continues as the clinician explains what hypnosis is and how hypnosis is experienced. The process then moves into reframing beliefs and labels that have been used by the patient in maintaining the dysfunctional behavior.

Many of the physiological markers of formal trance are often noticed during this pretrance experience. The patient is expecting trance to occur and is already entering into an altered state in preparation for trance.

The Role of Language

Language is inherent in how we learn. We automatically and unconsciously interpret the representational code of language to understand and apply meaning to our world. So the choice of language forms used by the patient and by the clinician are important to the change process.

We pay close attention to sensory-based language use. Language that is visual, kinesthetic, auditory, olfactory and gustatory are carefully noted, then used for improving rapport and facilitating change.

The Concept of Imprinting

We learn from repetition and from emotionally powerful experiences. When a thought, feeling or behavior is repeated, the unconscious is better able to accept that which is repeated as appropriate and valid, even if the behavior has a possible negative outcome. This is how we learn and establish habits, whether they are good or bad. We call this imprinting. We also learn from shock, trauma, extreme emotionality, serious illness and loss. These traumatic imprints initiate behaviors and emotions designed to reduce the trauma's effect on the individual. Such responses include anxiety, fear, depression, other emotional and psychological disorders.

Symptoms Are Seen as Attempts to Cope

We view those presenting problems that are labeled *Symptoms* as unconsciously initiated attempts to cope with imprints that are negative in nature. As they are repeated, these coping attempts become further imprinted and interpreted as dysfunctional.

Fight or Flight Response"

We postulate that most attempts to cope are initiated as a result of experienced anxiety due to the fight or flight response. The patient reacts either with an angry externalized coping behavior, or, if unable to externalize or run away, with an internalized response that may be expressed in some dysfunctional way. The chosen coping behavior is an attempt to alleviate the anxiety. Similar stressors repeat the anxiety and the chosen coping behavior. Repetition imprints the behavior and the experience, so they continue and are eventually perceived as dysfunctional.

Evolving Symptoms Create More Complex Dysfunction

As negative anxiety coping attempts are repeated, without resolution, they become more generalized and more complex and thus more dysfunctional. Anxiety that initially produced discomfort can evolve into avoidance when it becomes situational or object oriented. Eventually, with continued repetition of the anxiety experience in different situations, the avoidance behaviors can further generalize and evolve into agoraphobia. Anxiety that initially produced fear of future calamity may evolve into extreme obsessive or ritual behavior.

Treating the Initial Anxiety Rather Than the Evolved Complex Dysfunction.

The choice of different sets of criteria for classifying symptoms and dysfunctional behaviors has been used to establish different diagnostic labels for specific psychological disorders. These systematic efforts have led to the creation of different treatment protocols. In brief cognitive hypnosis, we have conceptualized dysfunctional behavior instead by determining the emotional and physiological response mechanism that operated originally as the patient first attempted to cope with a stimulus that was interpreted as threatening. This is in contrast to identifying the extended phobic or ritualistic behavior that evolved and became the later presenting problem as what needed to be addressed.

With this recognition, we are able to start at the beginning, and change the initial response on which later and more debilitating symptoms (i.e., dysfunctional coping behaviors) were built.

Simple Empty Habits

If the original circumstances that initiated the negative coping response are no longer present, and if the initial coping response has not evolved radically, although it may have become more intense, treatment may be simplified and shortened. The problem can be treated as a simple or empty habit that no longer serves a purpose. Therefore, it can be given up without substituting other dysfunctional behavior. This may be accomplished in a single visit.

Complex Habits

When dysfunctional behaviors continue to generalize and evolve because the original stressors are still present, or because intensification of the emotional response occurs, these exaggerated evolved coping mechanisms are labeled *complex habits*. They are complex negative behaviors that naturally take more than a single visit to resolve. These evolved more complex habits include overeating, agoraphobia, obsessive-compulsive rituals, alcohol and drug abuse, exacerbation of pain syndromes and aggravation of existing medical problems.

Choice of Induction

The ritual of the induction procedure that produces, or induces, the hypnotic trance state is viewed as separate from the trance state itself. It is a state of transition from the waking state, which may have some trancelike characteristics, into a more dissociated state. That dissociated state, the trance state, is characterized by a form of logic (called trance logic) that is less critical and judgmental than the form of logic associated with the waking state. Thus, in trance, the individual is more open to suggestion and change than in the waking state.

The choice of the induction procedure should be based on the needs of the patient and the particular problem to be resolved. However, in most cases, it should be short and uncomplicated. We avoid drawn out, complicated, elegant, inductions because we view them as uneconomical in regards to time and more often chosen to meet the needs of the clinician rather than those of the patient.

We also believe that the quicker the patient experiences relaxation and reduces the experience of anxiety, the more effective the treatment will be. Several preferred inductions have been included in this text that can be added to the practitioner's repertoire.

They include naturalistic inductions which are an extension of clinician-observed trancelike behavior before a formal induction has been initiated; inductions that are internally directed; inductions that are externally directed; inductions that do not include the teaching of self-hypnosis; and inductions that do include the teaching of self-hypnosis. All of these induction rituals are short and uncomplicated.

The choice of the trance induction is important because it should be tailored to meet the particular needs of the patient. In addition to being short and uncomplicated, inductions in the practice of brief cognitive hypnosis are direct and self-ratifying. They have built-in deepening mechanisms and access the sensory processing system of the patient.

The induction process involves redirecting the patient's focus of attention. As such, some induction procedures are designed to internalize the patient's focus of attention, others are designed to externalize it and still other induction procedures do both. If a change in mind and body function is what is called for, then an internalizing induction is indicated. However, if a release of emotional overlay is indicated, then an externalizing induction is indicated. If both goals are indicated, then the induction typically will be designed to both internalize and externalize. Also, many of our inductions are designed to add self-hypnosis or instant relaxation if appropriate.

The Importance of the Relaxation Experience

We believe that the experience of clinician-induced and self-induced relaxation, within the hypnotic construct, is a very important beginning to the change process. The reduction of emotional overlay and the building of a memory of physical and emotional comfort are important in helping the patient change from a negative mindset to one of positive expectancy. This allows for the establishment of a new memory that is a great relief from thoughts and feelings of suffering that the patient brought to the treatment setting. This new memory will be accessed again and again during the treatment process and strengthened until it automatically becomes the unconscious, and thus automatic memory of choice.

The Trance State

Because we assume that most of the work of change takes place during the waking state reframing process, we view the trance state as the more intense altered state where logic is set aside and suggestions, acceptable to the patient and appropriately presented, become fixed in place. Therefore, the state of trance can be relatively short, compared to the longer time involved for waking state reframing. Trance is the fixative or imprinter of change.

Self-Hypnosis

Our experience has shown that many simple or empty habits can be changed in a single visit, without self-hypnosis. For more complex problems, the teaching of self-hypnosis is essential. However, there are some occasions when the patient cannot or chooses not to practice self-hypnosis. When this situation arises, if the experience of deep relaxation occurs during clinician-initiated trance, self-hypnosis can be put aside, and more direct suggestions for change may be just as effective with many patients.

There are some important differences between our application of the use of self-hypnosis by the patient and that which is practiced by many clinicians.

No Self-Talk During Self-Hypnosis

First, we usually instruct the patient not to attempt to remember or repeat suggestions given during the office visit. These suggestions are often distorted or changed by the patient when self-administered during the self-hypnosis experience. Second, we have found that attempts to talk to one's self during deep relaxation often disturb the depth of the self-induced trance experience and its memory imprint, thus diminishing its effectiveness. We believe that the reexperiencing of deep relaxation originally produced during the trance state when in the clinician's office automatically reinforces the suggestions given by the clinician at that time. Therefore, no self-talk is necessary. Because suggestions do not become contaminated or subtly changed, this often shortens the length of time that is needed to help the patient change.

How Self-Suggestion is Employed

When it is determined that self-suggestion is appropriate, the patient is instructed to read carefully crafted, short, uncomplicated suggestions written by the clinician. These suggestions are read three or four times, silently or out loud, by the patient, before the initiation of self-hypnosis. Note, we say before, not during, the self-hypnosis trance experience. Contrary to common practice, we have found that repeating carefully scripted suggestions just before self-hypnosis is more effective than doing so during trance. As stated earlier, attempts to do self-talk during trance may reduce the effectiveness of the trance experience.

"Instant Relaxation" as an Immediately Available Coping Skill

The learning of Instant Relaxation skills, such as the Three Deep Breaths, Attention to Breathing, or Playing with or Holding a Marble, that we extensively covered earlier, can be an important adjunct to helping the patient deal with future situations that may be stressful. The use of these skills can also avert the fear of the return to old behavior. This is different from post-hypnotic cues or suggestions that are given to automatically feel relaxed. Our experience is that most post-hypnotic suggestions have a limited life span, unless they are frequently reinforced.

Because this form of instant relaxation is *consciously* evoked, we call it posttrance imprinting. Repeating these procedures eventually establishes them as automatic. Even the use of a marble can be imagined rather than real, and be just as effective.

IMPORTANT GENERAL REFRAMES

The "We Only Pay Attention to Events" Reframe

Change is recognized only in retrospect. Therefore, most patients may not be able to express improvement or change unless they are reminded of how things were when they started.

Reframe:

> We only pay attention to events. We don't pay attention to nonevents. When something is happening, we pay attention to it. When nothing is happening, there is nothing to pay attention to.

This is one of the reasons why people recognize change only in retrospect. If the patient is acting out dysfunctional behavior less often, when it is not happening it is not recognized as not happening. If nothing is happening, there is nothing to recognize, except in retrospect by comparison.

The "Illusion of Absolutes" Reframe

There is an "illusion of absolutes" that tends to prevent change. Patients often come to treatment convinced that they always do this or do that, whether it is smoking, or scratching, or being angry, or getting anxious, or freezing, or making mistakes, or whatever. As in the first reframe, the patient usually is not aware of when he or she is not doing it, so the patient establishes the belief that the problem is absolute, that it always happens, and that when it happens, it is all bad.

Reframe:

> The only absolute is that there are no absolutes.

It is important to question the patient who expresses the belief that the problem is always experienced and to get the patient's acknowledgment of the fact that sometimes the problem or symptoms are not being experienced. This can open the door to being able to place emphasis on the non-event, when the problem is not happening, as opposed to the event, when the problem had been happening.

The "Changing Labels Changes Beliefs and Behaviors" Reframe

What we call something leads to what we continue to do. Labeling something an *urge*, for example, implies that action is required to satisfy that urge. Changing the label to *memory* removes the requirement of action. Memories can go away very quickly, because no action is expected or required.

Reframe:

> The labels we place on the behavior we do dictate future behavior. What we call something leads to what we do about it. If we call something a *failure*, then we continue to repeat the behavior as if it were a failure. If we call it a *mistake*, we realize that mistakes can be corrected and so we haven't failed. We only made a mistake. So we can back off and start all over again and correct the mistake.

The "Changing Diagnoses Changes Treatment" Reframe

A good example of this important issue can be seen in the diagnosis and treatment of problems with alcohol. The problem of excessive alcohol intake is often labeled *alcoholism*. However, not everyone who has a problem with alcohol is an alcoholic. Some may be problem drinkers. If the diagnostic label is changed, the treatment process may be changed and the treatment outcome is therefore changed.

Reframe:

> Addictions and alcoholism cannot be cured. People who are labeled *addicts* or *alcoholics* can go into recovery, but they are considered to be in recovery forever. The alcohol or addiction rehabilitation and recovery process is long, complicated and arduous. Problem drinking and problem eating, on the other hand, as well as other problem behaviors, can often be dealt with successfully in a more focused and limited way, and in a shorter period of time.

Patients referred to treatment for driving under the influence (DUI) of alcohol can be helped to not drink when they are going to drive. They may still choose to drink, but not if they are going to drive. A program designed by JIZ many years ago, as part of New York State law involving counseling for those arrested for DUI, using self-hypnosis training, proved very effective in preventing future arrests, when compared to conventional alcohol treatment approaches.

The "Choices Mean No Longer Feeling Trapped" Reframe

It is our contention that insight alone does not change behavior. A change in beliefs, ways of thinking and the recognition that other choices are available allows changes of behavior to occur. Choices lead to change, because the recognition that there are choices means no longer feeling trapped.

Reframe:

> We are trapped only as long as we believe that we have no choices. Once we recognize that we have other choices and we make a choice, then we are no longer trapped.

Similarly, we are taught in childhood that "if at first you don't succeed, try, try again." Continuing to try something that isn't working will not make it work. However, recognizing that there are other choices, other ways of doing something, may allow for the possibility of success.

The "Harder You Try Not To" Reframe

Trying too hard not to think of or do something makes it harder to not think of it or do it. On the contrary, it makes it more likely that you will in fact continue to think of it or do it, and thus make the situation worse. "Trying not to" forces the thought or act to the conscious mind so that it becomes a preoccupation, a compulsive thought or act.

Reframe:

The harder you try not to think of or do something, the more difficult it becomes. Try not to think of a pink elephant. Go ahead, I dare you.

ESSENTIAL OVEREATING REFRAMES

The following reframes are the key ingredients of the brief cognitive hypnosis approach to problem eating.

On Losing Pounds

We will not be watching how many pounds you lose. You will not be weighing yourself. In any given day, you may be up or down 3 or more pounds based on how much fluid you retain. Usually at around 4:00 in the afternoon, you will weigh more than you did at 9:00 in the morning because of fluid accumulation during the day. We are more interested in how much more comfortably your clothes fit than in how many pounds you will have lost.

On Knowing When You're Full

The stomach does not signal you that it is full based on how much food you have eaten. The stomach does not signal the brain that is full based upon volume consumed. It is a time frame system. After a period of time, which varies with each person, a signal goes to the brain that says the stomach is full, no matter how much food you may have consumed. So, the slower you eat, the less you will have eaten, when your time is up and the stomach signals the brain that you are full.

On Recognizing the Messages of Your Body

You may have difficulty recognizing the messages of your body. Very often people with weight and eating problems misinterpret body signals as meaning they are hungry, even if they are not. For example, you may interpret the growling of your stomach as a sign that you are hungry, when in fact it is not. It may mean that you have swallowed too much air and your body is dealing with that. There may be other internal sounds and feelings of a similar nature that you are not consciously aware of that create the same mistaken impressions of hunger. We will help you correct these types of misunderstandings.

Why Diets Don't Work

Some people do lose weight from dieting. Almost any change in food intake will result in some weight loss for a short while, regardless of the particular diet. That is why there are so many different diets for weight loss. Many of them contradict each other, but they still bring about some weight loss temporarily. However, diets stop working after a while. They cause the dieter to become too preoccupied and worried about thoughts of pounds lost or gained, grams ingested and choice of foods that are supposed to be helpful. This preoccupation often becomes obsessive and increases anxiety and guilt when rituals that are prescribed are not exactly followed. With our approach, you will not be dieting. You will be changing the way you think about food and deal with food. You will be changing your eating behavior and habits.

There Are Weight Loss Plateaus

Even though you will not be weighing yourself, your body will know when you have lost enough weight to stop for a while. When you have lost 8 to 10 real pounds, not fluid, you will reach a plateau at which you will appear to stop losing weight for about a week to 10 days. You will continue to lose fluid during this time, so you may continue to feel your clothes feeling looser. This plateau is when your body makes whatever internal adjustments are needed to accommodate the change in weight. It is like going down a staircase and reaching a series of landings that are resting places in the descent. As you continue to change, you will reach these resting places and recognize them as helpful reenergizers rather than as problems.

SINGLE-SESSION SMOKING CESSATION REFRAMES

The single-session smoking cessation protocol is designed to accomplish all of the necessary steps of brief cognitive hypnosis in a single 1-hour session. For review and easy reference, these steps are outlined below:

1. Conduct the intake evaluation.
2. Reframe the distinction between the conscious and unconscious minds.
3. Explain what to expect when experiencing hypnosis.
4. Go over in detail the four U.S. Surgeon General's warnings that are listed on all cigarette packs sold in the United States. This involves explaining what they really mean, because they are compromises, and providing supporting facts and information.
   a. "Cigarette smoke contains carbon monoxide."

b. "Smoking causes lung cancer, heart disease, and emphysema, and may complicate pregnancy."

c. "Smoking by pregnant women may result in fetal injury, premature birth and low birth weight."

d. "Quitting smoking now greatly reduces serious risks to your health."

5. If you have access to British-made cigarettes include the warning "Smoking kills."

6. Read the article on the discovery of higher levels of Perrier in bottled water (see chapter 12).

7. Reframe the erroneous and misleading idea that "smoking relaxes me," and explain the true effects of the stimulant nicotine.

8. Reframe the erroneous and misleading idea that "cigarettes are addictive." Change the label *addiction* to *habit*.

9. Reframe the erroneous and misleading idea that when a person stops smoking, he or she will experience withdrawal symptoms. Change the label *withdrawal* to *stress reaction*.

10. Reframe the erroneous and misleading idea that hypnotic trance is a state during which the patient will "be under, and unconscious, and unaware, or asleep." This idea often leads the patient to ask the question, after "awakening" from the trance experience, "Why did I hear and remember everything that you said?" Clarify that the patient was not asleep, only relaxed, and the "doorway to the unconscious was open." Explain the importance of the conscious and unconscious minds in cooperating to change the smoking behavior to a nonsmoking behavior.

11. Reframe the concept of "urge" to "memory." This reframe addresses the question "What happens if I want to smoke after we are finished?" Help the patient to recognize that the thought of smoking is just a memory and *not an* urge. Help the patient relate this idea to the fact that the patient has already had the experience of thinking about smoking and not smoking. Elaborate on the idea that "you think about smoking more often than you actually smoke. So you don't smoke every time you think about smoking."

12. Employ the following reframe:

> We only pay attention to events. We don't pay attention to nonevents. Smoking is an event. We only pay attention to when we smoke. We don't pay attention to when we don't smoke. When we are not smoking, there is nothing to pay attention to.

13. Employ the reframe that "You cannot be nervous or stressed when you are relaxed." Instead, build on that notion and suggest to the patient that he or she will be able to automatically "borrow the feeling of relaxation by taking a few slow, deep breaths to bring calm."

Additional Comments

For some years, we have believed that society has gradually changed the meaning of words based on prevailing usage rather than original denotation. Often, the meaning of words is changed for economic reasons as well. In the July 22, 1996, issue of *U.S. News and World Report*, John Leo, in his column "On Society," wrote a fascinating clarifying article entitled "Thank You for Not Smoking." In his article, he made this point better than we could possibly have done.

Leo commented: 'Addiction Theory' was one of the grander social mistakes of the 1970s and 1980s. Every conceivable hard-to-shake habit was declared to be an addiction and therefore beyond the control of the newly defined and helplessly passive addict. Womanizers were revealed to be 'sex addicts,' and gamblers, joggers, daredevils and deadbeats were all labeled addicts as well" (Leo, 1996, p. 18).

In our search of the literature on smoking and nicotine, we noted that the earlier research called cigarette smoking "habituating." That label lasted until very recently, when the label was changed, without much explanation, to "addicting."

In his article, Leo (1996) wrote about alcoholism, by stating, "Alcoholism shed its aura of moral fault and moved from addiction to disease. Those of us who thought that heavy drinking often took place to escape or relieve conflict were told we had it backward: The conflict and stress are mostly a consequence of the drinking, not the cause" (p. 18).

Leo went on to say in the article:

James Prochaska of the University of Rhode Island's Cancer Prevention Research Center said, "The disease model is predicated on the idea that alcoholism is something that happens to you, and it puts us into a passive-reactive mode that doesn't help us prevent or solve the problem." This discussion has some obvious echoes in the debates about smoking. There is no longer any doubt that nicotine is physically addictive. But nobody seems to notice that smoking has been just as narrowly medicalized as drinking. The antismoking forces have the tobacco companies on the run for many reasons, but one is that they have succeeded in medicalizing a problem that is as much behavioral and psychological as it is medical. There's no mystery about why this is so. The argument over health effects has been the trump card. Seminars, conferences, and grants have all been dominated by medical people and technicians, most of whom seem absolutely certain a cigarette is nothing more than a nicotine delivery system. (p. 18)

This has very strong economic incentives, as we earlier suggested. Leo further stated, and we agree, that "people don't smoke just for nicotine. They smoke for a great array of nonchemical reasons, from depression and peer pressure to a courting of danger, or a belief that smoking equals liberation. Or because lighting up has become embedded in day-to-day life as a ritual, a way of punctuating a phone call, the end of a meal, the start of a difficult project" (Leo, 1996, p. 18). In other words, it has become a habit.

Leo ended his piece by pointing out that the passivity and poor outcomes that the researcher-psychologist James Prochaska noted among drinkers who were told that "alcoholism is something that happens to you" also is evidenced among smokers. "Addiction theory is a formula for no-fault, no-improvement misery" (Leo, 1996, p. 18), and passivity, we might add. If we are addicted, we can try, but we know we will fail, because we are addicted.

Labeling someone as addicted means that the person is not responsible. It tells the person who is labeled an addict that he or she is not in charge of his or her life. Therefore, it becomes an excuse for not being responsible or accountable for his or her actions. This in turn leads to the dysfunctional belief that nobody should expect that person to be responsible or accountable. What a dysfunctional absolute!

These types of dysfunctional beliefs often are imprinted as a result of being repeated as societal suggestions. They become accepted as "the truth" because they represent the expressions of acceptable authority and because they have been frequently heard and thus become imprinted. When a clinician can help a patient to think and feel differently via the reframing process, many of these negative and dysfunctional imprints can be changed. This increases the likelihood of successful outcomes in any kind of treatment.

References

Alden, P., & Heap, M. (1998). Hypnotic pain control: Some theoretical and practical issues. *International Journal of Clinical and Experimental Hypnosis, 46*(1), 62–76.

Alexander, F., & French, T. (1946). *Psychoanalytic therapy: Principles and applications.* New York: Ronald Press.

American Academy of Otolaryngology—Head and Neck Surgery. (2000). Snoring: Not funny, not hopeless. Patient Information and Education Web Page (www.entnet.org/snoring.html).

American Psychiatric Association. (1994). *Diagnostic and Statistical Manual of Mental Disorders* (4th ed.). Washington, DC: Author.

Antony, M. M., & Swinson, R. P. (2000). *Phobic disorders and panic in adults: A guide to assessment and treatment.* Washington, DC: American Psychological Association.

Bandler, R., & Grinder, J. (1979). *Frogs into princes: Neurolinguistic programming.* Moab, UT: Real People Press.

Bandura, A. (1976). *Social learning theory.* New York: Prentice-Hall.

Bandura, A., O'Leary, A., Taylor, C. B., Gauthier, J., & Gossard, D. (1987). Perceived self-efficacy and pain control: Opioid and nonopioid mechanisms. *Journal of Personality and Social Psychology, 53,* 563–571.

Barber, J. (1996). *Hypnosis and suggestion in the treatment of pain.* New York: W. W. Norton.

Bassman, S. W., & Wester, W. C. (1984). *Hypnosis, headaches and pain control: An indirect approach.* Columbus, OH: Ohio Psychology.

Bates, B. L. (1993). Individual differences in response to hypnosis. In J. W. Rhue, S. J. Lynn, & I. Kirsch (Eds.), *Handbook of clinical hypnosis* (pp. 23–54). Washington, DC: American Psychological Association.

Bateson, G., Jackson, D. D., Haley, J., & Weakland, J. H. (1956). Toward a theory of schizophrenia. *Behavioral Science, 1,* 251–264.

Beck, J. S. (1995). *Cognitive therapy: Basics and beyond.* New York: Guilford.

Beier, E. G. (1966). *The silent language of psychotherapy: Social reinforcement of unconscious processes.* Chicago: Aldine.

Benson, H., Arns, P. A., & Hoffman, J. W. (1981). The relaxation response and hypnosis. *International Journal of Clinical and Experimental hypnosis, 29*(3), 259–270.

Blanchard, E. B., Kim, M., Hermann, C., & Steffek, B. D. (1993). Preliminary results of the effects on headache relief of perception of success among tension headache patients receiving relaxation. *Headache Quarterly, 4,* 249–253.

Blankfield, R. P. (1991). Suggestion, relaxation, and hypnosis as adjuncts in the care of surgery patients: A review of the literature. *American Journal of Clinical Hypnosis, 33*(3), 172–186.

Bloom, P. B. (1994). Is insight necessary for successful treatment? Discussion of suggestibility and repressed memories of abuse. *American Journal of Clinical Hypnosis, 36*(3), 172–174.

Bower, G. H., & Hilgard, E. R. (1981). *Theories of learning.* New York: Prentice-Hall.

Bowers, K. S. (1976). *Hypnosis for the seriously curious.* New York: Norton.

Braid, J. (1843). *Neurypnology, or the rationale of nervous sleep considered in relation with animal magnetism.* London: Churchill.

Bromberg, W. (1959). *The mind of man: A history of psychotherapy and psychoanalysis.* New York: Harper.

Brooks, C. H. (1922). The practice of autosuggestion by the method of Emile Coué. New York: Dodd, Mead, and Company. (pp. 54–55).

Brown, D. P., & Fromm, E. (1987). *Hypnosis and behavioral medicine.* Hillsdale, NJ: Erlbaum.

Bryan, N. (1980). *Thin is a state of mind.* Minneapolis: CompCare.

Cameron-Bandler, L. (1978). *They lived happily ever after: A book about achieving happy endings in coupling.* Cupertino, CA: Meta.

Cannon, W. B. (1929). *Bodily changes in pain, hunger, fear, and rage (2nd ed.).* New York: Appleton.

Cautela, J. R., & Wisocki, P. A. (1977). The thought-stopping procedure: Description, application, and learning theory interpretations. *Psychological Record, 1,* 255–264.

Cheek, D. B. (1994). *Hypnosis: The application of ideomotor procedures.* Boston: Allyn & Bacon.

Chess, S., & Alexander, T. (1996). *Temperament: Theory and practice.* New York: Brunner/Mazel.

Clarke, J. H., & Reynolds, P. J. (1991). Suggestive hypnotherapy for nocturnal bruxism: A pilot study. *American Journal of Clinical Hypnosis, 33*(4), 248–253.

Clarkin, J. F., Yeomans, F. E., & Kernberg, O. F. (1999). *Psychotherapy for borderline personality.* New York: Wiley.

Clawson, T. A., & Swade, R. H. (1975). The hypnotic control of blood flow and pain: The cure of warts and the potential for use of hypnosis in the treatment of cancer. *American Journal of Clinical Hypnosis, 17,* 160–169.

Cochrane, G. (1987). Hypnotherapy in weight-loss treatment: Case illustrations. *American Journal of Clinical Hypnosis, 30*(1), 20–27.

Cochrane, G. (1992). Hypnosis and weight reduction: Which is the cart and which is the horse? *American Journal of Clinical Hypnosis, Vol. 35, No. 2,* 109–118.

Coe, W. C. (1993). Expectations and hypnotherapy. In J. W. Rhue, S. J. Lynn, & I. Kirsch (Eds.), *Handbook of clinical hypnosis* (pp. 73–94). Washington, DC: American Psychological Association.

Cohen, D. B. (1974). On the etiology of neurosis. *Journal of Abnormal Psychology, 83,* 473–479.

Conrad, S. W. (1954). The psychologic implications of overeating. *Psychiatric Quarterly,* *28,* 211–224.

Coué, E. (1922). *Self-mastery through conscious autosuggestion.* New York: American Library Service.

Council, J. R. (1999). Measures of hypnotic responding. In I. Kirsch, A. Capafons, E. Cardena, & S. Amigo (Eds.), *Clinical hypnosis and self-regulation: Cognitive-behavioral perspectives* (pp. 119–140). Washington, DC: American Psychological Association.

Crawford, H. J., Knebel, T., Kaplan, L., Vendemia, J. M. C., Xie, M., Jamison, S., & Pribram, K. H. (1998). Hypnotic analgesia: 1. Somatosensory event-related potential changes to noxious stimuli 2. Transfer learning to reduce chronic low back pain. *International Journal of Clinical and Experimental Hypnosis, 46*(1), 92–132.

DeGood, D. E., & Shutty, M. S. (1992). Assessment of pain beliefs, coping, and self-efficacy. In D. C. Turk, & R. Melzack (Eds.), *Handbook of pain assessment* (pp. 214–234). New York: The Guilford Press.

De Pascalis, V. (1999). Psychophysiological correlates of hypnosis and hypnotic susceptibility. *International Journal of Clinical and Experimental Hypnosis, 47*(2), 117–142.

DuBreuil, S. C., & Spanos, N. P. (1993). Psychological treatment of warts. In J. W. Rhue, S. J. Lynn, & I. Kirsch (Eds.), *Handbook of clinical hypnosis* (pp. 623–648). Washington, DC: American Psychological Association.

Dunlap. K. (1932). *Habits: Their making and unmaking.* New York: Liveright.

Eastwood, J. D., Gaskowski, P., & Bowers, K. S. (1998). The folly of effort: Ironic effects in the mental control of pain. *International Journal of Clinical and Experimental Hypnosis, 46*(1), 77–91.

Edmonston, W. E. (1981). *Hypnosis and relaxation: Modern verification of an old equation.* New York: Wiley.

Eimer, B. N. (1988). The chronic pain patient: Multimodal assessment and psychotherapy. *International Journal of Medical Psychotherapy, 1,* 23–40.

Eimer, B. N. (1989). Psychotherapy for chronic pain: A cognitive approach. In A. Freeman, K. M. Simon, L. Beutler, & H. Arkowitz (Eds.), *Comprehensive handbook of cognitive therapy* (pp. 449–465). New York: Plenum Press.

Eimer, B. N. (2000a). Clinical applications of hypnosis for brief and efficient pain management psychotherapy. *American Journal of Clinical Hypnosis, 43*(1), 17–40.

Eimer, B. N. (2000b, Summer). Hypnosis for the relief of pain: What's possible and what's not. *Psychological Hypnosis, 9*(2), 3–6.

Eimer, B. N., & Freeman, A. (1998). *Pain management psychotherapy: A practical guide.* New York: Wiley.

Eimer, B. N., & Hornyak, L. (2001, Spring). Forensic considerations when using hypnosis with post-accident personal injury patients: 10 essential guidelines. *Psychological Hypnosis, 10*(1), 11–15.

Ellenberger, H. F. (1970). *The discovery of the unconscious: The history and evolution of dynamic psychiatry.* New York: Basic Books.

Ellis, A. (1996). *Better, deeper and more enduring brief therapy: The rational emotive behavior therapy approach.* New York: Brunner/Mazel.

Erickson, M. H. (1948). Hypnotic psychotherapy. In *The medical clinics of North America* (pp. 571–583). New York: Saunders.

Erickson, M. H. (1961). Historical note on the hand levitation and other ideomotor techniques. *American Journal of Clinical Hypnosis, 3*, 196–199.

Erickson, M. H. (1980a). An hypnotic technique for resistant patients: The patient, the technique, and its rationale and field experiments. In E. L. Rossi (Ed.), *The nature of hypnosis and suggestion: The collected papers of Milton H. Erickson on hypnosis* (Vol. 1, p. 306). New York: Irvington.

Erickson, M. H. (1980b). Hypnosis in painful terminal illness. In E. L. Rossi (Ed.), *Innovative hypnotherapy: The collected papers of Milton H. Erickson on hypnosis* (Vol. 4). New York: Irvington.

Erickson, M. H. (1985). *Life reframing in hypnosis.* In E. L. Rossi & M. O. Ryan (Eds.), *The seminars, workshops and lectures of Milton H. Erickson* (Vol. 2). New York: Irvington.

Erickson, M. H., & Rossi, E. L. (1979). *Hypnotherapy: An exploratory casebook.* New York: Irvington.

Erickson, M. H., & Rossi, E. L. (1981). *Experiencing hypnosis: Therapeutic approaches to altered states.* New York: Irvington.

Erickson, M. H., Rossi, E. L., & Rossi, S. I. (1976). *Hypnotic realities: The induction of clinical hypnosis and forms of indirect suggestion.* New York: Irvington.

Evans, F. J. (1974). The placebo response in pain reduction. *Advances in Neurology, 4,* 289–296.

Evans, F. J. (1991). Hypnotizability: Individual differences in dissociation and the flexible control of cognitive processes. In S. J. Lynn & J. W. Rhue (Eds.), *Theories of hypnosis.* New York: Guilford.

Ewin, D. M. (1984). Hypnosis in surgery and anesthesia. In W. C. Wester II & A. H. Smith (Eds.), *Clinical hypnosis: A multidisciplinary approach* (pp. 210–235). Philadelphia: Lippincott.

Ewin, D. M. (1985, March/April). Hypnosis in medical practice: Putting the mind to work. *Medical Student,* 4–6.

Ewin, D. M. (1986). Hypnosis and pain management. In B. Zilbergeld, M. G. Edelstien, & D. L. Araoz (Eds.), *Hypnosis: Questions and answers* (pp. 282–288). New York: Norton.

Ewin, D. M. (1992a). Constant pain syndrome: Its psychological meaning and cure using hypnoanalysis. *Hypnos, 19*(1), 57–62.

Ewin, D. M. (1992b). Hypnotherapy for warts (*verruca vulgaris*): 41 consecutive cases with 33 cures. *American Journal of Clincal Hypnosis, 35*(1), 1–10.

Ewin, D. M. (1998). Rapid eye roll induction. In D. C. Hammond (Ed.), *Hypnotic induction and suggestion* (p. 49). Des Plaines, IL: American Society of Clinical Hypnosis.

Festinger, L. (1957). *A theory of cognitive dissonance.* Stanford, CA: Stanford University Press.

Fine, R. (1990). *History of psychoanalysis.* Northvale, NJ: Aronson.

Fourie, D. P. (1995). Attribution of meaning: An ecosystemic perspective on hypnotherapy. *American Journal of Clincal Hypnosis, 37*(4), 300–315.

Frank, J. D. (1974). *Persuasion and healing: A comparative study of psychotherapy.* New York: Schocken.

Frederick, C., & McNeal, S. (1999). *Inner strengths: Contemporary psychotherapy and hypnosis for ego-strengthening.* Mahwah, NJ: Erlbaum.

Fredericks, L. E. (2001). *The use of hypnosis in surgery and anesthesiology: Psychological preparation of the surgical patient.* Springfield, IL: Thomas.

Freeman, A., Pretzer, J., Fleming, B., & Simon, K. M. (1990). *Clinical applications of cognitive therapy.* New York: Plenum.

Frischholz, E., & Spiegel, H. (2000, February). *Hypnotizability assessment.* Workshop presented at the annual meeting of the American Society of Clinical Hypnosis, Baltimore.

Fromm, E., & Kahn, S. (1990). Self-hypnosis: The Chicago Paradigm. New York: Guilford.

Gatchel, R. J., & Blanchard, E. B. (Eds.). (1993). *Psychophysiological disorders: Research and clinical applications.* Washington, DC: American Psychological Association.

Gauld, A. (1992). *A history of hypnotism.* Cambridge, UK: Cambridge University Press.

Gravitz, M. A. (1994). The first use of self-hypnosis: Mesmer mesmerizes Mesmer. *American Journal of Clincal Hypnosis, 37*(1), 49–52.

Greenwald, A. G. (1992). New look 3: Unconscious cognition reclaimed. *American Psychologist, 47,* 766–779.

Grinder, J., & Bandler, R. (1976). *The structure of magic II: A book about communication and change.* Palo Alto, CA: Science and Behavior Books.

Grinder, J., & Bandler, R. (1981). *Trance-formations: Neuro-linguistic programming and the structure of hypnosis.* Moab, UT: Real People Press.

Haley, J. (1984). *Ordeal therapy.* San Francisco: Jossey-Bass.

Haley, J. (1986). *Uncommon therapy: The psychiatric techniques of Milton H. Erickson, M.D.* New York: Norton.

Hall, H. R. (1983). Hypnosis and the immune system: A review with implications for cancer and the psychology of healing. *American Journal of Clinical Hypnosis, 25,* 92–103.

Hanson, R. W., & Gerber, K. E. (1990). *Coping with chronic pain: A guide to patient self-management.* New York: Guilford.

Hartland, J. (1965). The value of ego-strengthening procedures prior to direct symptom-removal under hypnosis. *American Journal of Clinical Hypnosis, 8,* 89–93.

Hartland, J. (1971). Further observations on the use of ego-strengthening techniques. *American Journal of Clinical Hypnosis, 14,* 1–8.

Havens, R. A. (Ed.). (1992). *The wisdom of Milton H. Erickson: Hypnosis and hypnotherapy* (Vol. 1). New York: Irvington.

Haynes, S. N. (1992). *Models of causality in psychopathology: Toward dynamic, synthetic and nonlinear models of behavior disorders.* New York: Macmillan.

Hilgard, E. R., & Hilgard, J. R. (1994). *Hypnosis in the relief of pain* (rev. ed.). New York: Brunner/Mazel.

Holroyd, J. (1996). Hypnosis treatment of clinical pain: Understanding why hypnosis is useful. *International Journal of Clinical and Experimental Hypnosis, 44*(1), 33–51.

Hope, D. A., & Heimberg, R. G. (1993). Social phobia and social anxiety. In D. H. Barlow (Ed.), *Clinical handbook of psychological disorders* (2nd ed., pp. 99–136). New York: Guilford.

Humphreys, R. B. (2000). *The neurobiology of hypnosis.* Advanced workshop presented at the annual meeting of the American Society of Clinical Hypnosis, Baltimore.

Humphreys, R. B., & Eagan, K. P. (1999). *The autonomic model of hypnosis and its application in treatment.* Unpublished manuscript.

Hunter, M. E. (1987). Hypnosis in medical practice. In W. C. Wester (Ed.), *Clinical hypnosis: A case management approach* (pp. 96–112). Cincinnati: Behavioral Science Center.

Hunter, M. E. (1996). *Making peace with chronic pain: A whole-life strategy.* New York: Brunner/Mazel.

Imber-Black, E., Roberts, J., & Whiting, R. (Eds.). (1989). *Rituals in families and family therapy.* New York: Norton.

Johnston, M., & Vogele, C. (1993). Benefits of psychological preparation for surgery: A meta-analysis. *Annals of Behavioral Medicine, 15,* 245–256.

Kaplan, H. I., & Sadock, B. J. (1981). *Modern synopsis of comprehensive textbook of psychiatry* (3rd Edition). Baltomore: Williams & Wilkins.

Kelly, G. A. (1955). *The psychology of personal constructs* (Vols. 1 and 2). New York: Norton.

Kessler, R., & Whalen, T. (1999). Hypnotic preparation in anesthesia and surgery. In R. Temes (Ed.), *Medical hypnosis: An introduction and clinical guide* (pp. 43–58). New York: Churchill Livingstone.

Kihlstrom, J. F., Barnhardt, T. M., & Tataryn, D. J. (1992). The psychological unconscious. *American Psychologist, 47,* 788–791.

Kirsch, I. (1990). *Changing expectations: A key to effective psychotherapy.* Pacific Grove, CA: Brooks/Cole.

Kirsch, I. (1994). American Psychology Association definition and description of hypnosis: Defining hypnosis for the public. *Contemporary Hypnosis, 11,* 142–143.

Kirsch, I. (1999a). Clinical hypnosis as a nondeceptive placebo. In I. Kirsch, A. Capafons, E. Cardena, & S. Amigo (Eds.), *Clinical hypnosis and self-regulation: Cognitive-behavioral perspectives* (pp. 211–225). Washington, DC: American Psychological Association.

Kirsch, I. (Ed.). (1999b). *How expectancies shape experience.* Washington, DC: American Psychological Association.

Kirsch, I. (2000). The response set theory of hypnosis. *American Journal of Clinical Hypnosis, 42*(3, 4), 274–292.

Kozak, M. J., & Foa, E. B. (1999). *Mastery of obsessive compulsive disorder therapist guide.* New York: Academic Press.

Kraemer, H. C., Kazdin, A. E., Offord, D. R., Kessler, R. C., Jensen, P. S., & Kupfer, D. J. (1997). Coming to terms with the terms of risk. *Archives of General Psychiatry, 54,* 337–343.

Kroger, W. S. (1977). *Clinical and experimental hypnosis* (2nd ed.). Philadelphia: Lippincott.

LaCrosse, M. B. (1994). Understanding change: Five-year follow-up of brief hypnotic treatment of chronic bruxism. *American Journal of Clincal Hypnosis, 36*(4), 276–281.

Laing, R. D. (1965). Mystification, confusion, and conflict. In I. Boszormenyi-Nagy & J. Framo (Eds.), *Intensive family therapy.* New York: Harper & Row.

Langs, R. J. (1995). *The therapeutic interaction: Synthesis of the multiple components of therapy.* Northvale, NJ: Aronson.

Lankton, S. R. (1980). *Practical magic: A translation of basic neuro-linguistic programming into clinical psychotherapy.* Cupertino, CA: Meta.

Lankton, S. R., & Lankton, C. H. (1983). *The answer within: A clinical framework of Ericksonian hypnotherapy.* New York: Brunner/Mazel.

Leo, J. (1996, July 15/July 22). Thank you for not smoking: On society. *U.S. News and World Report,* p. 18.

Levitt, E. E. (1993). Hypnosis in the treatment of obesity. In J. W. Rhue, S. J. Lynn, & I. Kirsch (Eds.), *Handbook of clinical hypnosis* (pp. 533–554). Washington, DC: American Psychological Association.

Lewis, B. A., & Pucelik, F. (1982). *Magic demystified: A pragmatic guide to communication and change.* Lake Oswego, OR: Metamorphous.

Linehan, M. M. (1993). *Cognitive-behavioral treatment of borderline personality disorder.* New York: Guilford.

Maxmen, J. S., & Ward, N. G. (1995). *Essential psychopathology and its treatment.* New York: Norton.

McNeal, S., & Frederick, C. (1993). Inner strength and other techniques for ego strengthening. *American Journal of Clinical Hypnosis, 35*(3), 170–178.

Meichenbaum, D. (1977). *Cognitive-behavior modification: An integrative approach.* New York: Plenum.

Meichenbaum, D., & Turk, D. C. (1987). *Facilitating treatment adherence: A practitioner's guidebook.* New York: Plenum.

Melzack, R. (1999). Pain and stress: A new perspective. In R. J. Gatchel, & D. C. Turk (Eds.), *Psychosocial factors in pain: Critical perspectives* (pp. 89–106). New York: Guilford.

Melzack, R., & Torgerson, W. S. (1971). On the language of pain. *Anesthesiology, 34,* 50–59.

Moore-Ede, M., & LeVert, S. (1998). *The complete idiot's guide to getting a good night's sleep.* New York: Alpha.

Mutter, C. B. (1987). Hypnosis in psychotherapy. In W. C. Wester (Ed.), *Clinical hypnosis: A case management approach* (pp. 55–66). Cincinnati: Behavioral Science Center.

Palazzoli, M. S., Boscolo, L., Cecchin, G., & Prata, G. (Eds.). (1995). *Paradox and counter paradox: A new model in the therapy of the family in schizophrenic transaction.* Northvale, NJ: Aronson.

Peterson, C., Maier, S. F., & Seligman, M. E. P. (1995). *Learned helplessness: A theory for the age of personal control.* London: Oxford University Press.

Piaget, J., & Inhelder, B. (2000). *The psychology of the child* (rev. ed.). New York: Basic.

Powers, W. T. (1973). *Behavior: The control of perception.* Chicago: Aldine.

Raloff, J. (1996, November 30). How the brain knows when eating must stop. *Science News,* p. 343.

Reaney, J. B. (1987). Hypnosis in the treatment of habit disorders. In W. C. Wester (Ed.), *Clinical hypnosis: A case management approach* (pp. 305–324). Cincinnati: Behavioral Science Center.

Rosenbaum, J. F., Pollack, M. H., Otto, M. W., Bernstein, J. G. (1997). Anxious patients. In N. H. Cassem, T. A. Stern, J. F. Rosenbaum, & M. S. Jellinek (Eds.), *Massachusetts*

General Hopsital handbook of general psychiatry (4th ed., pp. 173–210). St. Louis, MO: Mosby.

Rossi, E. L. (1993). *The psychobiology of mind-body healing: New concepts in therapeutic hypnosis.* New York: Norton.

Rossi, E. L., & Cheek, D. B. (1988). *Mind-body therapy: Methods of ideodynamic healing with hypnosis.* New York: Norton.

Russ, W. (1987). Hypnosis in the treatment of obesity. In W. C. Wester (Ed.), *Clinical hypnosis: A case management approach* (pp. 183–196). Cincinnati: Behavioral Science Center.

Ruzyla-Smith, P., Barabasz, A., Barabasz, M., & Warner, D. (1995). Effects of hypnosis on the immune response: B-cells, T-cells, helper and suppressor cells. *American Journal of Clinical Hypnosis, 38*(2), 71–79.

Sanders, S. (1991). *Clinical self-hypnosis: The power of words and images.* New York: Guilford.

Seligman, M. E. P. (1975). *Helplessness: On depression, development, and death.* San Francisco: Freeman.

Selye, H. (1974). *Stress without distress.* New York: Harper & Row.

Selye, H. (1976). *The stress of life.* New York: McGraw-Hill.

Shutty, M. S., DeGood, D. E., & Tuttle, D. H. (1990). Chronic pain patients' beliefs about their pain and treatment outcomes. *Archives of Physical Medicine and Rehabilitation, 71,* 128–132.

Simonton, D. C., Matthews-Simonton, S., & Creighton, L. J. (1978). *Getting well again.* Los Angeles: Tarcher–St. Martin's.

Sluzki, C. E., & Ransom, D. C. (Eds.). (1976). *Double binds: The foundation of the communicational approach to the family.* New York: Grune & Stratton.

Sobell, M. B. (1978). *Behavioral treatment of alcohol problems: Individualized therapy and controlled drinking.* New York: Plenum.

Spiegel, H., & Spiegel, D. (1987). *Trance and treatment: Clinical uses of hypnosis.* Washington, DC: American Psychiatric Press.

Spires, S. (1990, January 25). Cigarettes have more benzene than Perrier. *Palm Beach Post,* p. 4A.

Stanton, H. E. (1993). Using hypnotherapy to overcome examination anxiety. *American Journal of Clinical Hypnosis, 35*(3), 198–204.

Steketee, G. S. (1996). *Treatment of obsessive-compulsive disorder.* New York: Guilford.

Surman, O. S., Gottlieb, S. K., & Hackett, T. P. (1972). Hypnosis in the treatment of warts. *Archives of General Psychiatry, 28,* 439–441.

Tarr, B. (1976). *Now you see it, now you don't! Lessons in sleight of hand.* New York: Vintage.

Teitelbaum, M. (1965). *Hypnosis induction technics.* Springfield, IL: Thomas.

Turk, D. C., & Flor, H. (1999). Chronic pain: A biobehavioral perspective. In R. J. Gatchel, & D. C. Turk (Eds.), *Psychosocial factors in pain: Critical perspectives* (pp. 18–34). New York: Guilford.

Turk, D. C., Meichenbaum, D., & Genest, M. (1983). *Pain and behavioral medicine: A cognitive-behavioral perspective.* New York: Guilford.

Turk, D. C., & Melzack, R. (1992). The measurement of pain and the assessment of people experiencing pain. In D. C. Turk & R. Melzack (Eds.), *Handbook of pain assessment* (pp. 3–14). New York: Guilford.

Turk, D. C., Okifuji, A., & Scharff, L. (1995). Chronic pain and depression: Role of perceived impact and perceived control in different age cohorts. *Pain, 61*(1), 92–102.

U.S. Surgeon General (1990). The health benefits of smoking cessation: A report of the Surgeon General. Washington, DC. Annual Surgeon General's Report.

Van Der Hart, O. (1982). *Rituals in psychotherapy: Transition and continuity.* New York: Irvington.

Vanderlinden, J., & Vendereycken, W. (1994). The (limited) possibilities of hypnotherapy in the treatment of obesity. *American Journal of Clinical Hypnosis, 36*(4), 248–257.

Vetter, H. J. (1969). *Language, behavior, and psychopathology.* Chicago: Rand McNally.

Walrond-Skinner, S. (1986). Double bind. In *Dictionary of psychotherapy* (pp. 102–103). London: Routledge & Kegan Paul.

Watkins, H. H. (1980). The silent abreaction. *International Journal of Clinical and Experimental Hypnosis, 28,* 101–113.

Watkins, J. G. (1978). *The therapeutic self.* New York: Human Sciences.

Watkins, J. G., & Watkins, H. H. (1997). *Ego states: Theory and therapy.* New York: Norton.

Watzlawick, P. (1978). *The language of change: Elements of therapeutic communication.* New York: Norton.

Watzlawick, P., Beavin, J. H., & Jackson, D. D. (1967). *Pragmatics of human communication.* New York: Norton.

Weisenberg, M. (1998). Cognitive aspects of pain and pain control. *International Journal of Clinical and Experimental Hypnosis, 46*(1), 44–61.

Wester, W. C. (Ed.). (1987). *Clinical hypnosis: A case management approach.* Cincinnati: Behavioral Science Center.

Wester, W. C., & Smith, A. H. (Eds.). (1984). *Clinical hypnosis: A multidisciplinary approach.* Philadelphia: Lippincott.

Wolpe, J. (1982). *The practice of behavior therapy* (3rd ed.). New York: Pergamon.

Woody, E. Z., Bowers, K. S., & Oakman, J. M. (1992). A conceptual analysis of hypnotic responsiveness: Experience, individual differences, and context. In E. Fromm & M. R. Nash (Eds.), *Contemporary hypnosis research* (pp. 3–33). New York: Guilford.

Zarren, J. I. (1996a). *Cognitive hypnosis for behavior change.* Unpublished manuscript.

Zarren, J. I. (December, 1996b). *Self-hypnosis in clinical practice.* Workshop presented at the annual meeting of the American Society of Clinical Hypnosis, Miami.

Zarren, J. I. & Eimer, B. N. (March, 1999). *Brief cognitive hypnosis.* Workshop presented at the annual meeting of the American Society of Clinical Hypnosis, Atlanta.

Zarren, J. I., & Eimer, B. N. (March, 2000). *A Single Session Smoking Cessation Program and Other Brief Behavioral Interventions.* Workshop presented at the Annual Meeting of the American Society of Clinical Hypnosis, Baltimore.

AUTHOR INDEX

SUBJECT INDEX

Absolutes
  illusion of, 97
  reframing concept of, 56–57
Absorption, increased, in hypnotic
    trance, 6
Acid secretion, of stomach, 52
Acute pain, chronic pain, treatment
    contrasted, 214
Addiction
  labeling behavior as, 32
  overuse of word, 249
  reframing, 31–32
Addiction theory, 277–278
Adjectives, for sensory system, 23
Adrenaline, 52
  smoking and, 248, 249
Advertising, 17
Agenda, of patient, 46
Aging of skin, cigarette smoking and, 247
Agoraphobia, 171, 268, 269
Alarm stage, in fight or flight, 101
Alcohol, smoking with, 259
Alcohol abuse, 32, 149, 162, 269
  case study, 163–168
Alcoholics Anonymous, as ritual, 109
Altered states, therapeutic application of,
    5
Alternative therapies, as ritual, 108
Alternatives, illusion of, 93–94, 95
Ambidextrous individuals, 53
Analgesia, acute procedural pain, 232
Ancillary help, in treatment,
    psychogenic aphonia, 28–29
Anesthesia, suggestions during induction
    of, 28
Anger
  case study, 201–206
  chronic, 212–239
  smoking cigarette in, 260–261
Anticipation, expectation, distinguished, 35
Anticipatory, use of word, 36
Anticipatory anxiety, 206

Anticipatory trance state, 36
Antidiuretic effect, smoking, 249
Anxiety, 122, 147–168, 169–211, 268
  anticipatory, 206
  evolving into avoidance, 268
  generalized, 103, 172
    case study, 182–185
  in patient, facial muscles, tension in,
      51
  performance, 173, 206–211
  public speaking, 206–211
  test, 206–211
Anxiety-based behaviors, 103–105
Anxiety disorders, common elements
    among, 171–172
Anxiousness, mild, 103
Aphonia, psychogenic, 18–19, 28–29
Appointment, initial, 13
Arms, rising, falling, induction trance
    script, 70–71
Arsenic, in cigarettes, 247
Athletes, anxiety control, 211
Attention
  focus of, internal, *versus* external, 62
  narrowed focus of, in hypnotic trance, 6
Atypical modes of thinking, facilitation
    of, in hypnotic trance, 6
Auditory sensory system
  primary, 23
  primary use by patient, 15
  processing information through, 22
Automaticity, 59–60
Autonomic nervous system, 51
  parasympathetic branch of, dominance
    of, in hypnotic trance, 6–7

Basic treatment plans
  more than one or two visits, 26–27
  one or two visits, 25–26
Behavior, as attempt to cope, 35–36
Behavioral manifestations of internal
    responses, 49

291

DATE DUE